Physician-Assisted Death in Perspective

Assessing the Dutch Experience

This book is the first comprehensive report and analysis of the Dutch euthanasia experience over the last three decades. In contrast to most books about euthanasia, which are written by authors from countries where the practice is illegal and therefore practiced only secretly, this book analyzes empirical data and real-life clinical behavior. Its essays were written by the leading Dutch scholars and clinicians who shaped euthanasia policy and who have studied, evaluated, and helped regulate it. Some of them have themselves practiced euthanasia. The book will contribute to the world literature on physician-assisted death by providing a comprehensive examination of how euthanasia has been practiced and how it has evolved in one specific national and cultural context. It will greatly advance the understanding of euthanasia among both advocates and opponents of the practice.

Stuart J. Youngner, MD, is the Susan E. Watson Professor and Chair of the Department of Bioethics at Case Western Reserve University School of Medicine. Trained as a psychiatrist, Dr. Youngner is a nationally and internationally recognized scholar in biomedical ethics. He has published extensively on topics including end-of-life issues, organ transplantation, and the definition of death.

Gerrit K. Kimsma, MD, MPh, is a practicing physician and philosopher and co-founder of the Department of Metamedicine at the Vrije Universiteit in Amsterdam. His present affiliation is with the Department of Philosophy and Medical Ethics of the St. Radboud University Medical Center in Nijmegen. He is a nationally and internationally recognized scholar in end-of-life issues and serves on the Boards of *Cambridge Quarterly of Health Care Ethics*, *Theoretical Medicine and Bioethics*, *Medicine HealthCare*, and *Philosophy*.

Physician-Assisted Death in Perspective

Assessing the Dutch Experience

Edited by

STUART J. YOUNGNER

Case Western Reserve University

GERRIT K. KIMSMA

St. Radboud University Medical Center, Nijmegen, the Netherlands

CAMBRIDGE
UNIVERSITY PRESS

CAMBRIDGE UNIVERSITY PRESS
Cambridge, New York, Melbourne, Madrid, Cape Town,
Singapore, São Paulo, Delhi, Mexico City

Cambridge University Press
32 Avenue of the Americas, New York, NY 10013-2473, USA

www.cambridge.org
Information on this title: www.cambridge.org/9781107007567

First published 2012

Printed in the United States of America

A catalog record for this publication is available from the British Library.

Library of Congress Cataloging in Publication data
Physician-assisted death in perspective : assessing the Dutch experience /
[edited by] Stuart J. Youngner, Gerrit K. Kimsma.
p. ; cm.
Includes bibliographical references and index.
ISBN 978-1-107-00756-7 (hardback)
1. Assisted suicide – Netherlands. 2. Euthanasia – Netherlands.
3. Assisted suicide – Moral and ethical aspects – Netherlands.
I. Youngner, Stuart J. II. Kimsma, Gerrit K.
[DNLM: 1. Euthanasia, Active, Voluntary – Netherlands. 2. Attitude
to Death – Netherlands. 3. Health Policy – Netherlands. 4. Physicians –
psychology – Netherlands. 5. Suicide, Assisted – Netherlands. WB 65]
R726.P484 2011
362.17′5–dc22 2011010907

ISBN 978-1-107-00756-7 Hardback

Contents

Contributors

Ron Berghmans, PhD, was trained as a psychologist at the University of Utrecht (1979) and received his PhD in bioethics at the Free University of Amsterdam (1992). He works in the Department of Health, Ethics and Society of Maastricht University. His major fields of interest are ethics in mental health care, care for dementia patients, mental capacity, neuroethics, end-of-life issues (euthanasia, assisted suicide), and research ethics. He has been a member of several committees of the Health Council of the Netherlands.

Boudewijn E. Chabot, MD, PhD, was trained as a psychiatrist and psychotherapist at the Erasmus University in Rotterdam and at the Institute of Psychiatry and Maudsley Hospital in London. He did research in psychotherapy at the University of Amsterdam and later specialized in psychiatry for the elderly. His name has been given to the Dutch Supreme Court case (1994) on physician-assisted dying in a psychiatric patient.

Chalmers C. Clark, PhD, is Adjunct Associate Professor of Philosophy, Union College, Schenectady, New York. His background is in naturalized epistemology and biomedical ethics. He received his PhD from the Graduate Center of the City University of New York (CUNY) and has been Visiting Scholar at the Institute for Ethics of the American Medical Association; Donaghue Visiting Scholar in Biomedical and Behavioral Research Ethics, Yale University; and Visiting Fellow at the Center for Philosophy and History of Science at Boston University. His interest is to extend epistemological holism into the domain of moral and political thought. The result has been research and publication in several interdisciplinary forms. Current work centers on trust relations in the professions (medicine expecially), the professions as stewards of public trusts, and the role that public trusts play in the basic structure of a free society.

Govert den Hartogh is Professor Emeritus of Ethics and Its History in the Department of Philosophy at the University of Amsterdam. He has also taught in the Faculty of Medicine and the Faculty of Law. He is the author of

Mutual Expectations, a Conventionalist Theory of Law (Springer 2002) and the editor of *The Good Life as a Public Good* (Kluwer 2000), and he has written many articles in moral, legal, and political philosophy and medical ethics. He is a member of the Dutch Health Council and of one of the Regional Review Committees for euthanasia. He is presently writing a book about medical and nonmedical decisions concerning the end of life.

John Griffiths held the chair in sociology of law in the Department of Legal Theory of the Faculty of Law of the University of Groningen from 1977 until his retirement in 2005. He studied philosophy (University of California, Berkeley) and law (Yale Law School) and taught law at, successively, Yale, the University of Ghana, and New York University before accepting his most recent appointment. His theoretical work in sociology of law has largely focused on the effectiveness of regulation. Most of his research and writing has dealt with problems of the regulation of euthanasia and other socially problematic medical behavior.

Cees M. P. M. Hertogh, MD, PhD, is professor of Geriatric Ethics at the EMGO Institute for Health and Care Research and in the Department of Nursing Home Medicine of the VU University Medical Center, Amsterdam. He is also working as a nursing home physician at the Vivium Zorggroep, Naarderheem, Naarden. His research focuses on ethical issues in the care and treatment of chronically ill elderly people using empirical research methods (empirical ethics). He has gained expertise in care ethics, qualitative research in ethics, end-of-life-decision making, euthanasia in patients with dementia, advance-care planning, and (decisional) capacity. He is also involved in an EC project that aims to develop guidelines for improving elderly participation in clinical research.

James C. Kennedy is Professor of Dutch History since the Middle Ages at the University of Amsterdam. He has specialized in postwar Dutch society, investigating the cultural changes of the 1960s and the advent of euthanasia policies in the 1970s and 1980s. He has also written extensively about political shifts in Dutch public life and the public role of religion in the modern Netherlands. He is currently working on *A Concise History of the Netherlands* for Cambridge University Press.

Gerrit K. Kimsma, MD, MPh, is a practicing physician and philosopher and co-founder of the Department of Metamedicine at the Vrije Universiteit in Amsterdam. He is a nationally and internationally recognized scholar in end-of-life issues and serves on the Boards of *Cambridge Quarterly of Health Care Ethics*, *Theoretical Medicine and Bioethics*, *Medicine HealthCare*, and *Philosophy*.

Johan Legemaate is a professor of health law at the Vrije Universiteit Amsterdam, and as chief counsel to the Royal Dutch Medical Association has been actively involved in Dutch developments and discussions regarding medical decisions at the end of life. Since September 2010 he has been a professor of health law at the University of Amsterdam (Academic Medical Center).

Bregje D. Onwuteaka-Philipsen is associate professor in the Department of Public and Occupational Health and the EMGO Institute at the VU University Medical Center in Amsterdam. She is program leader of the research program "Care and Prevention," one of the four research programs of the EMGO Institute for Health and Care Research. She also leads the research line "Public Health at the End of Life" at the Department of Public and Occupational Health. Since 1994, she has been involved in the Dutch nationwide studies on medical end-of-life decisions and evaluation of the regulation of euthanasia and physician-assisted suicide that takes place about every five years; she has been the project leader since 2001. She is author or co-author of more than 100 PubMed publications on end-of-life care. In 2008 she won a career award from The Netherlands Organisation for Scientific Research, which enabled her to develop the research program "The Patient Perspective in the Last Phase of Life: Personal Dignity, Preferences and Participation."

Hans Oversloot is a lecturer in the Department of Political Science, Leiden University. He studied history and political science at Leiden University. His research interests include Russian politics, political philosophy, and Dutch politics. He has published in *Acta Politica*, *The Review of Central and East European Law*, and the *Journal of Communist and Transition Studies*. More information can be found at http://www.fsw.leidenuniv.nl/politicologie/organisatie/medewerkers/oversloot.html.

Esther Pans has written a legal dissertation on the *Dutch Law on Euthanasia and Physician-Assisted Suicide* (Vrije Universiteit Amsterdam, 2006). This book analyzes the moral considerations underlying Dutch legislation and Dutch case law. She has written several articles on issues regarding the legal aspects of end-of-life decisions, such as physician-assisted suicide in case of dementia or being "weary of life." She is presently working as a health care–oriented lawyer in Amsterdam and is a member of the Civil Law Department of the Vrije Universiteit Amsterdam.

H. Roeline W. Pasman is a sociologist who works as a senior researcher at the EMGO Institute for Health and Care Research and the VU University Medical Center in Amsterdam. She has research experience in both qualitative and quantitative studies on end-of-life care. She wrote her thesis (2004) on forgoing artificial nutrition and hydration in nursing home patients. Currently, she participates in several (qualitative and/or quantitative) studies regarding end-of-life care, such as a large-cohort study of people with advance directives and an observational study regarding participation of patients in end-of-life decision making.

Mette Rurup is a senior researcher in the Department of Public and Occupational Health of the EMGO Institute for Health and Care Research of the VU University Medical Center. Her thesis (2005) was about requests for assisted suicide from people who are "weary of life" and the incidence and use of advance directives with patients with dementia. Her current research interests also include physicians' knowledge about opioids and pain management at the end of life, dignity at the end of life as perceived by patients in nursing homes, and the effect of advance directives.

Pieter J. J. Sauer is Professor of Pediatrics at the University of Groningen, Toronto, Canada. From 1986 to 1997, he was Professor of Neonatology in Rotterdam; in 1997 he became Professor of Pediatrics and Chairman in the Beatrix Children's Hospital, University Medical Center, Groningen. For many years, he has been interested in the ethical aspects of neonatology. He has published a number of papers on this topic, some on behalf of the Ethical Committee of the European Academy of Pediatrics.

Margo Trappenburg studied political science at Leiden University. She is associate professor in the Utrecht School of Governance at Utrecht University and holds an endowed chair at Amsterdam University. Her research interests include patient organizations, patient empowerment, euthanasia, the development of medical professional ethics, and contemporary political philosophy.

Agnes van der Heide, MD, PhD, is a medical doctor and epidemiologist. After getting her PhD in 1994 with a thesis on the assessment and treatment of early rheumatoid arthritis, she started working in the Department of Public Health at Erasmus Medical Center in Rotterdam. Her main research activities are in the field of end-of-life care and decision making. She has coordinated a large number of regional, national, and international empirical studies on the practice of euthanasia, palliative sedation, and care for the dying.

Marije van der Lee, PhD, works as head of the Science Department of the Helen Dowling Institute for psycho-oncology. Between 2000 and 2005, she studied the effect of depression on the risk for a request for euthanasia in terminally ill cancer patients and the consequences of depression and euthanasia on grief in the family members. She defended her dissertation "Before Death and Thereafter" in May 2005.

Evert van Leeuwen, PhD, is head of the section Ethics, Philosophy and History of Medicine of the Scientific Institute for Quality of Healthcare: IQ Healthcare at the Radboud University Nijmegen Medical Centre. He was a member of the Regional Euthanasia Committee in North Holland from 1999 to 2005. In 1999, he became a member of the Dutch Central Committee on Research Involving Human Subjects CCMO. He is on the editorial board of *Theoretical Medicine and Bioethics* (co-editor from 1995 to 2002) and is an International Board Member of the *Cambridge Quarterly of Health Care Ethics.*

A. A. Eduard Verhagen finished law school (health law) in 1987 and medical school at the University of Utrecht, the Netherlands, in 1991. He subsequently trained to become a pediatrician in Amsterdam (EKZ/AMC). He moved to Groningen in 2000, where he was appointed clinical director of the Paediatric Department of the University Medical Centre Groningen. Verhagen was one of the authors of the "Groningen Protocol," published in the *New England Journal of Medicine* in 2005. He finished his PhD on end-of-life decisions in Dutch neonatal intensive care units in 2009.

Heleen Weyers is a lecturer in Legal Theory at the University of Groningen. She teaches sociology of law, philosophy, and political science. She specializes in the history of the process of legal change concerning euthanasia in the Netherlands. Another main topic of her research is the emergence and effectiveness of smoking bans.

Henri Wijsbek works in the Department of Philosophy at the University of Amsterdam and at the Health Council of the Netherlands. He is interested in Dutch euthanasia practice, in particular how the unbearable suffering criterion should be applied.

Dick Willems is a former general practitioner and philosopher. He is Professor of Medical Ethics at the Academic Medical Centre of the University of Amsterdam. He has been a coordinator of the Center for the Development of Palliative Care at the Free University, Amsterdam. His research interests include ethical aspects of genetics, end-of-life issues, and home-care technology. He is the President of the Netherlands Association for Bioethics and Director of the Centre for Ethics and Health. He is a member of the Council for Public Health and Health Care (RVZ) and of the Ethics and Law Standing Committee of the Dutch Health Council.

Preface

Gerrit K. Kimsma

I have had a long-standing interest in end-of-life decision making in medicine. It started well before I began my career in the early 1970s as a teacher of medical ethics and philosophy at the Vrije Universiteit of Amsterdam and as a general practitioner working in a health center near Amsterdam.

I have witnessed and participated in all the phases of confrontation, acceptance, and integration of euthanasia in the Netherlands. I received my medical degree in 1974, the year of the "first" court case, and taught students and residents about the implications and what has followed since. I ended the unacceptable suffering of a terminal patient with a brain tumor by injection in 1977; this was my first time, and it was during a period when there was neither unanimity about the practice nor regulations that would protect a physician. I have reported all my cases except this first one, and I still feel ambivalent about it. It was justified but troublesome because of the legal risks and the mixed emotions I felt. This ambivalence has never left me and is revived each time I receive a request to help someone to die.

My motivation was based on a conviction that people at the end of their lives should not suffer unnecessarily. In general, I believe that this type of suffering serves no real purpose, except to remind us of the tragic and vulnerable side of life. As a physician, I have observed that suffering may be part and parcel of diseases; nowadays, however, the well-intended but often damaging interventions of medicine may actually increase suffering. Although medicine is intended to address the cause and nature of diseases, in so doing it changes the accompanying suffering and often extends it in unforeseen ways. My personal conviction coincided with an emerging cultural discomfort with the medicalization of death and dying and a growing belief that how one dies should be a personal choice. I shared the belief that the medical profession alone is incapable of making this choice and that patient input is essential but not, by itself, decisive.

I have always maintained the position that physician-assisted death (PAD) should respect the moral position of physicians because they are not just the "means" of fulfilling a request; rather, they are moral agents with their own professional responsibilities, emotions, and consciences. PAD is a relational process that involves at least two individuals. It is not just an intervention to help someone die.

This friction between death under the guidance of medical technology and the option of autonomous choice has been the motivating force behind Dutch end-of-life decision making and much of what has happened since the seventies in the Low Countries. I found the Dutch national investigation on medical practices at the end of life to be brave and extremely enlightening because it did away with a lot of speculation and furnished facts. These investigations were the start of cooperative efforts between the government and the medical profession, resulting in the development of programs for euthanasia consultants and review committees. I have been intimately involved in these programs as an independent consultant, even before the new acts. I have been a teacher in the Royal Dutch Medical Society for the Advancement of Medicine (RDMA) programs for consultants since 1997. I was also a physician-member of a Euthanasia Review Committee for twelve years after 1998 (after the new acts were passed) that determines whether it is legal to end an individual's life.

From early on I have been aware of the "open ends," risks, and dangers of these irreversible interventions by physicians. Chris Ciesielski-Carlucci and I interviewed families for the first time after the acts were passed. David Thomasma, Thomasine Kushner, and I interviewed physicians who ended the lives of their patients. We published *Asking to Die: Inside the Dutch Debate about Euthanasia* (Kluwer Academic Publishers, Dordrecht/Boston/London) in 1998 in order to open up public debate about the personal and private consequences of physician-assisted death.

I was and still am impressed by the personal involvement of physicians with their patients and families, and can assure people that they are not being or becoming indifferent, as some feared. On the contrary, everyone we interviewed was deeply touched by these decisions. As a consultant, I have witnessed the courage and strong convictions of patients who ask for an end to their suffering. I am struck by the depth of involvement of all the participants in physician-assisted dying. I have seen no hints of routinization, callousness, or a "slippery slope"; there are no studies that reflect such developments.

Even though these personal experiences and small-scale research activities were inspiring, there was reason to doubt whether they were representative or complete. There was a need for more comprehensive empirical and theoretical research on many aspects of medicine at the end of life in order to grasp the total picture of PAD.

So it was more than a lucky coincidence that Stuart J. Youngner, who is an interested but critical observer of "Dutch euthanasia," expressed an interest similar to mine. Our professional partnership in teaching, our friendship, and our intellectual curiosity inspired this book, which is intended to present the next phase in Dutch empirical, legal, and ethical developments. This book includes information on how Dutch professionals of all ranks respond to the challenges of a "permissive system." It demonstrates how they confront the "new" borders of suffering, both at the end of life, such as with Alzheimers' patients and the elderly who are "tired of living," and at the beginning of life, such as in the extremely problematic issues of neonatology.

I acknowledge that the system may not be perfect, that reporting may not be a hundred percent, and that Euthanasia Review Committees (ERCs) conclude that the PAD has not been "careful" in a small minority of the cases. Nevertheless, the existence of an option for patients to be allowed to die when they choose has increased the humaneness of death and made its acceptance easier, in spite of the enormous grief for anyone whose end has come and the grief of his or her dependents.

Preface

Stuart J. Youngner

I have had a long-standing interest in end-of-life decision making within the United States. It began with my career in the early 1970s as a consultation-liaison psychiatrist, working primarily in the medical and surgical areas of the hospital.

Psychiatry had gained credibility during this period by identifying clinical depression as a potentially lethal disease. Epidemiological studies confirmed that most suicides took place in the context of mental illness and could often be prevented with timely intervention. The perception that depression was, in fact, a public health problem led to the establishment of a national network of suicide prevention centers. This, and the development of new drugs that could often effectively treat serious depression, provided new recognition and prestige for the field of psychiatry.

Another seemingly unrelated development occurred during this same period. The first intensive care units were opening in American hospitals – that is, an impressive concentration of "lifesaving equipment" and specially trained medical personnel brought together in special areas in the hospital to salvage lives that would previously have been lost. I took an interest in the psychological and social issues raised by intensive care – issues that affect patients, families, and health professionals alike. A new problem became apparent very quickly. Sometimes critical illness could not be reversed by lifesaving machines, pharmaceuticals, and invasive monitoring. Sometimes people lingered in a technological limbo in which suffering, indignity, and isolation seemed to overwhelm the noble goals of medicine.

In this context, a national discussion began concerning when death was the least worst alternative. After decades of court cases, legislation, news stories, editorials, movies, and books, American society seems to accept, though somewhat uneasily at times, that allowing death to come may sometimes be the better alternative. The social and legal discussion has focused largely on the claim that passively allowing death to come is sometimes acceptable and even desirable, whereas "actively" ending a patient's life is *never* acceptable. Phrases such as "letting nature take its course" are used to characterize what is judged to be acceptable behavior; unacceptable behavior is branded with the socially toxic words "killing" and "suicide." In fact, the toxic words were used initially to characterize the consideration of forgoing almost every lifesaving intervention. Withdrawal of fluids and nutrition can still evoke passionate accusations of "killing," as the 2005 Terri Schiavo case illustrated.

Most psychiatrists used to see patients in their offices or in psychiatry units where they sought help for depression. These psychiatrists never ventured into an intensive care unit or cancer ward, where patients were increasingly faced with the terrible choice of life burdened either by invasive medical technology or by the diminished state in which "rescue" technology had left them. Here, death was never the first choice. The first choice was cure or recovery to an acceptable state. Unfortunately, that choice was often not available; death appeared the best choice available to many. Although this reality was accepted by a growing number of health professionals and the American public, psychiatry clung to the rigid belief that a wish to die was *always* a product of mental illness. Psychiatry's newly found ability to understand and treat suicidal ideation and behavior as symptoms of depression too often blinded it to the plight of this new group of patients who often (though not always) chose death rationally.

Throughout our national debate about end-of-life decisions (from do not resuscitate [DNR] orders and stopping fluids and nutrition to turning off ventilators), opponents argued that we were heading down a slippery slope to the lethal injection, where there was no ambiguity between killing and letting die. They were right. Once we accepted the notion that death could be the least worst alternative and that it was cruel to keep people alive in these situations against their wishes, it was a matter of time until we considered the lethal injection.

I have often found the most vocal American critics of Dutch euthanasia to be a bit shrill and doctrinaire. They have sometimes resorted to attacking the Dutch character. The more I learned about euthanasia in the Netherlands, the more I was impressed by the thoughtfulness, the evidence-based policy, and the transparency with which it is implemented. Are there problems? Of course. But the Dutch take them seriously. Is the Netherlands heading down a slippery slope to Nazism, as some of its critics have suggested? Hardly. I view the Netherlands as a healthy, bourgeois, liberal democracy with a strong sense of social solidarity that I envy.

My own views on active euthanasia (the lethal injection by a physician) are complicated. While I am intellectually comfortable with its moral logic, I am psychologically (or culturally) uncomfortable with it. I have been asked by patients but have never complied – even in situations where I thought it would be very reasonable. Fortunately (or unfortunately), I have never practiced in a setting where lethal injection was socially and legally permissible. If I did, I cannot predict what I would do.

Putting this book together with Gerrit K. Kimsma has been a great learning experience. It has not, however, made it any easier for me, as a physician, to contemplate giving a patient a lethal injection. Perhaps that discomfort, which is shared by many physicians who practice euthanasia in the Netherlands, is a reassuring take-home message from this book.

Introduction

Stuart J. Youngner and Gerrit K. Kimsma

This book affords those Dutch who have conceived, studied, regulated, and practiced Dutch euthanasia the opportunity to tell their stories in one place in their own voices. Most persons who have written about physician-assisted death (PAD) have lived in countries and cultures in which PAD is illegal and members of the medical professions are strongly opposed to it. This "limitation" results in speculation rather than analysis. The Dutch have now had experience for more than three decades, allowing an unparalleled opportunity to study and reflect about PAD both statically and as its practice unfolds over time in a specific social and cultural context.

Together, we identified and interviewed potential authors and, with them, shaped the content of the book. They were, without exception, enthusiastically cooperative and trusting. Our focus was on the practice of PAD and, therefore, we did not include authors (inside or outside of the Netherlands) who find PAD in general or Dutch PAD in particular morally unacceptable. Therefore, what follows does not serve as a representative or "balanced" discussion of the moral acceptability of PAD in general or Dutch PAD in particular. Nor was it intended to do so. We do hope that the reflections and experiences provided in this book will make a valuable contribution to the ongoing discussion of PAD for supporters and critics alike.

In using the term *physician-assisted death* (PAD), we mean to include two behaviors. The first is the unambiguous and intentional ending of a patient's life by a physician, of which lethal injection is emblematic. The second is physician-assisted suicide, in which a physician intentionally provides the patient with the medical means to end his or her life. When the Dutch use the term *euthanasia*, they have something more restricted in mind (see Chapter 2 by Johan Legamaate). In the Netherlands, euthanasia has a specific social and legal meaning, that is, PAD with specific conditions, such as voluntariness, unbearable suffering, and certain procedural requirements. We have tried to standardize the language in the chapters that follow to avoid confusing the reader.

The first section of the book includes "Background and History." Contemporary historian James C. Kennedy provides a unique interpretation concerning how and why the PAD practice developed in the Netherlands at a particular point in history. He emphasizes the "anti-taboo" culture of the 1970s and 1980s, and the importance the Dutch have historically attached to *bespreekbaarheid* (the freedom to speak openly). Judicial expert Johan Legemaate discusses the importance and ongoing problems of the Dutch classification just mentioned. His discussion of palliative (or terminal) sedation suggests the persistent problem of the active/passive distinction, even in the Netherlands. In the first of her two chapters, Heleen Weyers, a sociologist of law, traces the political, legal, and social practices that shaped the current Dutch law and practice of euthanasia, including a discussion of the key legal cases. Next, lawyer Esther Pans explicates the moral underpinnings of the Dutch euthanasia law, emphasizing the importance of beneficence relative to autonomy. In her second chapter, Heleen Weyers examines positions taken by organizations representing physicians, patients, and religious denominations and how they have evolved over time. Finally, political scientists Margo Trappenburg and Hans Oversloot identify three strands in the Dutch social fabric: the consensual character of the Dutch social and political culture; the Dutch health-care system, in particular the system of general practitioners; and the trust that Dutch patients have in their doctors. They argue that these strands allow the Dutch system to be both liberal and moderate. They also discuss how recent social and political developments may threaten the stability of these strands.

The next section, "Regulation and Practice Deficiencies," contains four chapters written by social scientist researchers who have either conducted the primary government studies or written extensively about them. Bregje D. Onwuteaka-Philipsen and Agnes van der Heide, leaders of the next generation of government studies, address the issues of unreported cases and cases in which there was no specific request for euthanasia – two issues that have motivated a great deal of the criticism of Dutch euthanasia. H. Roeline W. Pasman deals with the interesting question of cases in which physicians refuse requests for euthanasia. Finally, John Griffiths, a supporter of Dutch euthanasia in general, suggests some gaps in the methodology of the research to date.

Experience and information from early studies led the Dutch to make serious efforts to monitor and improve their system of euthanasia. In the section "Quality Assurance," two of these efforts, a systemic approach to consultation and a nationwide review process, are described and analyzed by Gerrit K. Kimsma and philosopher Evert van Leeuwen. Next, physician-philosopher Dick Willems reports on the development of palliative care in the Netherlands in relation to euthanasia.

The section "Learning from the Practice" includes seven chapters that address difficulties identified in the course of the actual practice of Dutch euthanasia. Geriatrician-philosoher Cees M. P. M. Hertogh describes the problem of advance directives and euthanasia for persons with advanced dementia.

Here, physicians have put the brakes on a practice that was allowed by law. Psychologist Ron Berghmans addresses the problem of competence to request euthanasia in patients with early Alzheimer's. Health services researcher Mette Rurup explores the problem of "weariness of life," that is, when patients without a clearly identified medical cause for their suffering request euthanasia. The Dutch courts have forbidden this practice. Kimsma and Chalmers C. Clark describe the impact of euthanasia on physicians by reviewing empirical studies and suggesting that the term *medical friendship* describes the ideal context for euthanasia. In contrast to some who argue that physicians "should never kill patients," they suggest that *only* physicians should do it. Psychologist Marije van der Lee discusses the complicated issue of depression and its relationship to requests for euthanasia, concluding that depression must be taken very seriously but that it hardly characterizes all requests. Pediatrician Pieter J. J. Sauer and pediatrician-lawyer A. A. Eduard Verhagen address the Groningen Protocol, which sets conditions for ending the lives of newborn infants with severe congenital abnormalities. This practice does not count as Dutch euthanasia because, obviously, infants cannot give consent. It has, therefore, stirred considerable controversy around the world. Is it the beginning of a slippery slope in the Dutch end-of-life practice? The authors address this and other questions. Finally, psychiatrist Boudewijn E. Chabot reports on his study of the hastening of death through voluntary cessation of fluids and nutrition in the Netherlands – a practice that is surprisingly common. This is the first such study reported in the world literature.

According to Dutch practice and law, patients who receive euthanasia must demonstrate "unbearable suffering." In the next sections, Henri Wijsbeck and Kimsma explore this key but quintessentially subjective term, philosopher Wijsbeck in a more theoretical way and Kimsma from the perspective of actual practice.

The book concludes with chapters by two senior scholars and longtime commentators on euthanasia in the Netherlands. Theologian Govert den Hartogh judges the success of the Dutch system of euthanasia on its own terms. Specifically, he addresses the rate of reporting, euthanasia without specific request, effectiveness of the review committees, and the newly emerging issue of the classification of terminal sedation. In her final chapter, Trappenburg echoes some of the concerns that she raised in her earlier contribution about changes in the fabric of Dutch society. In contrast, euthanasia policy is, she concludes, "something we really did right."

PART I

BACKGROUND AND HISTORY

I

The Lateness of the Dutch Euthanasia Debate and Its Consequences

James C. Kennedy

In 1932, the Dutch physician Gerrit Arie Lindeboom (1905–1986) observed in an obscure journal that the "moderne mensch" now found it within his reach to bring the old dream of human autonomy into actual practice. That is why Lindeboom wrote:

> Life now must be well-regulated; every disturbance, every roughness must be eliminated, and the course of human life must be characterized by *eugenese* [a good beginning], *eubiose* [a good life] and *euthanasie* [a good death].
>
> And euthanasia seeks death in order to bring a worthy end to a worthy human life, and wishes at every cost to spare it from the frightful aspects of struggle and suffering.[1]

Lindeboom, himself a Calvinist, urged his coreligionists to resist this trend toward embracing euthanasia. He urged Christian doctors to help their patients to fully face the death that awaited them through a palliative approach, directed at both body and soul, instead.

Lindeboom's article is interesting in several respects. It reveals the ethical interests of a physician who in the 1950s would write the ethical guidelines for the Dutch medical profession. More specifically, it shows a man interested early on in a subject that would command his attention only in his later years: In the 1970s, this Free University professor emerged as a leading opponent of the rapidly ascendant support for euthanasia. Quite in contrast with the situation in the seventies, however, four decades earlier Lindeboom had found no serious public opponents in the Netherlands to contest his Christian vision of a good death. As Aldous Huxley did in his own way in *Brave New World* (1931), Lindeboom noticed the cultural shifts in Western society: a new relationship to technology and the emergence of a new morality that was changing the way people thought about life itself. But the shift signaled by Lindeboom made almost no impression on Dutch public or medical discourse until the 1960s, when the thrust of the discussion quickly moved in a direction that appalled Lindeboom and the dwindling number of like-minded souls.

It is striking, then, that a country whose public debate and policies on euthanasia exhibited – for good or for ill – such a degree of openness since roughly 1970 should have been so silent about the subject prior to the changes brought about by the 1960s. That says little, of course, about actual practice, only the debate.[2] This silence can be partly attributed to an international pattern: In many countries, the 1960s served as the starting point for sustained public discussion about such matters. Only then and in subsequent years did the convergence of the "rights revolution" and critique of the medical establishment and its power provide important stimuli for public debate – though of course this debate has been livelier in some countries than in others.

Nevertheless, in several countries there was public debate about the permissibility of euthanasia (both voluntary and involuntary). Germany is perhaps the most infamous example, but in fact it was primarily in Great Britain and the United States (where it was known as "mercy killing") that such discussions took place throughout much of the twentieth century. Although they did not succeed, the first legislative attempts to sanction active, voluntary euthanasia took place in the American Midwest in states such as Iowa, Nebraska, and Ohio shortly after the turn of the century.

During the 1930s, pro-euthanasia societies came into being in both the UK and the United States. These early societies emphasized the voluntary nature of euthanasia, for example, as the Euthanasia Society of America did in its 1938 publication *Merciful Release*.[a,3] Polls in 1939 suggested high rates of support among the American population; according to one source, 90% of New York doctors who were surveyed supported legalization of voluntary euthanasia.[4] Ten years later, in 1949, Hermann Sander, a doctor in New Hampshire was acquitted of murder after he injected air into a vein of an unconscious and dying woman – but not before impassioned defenders and detractors wielded many pens against each other.[5]

Britain led Europe in efforts to legalize euthanasia.[6] In the mid-1930s, Lord Ponsonby introduced legislation in Parliament supporting voluntary euthanasia, gaining the support of a third of the House of Lords.[7,8] After the Second World War, too, the British Parliament strenuously debated euthanasia in 1952 and again in 1969 before ultimately rejecting legalization.[6,8,9]

By the early twentieth century, various countries elsewhere in Europe – for example, Norway – had made allowance in their penal codes for doctors performing euthanasia, reducing the penalty for conviction. In Germany, there was substantial discussion about euthanasia as early as the late nineteenth century, which reached its greatest intensity in the 1920s. Although much of this debate advocated the involuntary euthanasia of "useless mouths" on the grounds of social utility, some of it also was concerned with honoring the requests of those who wished to die. National socialism played little, if any, direct role in these debates.[10]

[a] For a Dutch-language summary, see 3. Jongsma 1968.

Debate continued on both sides of the Atlantic into the 1950s and 1960s in both the popular press and more academic forums. But it picked up in the last half of the 1960s, and the 1970s was dubbed "the age of thanatology" – ostensibly following the sexual revolution. Humane treatment of the dying became a concern where people were living longer – sometimes longer than they wanted – and expecting better treatment for themselves and their loved ones. By 1972, the U.S. Senate was holding hearings on "death with dignity."[11]

None of this led, however, to legislation legalizing euthanasia. The failure of the Anglo-American world to develop a euthanasia regime has to do with several different factors, including, at the very least, different understandings of law, the substantially different position of general practitioners in contrast with the Dutch *huisarts*, different systems of political regulation of medical practice, and, perhaps most fundamentally, the ways in which these different societies think about power, specifically in regard to the patient–physician relationship and the extent to which the physician can be trusted to act in the interests of patients. But as I shall argue in the remainder of this chapter, it also has something to do with the distinct relationship of the Netherlands to the broader history of the twentieth century and the unique lessons the Dutch drew from it.

WHY THE DUTCH NEVER TALKED ABOUT EUTHANASIA BEFORE THE 1960S

Dutch physicians shortened the lives of suffering patients in the decades prior to the 1960s,[12] but public debate in the Netherlands over this topic barely existed. In contrast, "euthanasia" became a topic of public discussion in the early twentieth century in some Western countries, most notably Germany, Britain, and the United States. This was particularly noticeable after the First World War.

In the first place, the carnage of the First World War encouraged the "reappraising [of] ethical precepts concerning the sanctity of life and the extent to which it was deemed acceptable to interfere with divine providence," inasmuch as traditional understandings of Christian death and burial, for instance, were weakened by the wartime experience.[6,13] Moral outlook was often consciously shaped by Darwinian thought, and more particularly an interest in eugenics, including, in the years after the war, an interest in "negative eugenics" programs that through sterilization – or mercy killing – might reduce the social and economic burdens of society.[6,11]

These influences were weaker in the Netherlands. Of course this country, too, had witnessed a sharp process of "dechristianization" in the early twentieth century, as large numbers of socialists and freethinkers formally broke with the church. But if the First World War left its mark on Dutch intellectual life, the moral world of the Dutch had not been as radically shaken by a war in which the Netherlands managed to remain neutral. More important, in contrast to Germany and Britain, the decline of a once-dominant Christian moral world had been checked for the time being by powerful religious movements, Catholic and Protestant, that opposed the new ethical outlook (as Lindeboom illustrates).

The social scientist Dick Meerman has shown how euthanasia (variously defined) generated much English and German literature after 1870, but very little within the Netherlands itself. In 1923 the freethinker and writer Max Greeve made a case for euthanasia in a pamphlet, but no one followed him in championing this cause.[10,14] Meerman suggests that discussions about euthanasia were subsumed under discussions about abortion,[10] but a more obvious explanation is that the power of orthodox Christianity in the Netherlands discouraged open discussion. Dutch eugenicists, in contrast to their German, American, and English counterparts, never made much headway in prewar Holland because of the strength of the country's religious subcultures, which may explain why euthanasia – often associated in the early days with other eugenicist concerns – seldom was discussed.[15] Moreover, regardless of religious belief, the Dutch medical profession remained hostile to euthanasia.

In the second place, research-driven, state-directed medicine was weaker in the Netherlands than in Germany or the United States. The rise of the research universities, which were far more extensively developed in those countries than anywhere else, sometimes went hand in hand with initiatives at social engineering. Although the United States never did legalize euthanasia, and although Hitler waited until the Second World War to implement mass murder under the guise of mercy killing, some of the proponents of mercy killing envisaged an important role for the medical profession and the state in achieving their aims.[12] In the Netherlands, however, political commitment to a strong, assertive nation-state was weaker, and government was seen as facilitating private (and often religious) initiative. Indeed, many of the asylums were created and run by various religious organizations, which showed little interest in eugenics generally or euthanasia more particularly.

Finally, it should be noted that in the United States and Great Britain, the calls for euthanasia (again, in both its voluntary and nonvoluntary forms) were often made by what might be called the radical dissenting tradition: liberal Protestants, including Unitarians, and those associated with humanist organizations.[12] (The Episcopalian priest-cum-atheist Joseph Fletcher, the famous father of "situation ethics," is a striking American example of this pattern.) In the United States, some of these religious progressives were closely tied to the Progressive political movement of the early twentieth century. These groups, more than others, determined both the membership and orientation of the voluntary euthanasia associations that sprang up in both countries in the 1930s. Although limited in number, their members were generally well educated and articulate, enjoying access to the cultural and political establishments of their respective countries.

By the 1970s and 1980s, Dutch humanists and liberal Protestants would take an important public role in championing euthanasia (the Protestant ethicist-theologian Harry Kuitert's life and role in the euthanasia debate in some ways parallel Fletcher's trajectory). As early as the 1950s, the Humanist Society would try to put euthanasia on the agenda as an ethical issue,[16] but prior to the Second World War the Netherlands did not really have the equivalent of the well-organized, liberal "ethical culture" in place in America and Britain. Perhaps the closest expression published in Dutch came from M. C. van Mourik Broekman, a liberal Protestant theologian, who might have been influenced in his thought by his co-religionists in Britain. Writing during the war and posthumously published in 1946, he suggested that a doctor performing euthanasia might not always deserve moral condemnation:

> No one should cast a stone ... on him who on exception and in empathy with the sufferer, directly or indirectly, offers a release from the suffering. It is good that public opinion keep euthanasia at bay, where a natural sense and a metaphysically directed consciousness induce great reticence in desiring euthanasia for oneself or others.... Whenever a humanitarian sense influences Christian morality, which is mild in its judgment, there is a danger that morality will be weakened, but it is also more just and realistic in judgments concerning human need.[17]

But such carefully expressed sentiments never translated into an organization or movement for the practice of euthanasia in the Netherlands; that would have to wait until the early 1970s.

THE DUTCH DEBATE AS A "NEW" DEBATE

The absence of a debate over euthanasia in the Netherlands prior to the 1960s was important for the quality of the debate that began with the cultural changes of that decade. In the remainder of this chapter, I want to outline three historical dimensions of the euthanasia debate in the Netherlands that help explain why the Dutch came to see euthanasia as morally acceptable. These considerations cannot, of course, offer a complete explanation for why the Dutch developed the practice as they did, which has much to do with how the political and social system tries to channel potentially disruptive practices rather than to forbid them. The Dutch legal system played an important part in the changes.[18] But these historical dimensions do help shed light on how the Dutch were able to conceive of euthanasia in terms that rendered them open to the practice.

In the first place, the Dutch debate was relatively free of arguments that underscored the social, in addition to the individual, benefits of legalized euthanasia – arguments that would have made it vulnerable to the charge that proponents were insufficiently interested in the voluntary nature of euthanasia. Social arguments were certainly present in the Netherlands, but they appeared briefly around 1970, only to disappear shortly thereafter. In this respect, and unlike their American and British counterparts, the late arrival of the Dutch euthanasia movement spared the movement from having to face a past of less-than-cautious discussion of the terms under which the recipients of compassion might be released from this life.

In the second place, the absence of a powerful eugenicist movement, a coercive medical establishment, and totalitarian dictatorship allowed the Dutch, after some discussion, to perceive euthanasia as they sought to regulate it as completely disanalogous to the Nazi situation.

Finally, and most importantly, the Dutch saw the allowance of euthanasia not at all as a return to a dark past but as a break with the narrowness of their past: The proponents of liberalization had the sense that they were dealing with an issue that, before their own pioneering role, had not yet been openly discussed. That sense of breaking with a history of silence gave additional energy to the Dutch euthanasia movement. In a word, the Dutch felt that the excesses and missteps of the past were not *theirs* and not particularly relevant for the present. Rather, by opening debate, the Dutch understood themselves to be drawing quite a different lesson from their own past, criticizing the shortcomings of a religious and moral system that seemed now, to many of them, hypocritical and untruthful.

The Social Utility of Euthanasia

It is, of course, important to ask: Was there really no nexus between the debates held by the British and Americans prior to the 1960s and the Dutch debate thereafter? The arguments made for voluntary euthanasia were much the same. But one notable feature of the Dutch debate has been its emphasis on the right to die as a *voluntary* act, and the focus of their discussion in the 1970s and 1980s on the rights of mentally capable patients to choose their own death. In contrast to the United States, where much of the debate centered on the fate of comatose patients like Karen Ann Quinlan and Nancy Cruzan, the Dutch focused on patients who possessed decision-making capacities. More broadly, the Dutch debate has conceived of euthanasia as an *individual* decision that, in theory, has nothing to do with the interests of *society,* unlike the position of the early Anglo-American euthanasia societies.

The early years of the Dutch euthanasia debate – from the late 1960s to the mid-1970s – do, however, show some signs of the older concern for the social value of euthanasia – not in eugenicist terms, but in respect to the challenge of allocating scarce resources that would only grow worse in the future. There was perhaps no Western country more consumed with the overpopulation "problem" than the Netherlands in the 1960s and early 1970s. Warnings about high birth rates were both frequent and dire.[b,19] It is not surprising, therefore, that a concern about overpopulation would play some role not only in the abortion debate[c,20,21] but in the euthanasia debate as well.[11]

[b] For a rather militant example of this, see, for instance, 19. Drogendijk 1974.

[c] Scholars investigating the history of the modern abortion debate are divided on how great a role these neo-Malthusian concerns played, with Joyce Outshoorn realizing the significance that Jan de Bruijn attaches to it (see 20. Outshoorn 1984, and 21. de Bruijn 1979).

The issues of euthanasia and overpopulation met each other most clearly in what was sometimes called the *bejaardenvraagstuk,* the problem of the elderly. By the 1960s, the growing number of older people, and the challenge of providing and funding care for them, had come to be seen as a social problem.[22] By the early 1970s, the growing problem of too many old people in the future was a topic of considerable debate, and that debate also included "euthanasia" (variously defined).[23] The Dutch weekly *Haagse Post* had noted: "In 1970 increasing numbers of people in overpopulated Holland are seeing that ending purposeless human life can be done out of compassion."[24] In 1975 the recently established Voluntary Euthanasia Foundation noted with concern that Dutch society was showing an active interest in "euthanizing" people who experienced, in the eyes of many, "a life without purpose," whose "large number constitute a heavy burden on society."[25]

The costs of health care in the Netherlands rose some 450% from 1963 to 1972.[26] In general, this seemed to put into question by the early 1970s whether the Dutch could afford to keep alive everyone for whom that was technologically possible. The Protestant ethicist at the University of Groningen, P. J. Roscam Abbing, argued that keeping people alive at any cost would mean that the whole national budget would have to be spent on health.[27] In particular, expensive technology that would not be available for everyone meant, at the very least, that "passive euthanasia" was unavoidable. Medical decisions would have to be made – indeed, were already being made – that consigned some people to this kind of euthanasia, and this trend would only become more pronounced in the future.[d,28]

Two early and prominent proponents of euthanasia in the Netherlands had themselves been vocal and active in combating overpopulation. Hendrik Jan van den Berg's objections to the "power" of medicine (*medische macht*) stemmed in part from the fact that this power enabled too many people to live too long and too badly. His hugely popular *Medische macht en medische ethiek* (Medical power and medical ethics), published in 1969 and continually reprinted in the 1970s, articulated at the same time the right of the patient to end his or her own life and the duty of doctors to end the lives of those who were suffering unjustifiably. In 1969, van den Berg added that medical power had doomed "countless people" to further existence who otherwise would have died much earlier, with "calamitous" results, including a rising suicide rate among older people and "the quickly increasing overpopulation of our country." Under these conditions, he maintained, a change in medical ethics was unavoidable.

The other key figure was Pieter Muntendam, who became the chairman of the Dutch Association for Voluntary Euthanasia (NVVE) in early 1976 at the age of 74, and who would play an essential role in giving the new organization a

[d] The views of state secretary A. J. H. Bartels in 1968, quoted in 28. van Berkestijn and Treffers 1971, are particularly interesting.

respectable and moderate face. A medical doctor and longtime public servant, Muntendam had been a driving force in the 1960s to reduce world population and in the early 1970s would chair a government commission charged with examining the issue.[e,29] It was perhaps natural for Muntendam, as an expert in what at the time was called "social medicine," to be interested in the "social" aspects of euthanasia, including its economic aspects. For Muntendam in particular and the NVVE in general, it was clear "that voluntary euthanasia ... must constitute a natural part of the question [of how to treat the] elderly."[30] For Muntendam, this meant that debate about euthanasia must necessarily take on the economic challenge of an aging population. For him, the primacy of the individual's right to choose when to die did not preclude discussion of wider economic and social issues.[31,32]

We can draw two conclusions from this evidence. First, the early years of the Dutch euthanasia movement showed some of the same interest in the macro-level, societal dimensions of euthanasia that had long characterized the Anglo-American euthanasia movements. The individual's right to die and society's welfare were conceived as moving in the same direction, though how the interests of the two were related was seldom articulated.

Second, it is striking how quickly this discourse declined, even though it did not entirely disappear. One reason (there are several) is that various leaders of the euthanasia movement acted decisively to interpret euthanasia purely as an individual choice. Later proponents of euthanasia would drop discussion of the socioeconomic aspects of euthanasia altogether. In 1976, pro-euthanasia advocates Andries and Truus Postma-Van Boven said that economic motives should never be used as an argument for letting people die, and by the end of the decade this had become the movement's standard response to the issue.[33] Henk Leenen, a highly influential professor of health law, stressed *voluntary* euthanasia when he took a leading role in the campaign for legalization in the late 1970s, a very conscious effort to excise the pro-euthanasia camp of socio-economic motivations.[34] During the last half of the 1970s, social and economic arguments for euthanasia were fast disappearing, and before long euthanasia discourse was almost wholly defined in terms of an individual decision that had nothing to do with society per se. John R. Blad, a scholar in the field of legal change and member of the Dutch Association for Voluntary Euthanasia, wrote in 1996 that none of the "social" arguments for euthanasia had "survived the critical test of democratic discussion."[35]

Dutch Euthanasia versus Nazi "Euthanasia"

The Dutch debate over euthanasia showed little interest in the British and American experience, but it was forced to confront the most negative legacy of

[e] The commission's report says nothing about euthanasia, and the most direct connection he made was that quality of life should now receive more emphasis than the quantity of life (see 29. Muntendam et al. 1977).

the past: Nazi mass murder as a form of "euthanasia." The charge that Dutch-style euthanasia, at least in some of its aspects, revisited Nazi practice and that Dutch proponents of euthanasia were driven chiefly by a desire to rid society of useless people continues to haunt Dutch euthanasia debate into the twenty-first century. Discussions in the Netherlands from the late 1960s to the early 1970s often brought up the Nazi example.[36,37] The sociologists reported in the early 1980s that if they had heard it at all, older people often had negative associations with the word *euthanasia,* linked as it was with the Third Reich.[f,38] It would take decades before the word was sanitized of its primary association with Nazi Germany.

Moreover, opponents of euthanasia would increasingly use the example of Nazi practices to highlight what they saw as the dangers of Dutch euthanasia practice. Law professor C. I. Dessaur's 1986 *Mag de dokter doden?* (May doctors kill?), published after the pro-euthanasia consensus in the Netherlands was already achieved, is the best-known example of this kind of effort.[39] Perhaps the fact that Dessaur was Jewish made it harder to discount her charges, lest her critics appear insensitive to what Jews had experienced in the Holocaust. There were also the occasional anti-euthanasia histories, such as those published by the dermatologist I. van der Sluis and Lindeboom in the 1970s, which cast euthanasia within a wider and more sinister pattern of modern medical eugenics.[g,8,40]

Not surprisingly, Dutch proponents of euthanasia were indignant at being tarred with the Nazi brush, which they felt was a wholly unjust characterization. Later opponents of euthanasia would complain that any comparison between the Dutch and German experience (both before and during the Nazi period) was taboo in the Netherlands and that proponents of euthanasia were more than a little sensitive to the charge.[41,42] In 1984, lawyer H. A. H. van Till-d'Aulnis de Bourouill, an early proponent of liberalizing euthanasia and the secretary of the Voluntary Euthanasia Foundation, said that it was good to occasionally hold up the mirror of the Nazi regime so as to remind contemporary society not to put pressure on people to end their lives or end the lives of those unable to speak for themselves.[43] A year later, she decried the proposal of the government study commission on euthanasia (the State Commission on Euthanasia) to euthanize coma patients without their permission precisely on the grounds that this was the kind of thing done in the Third Reich.[44] Thus, the negative example of Nazism remained in the background of the discussion, always prompting proponents to stress the voluntary nature of their proposals and helping set boundaries for what was, and was not, permissible.

If the Nazi example was the most persistent memory of the past, however, it was at the same time the most easily discounted. Many prominent figures

[f] Nursing homes were resistant to the very notion of euthanasia (see 38. Verhoef and Hilhorst 1981).

[g] More substantial historical studies would follow a decade or more later (see 7. Eijk 1987, and 10. Meerman 1991).

who favored liberalizing euthanasia were in fact pretty confident that what they were proposing had nothing to do with what the Nazis had done. Critics of van den Berg's *Medische macht* might raise the specter of Nazism, as did one reviewer in *De Groene Amsterdammer* in 1969, who warned readers that van den Berg's proposal for doctors to save only life that was "purposeful" might be abused by, as she saw it, ethically impressionable people, as had been the case in Nazi Germany.[45] But van den Berg himself had already dismissed any such connection, saying that the spectre of Nazism ought *not* to be brought up as a reaction to his heartfelt plea for putting an end to lives without purpose.[46] Jan Menges, a Dutch physician whose *"Euthanasie" in het Derde Rijk* (1972) would be the only major Dutch-language study of German practice for over two decades, issued a foreword in which he laid out the differences between illegitimate Nazi "euthanasia" and the legitimate forms of contemporary euthanasia.[47]

Others concurred. The television producer Henk Mochel took on the challenging task of showing that euthanasia in the 1970s was quite different from the type practiced by the Nazis.[48] The time seemed ripe to point this out. The span of a quarter century since the Nazi atrocities, said the theologian-ethicist P. J. Roscam Abbing in 1972, enabled people to distinguish between practices that were an "abomination" and "responsible" euthanasia.[49] For some, it became essential, in fact, that the Dutch be able to distinguish between the two types of euthanasia. In the early 1980s, Harry Kuitert, the Protestant theologian and ethicist who would subsequently play a highly influential role in the discussions, stressed that euthanasia as such had *nothing* to do with Nazi practices and that if people were going to prevent technology from having the last word at the end of life, it was necessary to break through the taboos created by the legacy of the Third Reich.

Doubtless these taboos prevailed in the minds of many Dutch, even into the 1980s and 1990s; for some proponents of euthanasia, such connections could not easily be dismissed. But by and large, even the specter of the Nazis did not inhibit the Dutch debate. Dutch culture and medical practice looked too different for that to be very convincing, at least to most Dutch people.[h,50] Further, as anti-euthanasia journalist Chris Rutenfrans has argued, the Nazi past was not *Dutch* history. According to him, the fact that the Dutch had not had any kind of prewar euthanasia movement (or, I would add, many negative experiences with authoritarian medicine in the mid-twentieth century) made them "naive" for the "dangerous road" they had chosen to tread in the previous few decades.[51] One might counter, of course, that the Dutch were less encumbered by a past that did not speak, and could not speak, to their situation. Whatever the truth, the *relative* ease with which the Dutch managed to free themselves from the Nazi question seems part of a more general pattern in

[h] Many orthodox Protestants were too suspicious of their doctors' intentions to take at face value their commitment to *voluntary* euthanasia.

their euthanasia discussion, namely, the assumption that this was a *new* problem that would have to be solved in *new* ways.

Breaking with the Dutch Past

The Dutch have often defended their euthanasia policy as one that above all has made death and thus the issue of ending life *bespreekbaar,* that is, "discussable." That word itself, which originated in the 1960s, says a great deal about the moral impulse that allowed the Dutch to choose in favor of euthanasia with greater moral certainty than other countries.

To say that the Dutch tried to make death *bespreekbaar* is not to deny that talking openly about death was a theme throughout the West in the 1960s and 1970s. That the "discussability" of death is not exclusively a Dutch phenomenon is evidenced by the fact that it was not Dutch but American scholars who first conceived of death as a taboo subject that had to be overcome, and a British scholar, John Hinton, who published the first book on dying (in 1967) that the Dutch were to use in their own debate.[52,53] Moreover, Dutch proponents of openness toward death and dying in the 1970s remained heavily indebted to international literature on the subject. The greatest apostle to preach a new openness to death was the Swiss-American Elizabeth Kübler-Ross, who was widely read not only throughout Western Europe and North America but also in the Netherlands, though Kübler-Ross herself opposed euthanasia.

The Dutch were seldom the first to raise any controversial issue or problem. The agenda for any given social and moral problem was usually launched elsewhere, including the taboo of death and, as we shall see in the next chapter, of euthanasia itself.

In what way, then, were the Dutch different from others in respect to discussing difficult or taboo subjects? It appears that the Dutch were as zealous in throwing off the unyielding norms of yesteryear as any culture in Europe, and of putting a new ethical premium on morality governing a range of issues concerning sex and death that were formerly taboo.[54] In any event, the Netherlands changed radically after 1960. The internationalization of Dutch politics, the sudden boom in the economy, and the creation of a postwar welfare state rapidly transformed Dutch society, which had been among the most religious and traditional in Western Europe up to that point. In this flux, many Dutch questioned why "old-fashioned" ideas about life and death, increasingly experienced as arbitrary and repressive, should be maintained in a "modern" world. Because the isobars of change were particularly dense in the Netherlands, the distance between tradition and modernity was perhaps felt more acutely than in many other parts of Europe. "Old" ways of thinking were attacked on all sides. Even many of those who held onto their religious convictions over the course of the 1960s frequently felt compelled to reorient their beliefs. Near the top of the agenda for many Dutch was to part with the silence and hypocrisy that ostensibly had characterized the world before 1960.

The Dutch, then, were not primarily trying to work out the problematic histories of others. They were, rather, trying to find a way to move beyond their own morally confined and old-fashioned past. As traditional values declined and fell under intense scrutiny, there was also a collective feeling that all morals, mores, and taboos were falling away, and that the standards of human conduct would all have to be renegotiated. It seemed that human beings would have to develop new sensibilities in a new age, such as daring to question taboos that protected an old-fashioned and no longer viable morality.[55]

This new orientation seemed to be most clearly expressed by religious and humanist groups seeking to restate the meaning of death, as conventional Christian morality came under pressure in a society where many believers were rapidly rejecting the moral discipline they had hitherto followed. There were also parallel developments within the medical world, both influencing and influenced by these developments. In medicine, too, there was a growing reaction against muzzling any discussion of death. The social scientist Cas Wouters, who has written about changing norms governing sex and death, argues that by the 1950s, as the medical hierarchy softened, as "personal involvement" replaced "calling" as an ideal, and as the distinction between sickness and wellness blurred, nurses were beginning to identify more strongly with their patients. This trend meant that nurses and patients were more able to speak openly with each other.[56] Although the emphasis on patient rights would have to wait until the late 1970s, this emergent "culture of discussion" challenged the medical regime in most hospitals, where nurses and doctors had avoided discussions about death because they were themselves incapable of broaching the subject, because they thought it would demoralize their patients, or simply because the efficiency model of the "health factory," as one critic called it, would not allow for it.[i,57]

The increasing insistence that death and dying be more openly discussed at the bedside than had previously been the case is perhaps best evidenced in the success of J. J. Buskes's *Truth and Lie at the Sickbed*, which went through eight printings in the decade following its release. Buskes, a prominent Protestant clergyman, argued that our inability to talk about illness and death had rendered those who were sick and dying *onmondig*, literally "without mouths." But doctors, nurses, pastors, and family members had the moral obligation to speak frankly and honestly to the patient about his condition and desires. They had the obligation to be open with the patient about difficult treatment options as well. This obligation did not always mean telling the unvarnished truth, but it did mean rejecting the systemic lies and evasions too typical of the hospital culture.[58] Toward the end of the 1960s, it became something of a commonplace to say that the taboo that the healthy had placed around death had made it difficult for patients to make their own feelings and desires *bespreekbaar*. "Our

[i] The phrase comes from J. J. Buskes (see 57. Buskes 1975).

dying are being silenced to death," an editorial in *Nieuwe Revu* pronounced in 1969.[58] This made it all the more urgent to speak truth at the bedside.[59]

One might argue that putting away taboos and making everything open to discussion was particularly important in a society that had always put a primacy on talking and that now set out, with particular energy, to dismantle what had come to be perceived as an outdated moral consensus. The taboos around death, with all their practiced piety, had for too long served as a reason not to face – not to discuss – that which must be discussed. "Reverence" was one concept sometimes associated in the 1970s with an unhealthy silence and seen as a virtue that had been too dominant in the past. Kees Trimbos, a former Catholic turned progressive and a highly influential psychiatrist, decried the resistance to research on "assistance to the dying" on the grounds of "reverence" for dying patients and their families:

> I was raised with a surfeit of reverence; reverence for nature and for the supernatural, for dying, for the dead, for the newborn child and the unborn child, for life, for old age ... for my father and mother, for my body ... for my guardian angel, for priest, bishop and pope, for authority, for my superiors and who knows what else.
>
> I have now lost all that reverence and don't understand why I must have more reverence for a dying person than research about dying. Reverence is a worn-out and dilapidated concept that has been abused countless times and may no longer serve as a weapon in serious discussions on ethical problems.[j,60]

This rejection of reverence went hand in hand with the sense that human beings, in having left absolute morality and taboos behind them, had taken on new and heavy responsibilities. Society had now grown to adulthood, said the authors of one 1972 study on death, and the future would be characterized by a new level of "shared responsibility," not least in facing death and those who were dying.[61] The physicians' journal *Medisch Contact* was full of such themes in the first half of the 1970s, as was P. J. Roscam Abbing's authoritative book *Increased Responsibility*, an ethical handbook on difficult medical decisions, including euthanasia.[50] Taboos could no longer – should no longer – shape decisions; human beings, in the spring of their adulthood, should put childish things behind them and take on the mantle of maturity.

For many, breaking with the taboo of openness concerning death had everything to do with the acceptance of euthanasia. In 1975, C. Leerling, director of the Catholic nursing home Regina Pacis in Arnhem and an early proponent of euthanasia, emphasized the advantages of "talking about death." He explained: "If we are more accepting of death we shall stand freer in relationship to it and can give people of advanced age the opportunity to die a good death."[62] Physician and popular writer Ivan Wolffers, speaking more generally,

[j] It is interesting to note that Trimbos was criticizing the reservations of Muntendam and J. F. Rang to research of the dying – scholars hardly opposed to euthanasia (see 60. Trimbos 1776).

made a similar point: that until we face death we are not ready for an "open discussion" about euthanasia.[63] Whatever the connection between the acceptance of death and the acceptance of euthanasia, many proponents believed that the two were inseparably linked. Pieter Admiraal, an anesthetist, outspoken humanist, and author of the 1980 "how to" pamphlet informing doctors about performing euthanasia, expressed his opinion in 1983 that the taboo to overcome was not that surrounding euthanasia but around death itself.[64]

An additional reason why many Dutch of the 1970s thought that the taboos surrounding death and euthanasia should be broken was that doctors were *already* euthanizing patients behind the scenes. The issue of "crypto-euthanasia" was dramatically brought to life in the 1973 trial of the physician Truus Postma-Van Boven, who had euthanized her own mother (at the mother's request) in 1971. There was a widespread sense that physicians should not have to lie about what they actually did and should be able to admit their deeds openly. "It shouldn't happen sneakily," Dr. Postma-Van Boven told an interviewer after her trial.[k,65]

The Dutch insistence that a taboo covered secret forms of euthanasia – simply intolerable in this age of openness – seems to reflect a peculiarly Dutch preoccupation with a certain kind of truth telling in regards to euthanasia. Breaking the taboo was not only good medical policy but also a moral step forward, the argument ran. Mochel saw talking about euthanasia as a way to protest and combat the "dogmatism and legalism that protect the medical class from uncertainty."[48] The Dutch weekly *Elsevier* argued that the change toward euthanasia had less to do with changed opinion than with a simple willingness to talk about it, and then added, "the sought-after death is emerging from the domain of the taboo, the domain of stigmatization and secrecy, of damnation and medieval certainties."[66]

Dutch anti-taboo culture of the 1970s and 1980s, then, placed hypocrisy at the top of the list of sins, and to break the taboo of euthanasia was to wage war against hypocrisy. Klazien Sybrandy, the maverick pro-euthanasia activist who helped found the NVVE, wrote with her compatriot and euthanasia activist Rob Bakker that the guilt surrounding euthanasia was not about motives or deeds but about *lying*.[67] Strikingly, many doctors would voice their own moral anguish with having to lie on the death certificate and elsewhere in order to avoid prosecution; they would argue that one of the advantages of legalization could be to unbind the consciences of conflicted doctors. At the same time, there was hostility toward the "hypocrisy" of doctors in euthanizing patients and not reporting it as such.[68]

In summary, the pro-euthanasia movement drew moral strength from the particularly strong anti-taboo culture of the 1970s and 1980s, with its emphasis

[k] Wim Ramaker thought this quotation so poignant, or so central to the whole interview, that his published interview bears it as its title (see 65. Ramaker 1973).

on breaking with the morality of the Dutch past, rejecting "hypocritical" and unquestioned practices in favor of truth telling and *bespreekbaarheid,* to make matters "discussable." The moral ambiguities in euthanasia (and assisted suicide) were given greater clarity through the conviction that taboo breaking toward sex and death in particular was good, and that taboo breaking in respect to euthanasia, with its promise of less hypocrisy and more openness, must also be good. This powerful cultural impulse helps explain why, in contrast to other countries, the Netherlands, relatively early on and with a high sense of moral confidence, dared to openly adopt the practice of euthanasia.

References

1. Lindeboom, Gerrit A. 1932. Euthanasie. *Predikant en dokter* 2: 207.
2. The, Anne-Mei. 2009. *Verlossers naast God, Dokters en euthanasia in Nederland.* Amsterdam: Thoeris.
3. Jongsma, M. W. 1968. Verlenging en verkorting van het leven. In *Recent medisch ethisch denken*, ed. L. H. Th. S. Kortbeerk, 131–133. Leiden: Stafleu's.
4. Meier, Henk J. 1968. *Menswaardig sterven: Euthanasie in discussie*. Hilversum: P. Brand.
5. Filene, Peter G. 1998. *In the Arms of Others: A Cultural History of the Right-to-Die in America.* Chicago: Ivan R. Dee.
6. Kemp, Nick. 2002. *Merciful Release: The History of the British Euthanasia Movement.* Manchester: Manchester University Press.
7. Eijk, Willem Jacobus. 1987. *De zelfgekozen dood naar aanleiding van een dodelijke en ongeneeslijke ziekte. Een medisch-historisch en medisch-ethisch onderzoek ten behoeve van een Rooms-Katholiek standpunt inzake euthanasie.* Bruges: Tabor.
8. Sluis, I. van der. 1979. *Het recht om grootmoeder te doden.* Amsterdam: Saint Jacques.
9. Ezekiel J. Emanuel. 1998. "Why Now?" In *Regulating How We Die: The Ethical, Medical and Legal Issues Surrounding Physician-Assisted Suicide*, ed. Linda L. Emanuel, 189. Cambridge, MA: Harvard University Press.
10. Meerman, Dick. 1991. *Goed doen door dood te maken. Een analyse van de morele argumentatie in vijf maatschappelijke debatten over euthanasie tussen 1870 en 1940 in Engeland en Duitsland.* Kampen: Kok.
11. Dowbiggin, Ian. 2003. *A Merciful End: The Euthanasia Movement in Modern America.* Oxford: Oxford University Press.
12. The, Anne-Mei. 2009. *Verlossers naast God.* Amsterdam: Thoeris.
13. Dowbiggin, Ian. 2005. *A Concise History of Euthanasia: Life, Death, God and Medicine*. Lanham, MD: Rowman & Littlefield.
14. Greeve, Max. 1923. *Zelfmoord, met ideeën betreffende eene wettelijke regeling.* The Hague: Haga.
15. Noordman, Jan. 1989. *Om de kwaliteit van het nageslacht. Eugenetica in Nederland, 1900–1950.* Nijmegen: SUN.
16. Flokstra, Tjeerd, and Sjoerd Wieling. 1986. *De geschiedenis van het Humanistisch Verbond, 1946–1986*. Utrecht: De Walburg Press.
17. Mourik Broekman, M. C. van. 1946. *Beschikkingsrecht over leven en dood. Zedekundige opstellen over actueele vraagstukken* The Hague: Leopolds.

18. Weyers, Heleen. 2004. *Euthanasie. Het process van rechtsverandering.* Amsterdam: Amsterdam University Press.
19. Drogendijk, A. C., Jr. 1974. Op de grens van soort en individu. *Medisch Contact* 29: 505–509.
20. Outshoorn, Joyce. 1984. *De politieke strijd rondom de abortuswetgeving in Nederland, 1964–1984.* Den Haag: VUGA.
21. Bruijn, Jan de. 1979. *Geschiedenis van de abortus in Nederland.* Amsterdam: Van Gennep.
22. Jörg, A. J. 1968. *Wat gaat ons de toekomst aan? Zes orientaties ten aanzien van de naaste toekomst.* The Hague: Boekencentrum.
23. Zonneveld, R. J. 1974. Oud worden in onze maatschappij. In *Oud worden, oud zijn*, ed. D. W. van Bekkum et al., 18. Deventer: Van Loghum Slaterus/Stichting Bio-Wetenschappen en Maatschappij.
24. Aalders, Marius. 1971. Het recht om te sterven – een goed recht. *Haagse Post*, January 27.
25. Stichting Vrijwillige Euthanasie. 1975. *De dood komt soms te laat.* Lochem: De Tijdstroom.
26. Kosten gezondheidszorg tussen 1963 en 1972 gestegen met ongeveer 450%. 1975. *Medisch Contact* 30: 683.
27. Herbergs, Ben. 1984. *Laat me sterven voor ik wakker word … tien jaar strijd om het recht op een menswaardig levenseinde.* Amsterdam/Brussels: Elsevier.
28. Berkestijn, Hans van, and Flip Treffers. 1971. Het recht op de dood. *Groene Amsterdammer*, January 9.
29. Muntendam, P., et al. 1977. *Bevolking en welzijn in Nederland. Rapport van de Staatscommissie Bevolkingsvraagstuk vastgesteld te Leidschendam December 1976.* The Hague: Staatsuitgeverij.
30. NVVE (Nederlandse Vereniging voor een Vrijwillig Levenseinde). 1976. "Oud worden – oud zijn." *NVVE Kwartaalblad* 2, (April).
31. NVVE (Nederlandse Vereniging voor een Vrijwillig Levenseinde). 1976. "Prof. Muntendam en de euthanasiewetgeving." *NVVE Kwartaalblad* 2, (April).
32. Muntendam, P. 1982. Euthanasie, weer terug in de taboesfeer? *NVVE Kwartaalblad* 8, (September).
33. Jansma, Klaas. 1976. Term euthanasie misbruikt bij proces tegen Frans H. *Het Parool*, May 8.
34. Interview with Henk Leenen, Amsterdam, June 6, 2000.
35. J. R. Blad. 1996. *Abolitionisme als strafrechtstheorie: Theoretische beschouwingen over het abolitionisme van L. H. C. Hulsman*, 325. Deventer: Gouda Quint.
36. Jongsma, M. W. 1968. Geneeskunde en ethiek. In *Om de mens. Ethiek in wetenschap en beroep*, ed: P. J. Roscam Abbing 1968, 87. Leiden: A. W. Sijthoff. – Jongsma. 1968. Verlenging en verkorting van het leven. In *Recent ethisch medisch handelen*, ed. L. H. T. S. Kortbeek, 134. Leiden: Stafleu. – J. Th. R. Schreuder. Het recht om te sterven. 1968. In Kortbeek, 155.
37. Schreuder, J. T. R. 1968. Het recht om te sterven. In *Recent medisch ethisch denken*, ed. L. H. Th. S. Kortbeek, 155. Leiden: Stafleu.
38. Verhoef, Marja J., and Henri W. A. Hilhorst. 1981. *De "zachte dood" in de praktijk. Stervensbegeleiding en en euthanasie in het verpleeghuis.* Lochem: De Tijdstroom.

39. Dessaur, C. I., and C. J. C. Rutenfrans. 1986. *Mag de dokter doden? Argumenten en documenten tegen het euthanasiasme*. Amsterdam: Querido.
40. Lindeboom, Gerrit A. 1978. *Euthanasie in historisch perspectief.* Amsterdam: Rodopi.
41. Goud, Johan. 1995. Ethische ficties. In *Als de dood voor het leven. Over professionele hulp bij zelfmoord*, ed. Hans Achterhuis et al., 29. Amsterdam: G. A. van Oorschot.
42. Croughs, R. W. M. 1988.Euthanasie: Een vergelijking van de huidige discussie in Nederland met de discussie in Duitsland vóór 1933. In *Gebroken wereld. Zwakzinnigen zorg en de vraag naar euthanasie*, ed. J. Stolk, 104. Kampen: Kok.
43. Pols, Bram. 1984. Secretaris van de Stichting Vrijwillige Euthanasie: Nieuwe wetgeving is onnodig. *Trouw*, February 29.
44. Till-d'Aulnis de Bourouill, H. A. H. van. 1985. Patiëntenrecht en het artikel 292 bis van de Staatscommissie Euthanasie. *Medisch Contact* 43: 1347.
45. Mey, C. Wennen van der. 1969. Medische ethiek ter discussie. *Groene Amsterdammer*, October 4.
46. Berg, J. H. van den. 1969. *Medische macht en medische ethiek*, 47. Nijkerk: Callenbach.
47. Menges, J. 1972. *"Euthanasie" in het Derde Rijk*. Haarlem: De Erven Bohn.
48. Mochel, Henk, ed. 1972. *Een milde dood. Gedachten en een verslag van een televisieserie over euthanasie*, 12–13. Kampen: Kok.
49. Roscam Abbing, P. J. 1972. *Toegenomen verantwoordelijkheid. Euthanasie – Eugenetiek – Moderne biologie. Medisch-ethische beschouwingen*. Nijkerk: Callenbach.
50. Kuiper, Roel. 2000. *SISWO presentation*, Amsterdam, June 30.
51. Rutenfrans, Frans. 1997. Alles onder controle, eerst het water, nu de dood. *De Gids* 160 (7/8): 586.
52. Glaser, B. G., and A. L. Strauss. 1965. *Awareness of Dying*. Chicago: Aldine.
53. Hinton, John. 1967. *Dying.* Harmondsworth: Penguin Books.
54. Kennedy, James. 2002. *Een weloverwogen dood. Euthanasie in Nederland.* Amsterdam: Uitgeverij Bert Bakker.
55. Interview with Cor Spreeuwenberg, Maastricht, June 29, 2000.
56. Wouters, Cas. 1990. *Van minnen en sterven*. Amsterdam: B. Bakker.
57. Buskes, J. J. 1975. *Waarheid en leugen aan het ziekbed* [Truth and lie at the sickbed]. Baarn: Ten Have.
58. Onze stervenden worden doodgezwegen. 1969. *Nieuwe Revu*, July 19.
59. Menges, L. J. 1971. De waarheid aan het ziekbed. In *Over dood en sterven*, ed. Heije Faber, 61–70 Leiden: Universitaire Pers Leiden.
60. Trimbos, Kees. 1976. Sterven en onderzoek. *Maandblad voor Geestelijke Volksgezondheid* 31: 103.
61. Thia, A. J. H. Dens, and L. A. A. Bakker. 1972. *Doodgaan is nog geen sterven.* Baarn: Het Wereldvenster.
62. NVVE (Nederlandse Vereniging voor een Vrijwillig Levenseinde). 1976. "Praten over sterven." *NVVE Kwartaalblad* 2 (January).
63. Wolffers, Ivan, and Waldemar Post. 1979. *Een eindje mee lopen*, 91. Baarn: Ambo.

64. NVVE (Nederlandse Vereniging voor een Vrijwillig Levenseinde). 1983. Lustrum congres: Euthanasie in de praktijk. *NVVE Kwartaalblad* 9 (December).
65. Ramaker, Wim. 1973. *Er is een tijd om te sterven*, 108. Kampen: Kok.
66. Luijk, Henk van. 1980. De ethiek van de gezochte dood. *Elseviers* 9 (March 1).
67. Sybrandy, Klanzien, and Rob Bakker. 1984. *Zorg jij dat ik niet wakker wordt? Vrijwillige euthanasie in de praktijk.* Amsterdam: Anthos.
68. Dekker, A. 1982. Euthanasie: ethische aspecten. In *Euthanasie. Medische, ethische en juridische aspecten*, ed. A. Dekker, G. E. Mulder, and D. Post, 37. Kampen: Kok.

2

Classifications and Definitions

Dutch Developments

Johan Legemaate

INTRODUCTION

Classifications and definitions play an important role in the debate on medical intervention in end-of-life treatment, both in the Netherlands and internationally. They can also play an important role in clarifying the standards and requirements for due care that have to be observed in certain forms of medical intervention in the end-of-life phase. Classifying and defining the nature of these interventions and what they entail thus enables a better understanding of what actions are actually involved, as well as the degree of ethical, legal, or social control that is desirable or necessary. That is one side of the issue. The other side is that classifications and definitions can play a guiding role, and indeed it is often with that purpose in mind that they are introduced and formulated. This is because they draw a distinction or line between, for example, those forms of intervention that are considered acceptable and those that are not. To that extent, they cannot be viewed separately from the views and intentions of the people or organizations putting these classifications and definitions into words. Both elements – the structuring and the guiding sides – are clearly recognizable in the debate surrounding medical intervention in the end-of-life phase.

This chapter analyses the way in which classifications and definitions in the Netherlands have influenced both day-to-day practice and regulations on medical intervention at the end of life.

HISTORY: PHASE I

The need for a distinction between different forms of medical intervention in the end-of-life phase arose in the Netherlands in the early 1970s.[1,2] The first occasion on which a Dutch court ruled concerning active termination of a life by a doctor was in 1973 in the *Postma* case, which triggered extensive discussions both within and outside the medical profession. The *Postma* case occurred at a time when the limits of medicine were increasingly being questioned. And these questions were very clearly reflected in the ruling when the judge concluded that the average physician in the Netherlands no longer believed that a patient's life should be prolonged until the bitter end; this was one of the reasons why the court ruled that it was conceivable and acceptable in certain circumstances for a doctor actively to terminate a life.

This new reality demanded new terminology. Although the term *euthanasia* immediately became important in this respect, it also created problems; it was a term that had traditionally had a broad meaning in the sense of a good or merciful death. This resulted in the decision by the Dutch right-to-die association, established in 1973 in the wake of the *Postma* case, to call itself the Dutch Association for Voluntary Euthanasia (Nederlandse Vereniging voor een Vrijwillige Euthanasie). The common definition of euthanasia in use until then had not included this element of *voluntariness*. Traditionally, "euthanasia" had also included situations in which life was terminated without the request of the person concerned. Similarly, no distinction had normally been made between direct and indirect forms of terminating life, as the term was also used in situations in which a patient died after a decision to withdraw ineffective treatment. These situations were referred to as "passive euthanasia."

In other words, euthanasia can be active but also passive, direct but also indirect, and voluntary but also involuntary. We come across all these terms and descriptions in the debate that arose in the Netherlands in the 1970s.[1,3]

HISTORY: PHASE 2

Toward the end of the 1970s, there were increasing calls for the ending of life at a person's request not only to be accepted but also to be permitted by law. And this development was the primary factor prompting a reassessment of the terminology that had been used in the debate until then. Statutory regulations on terminating life on request would clearly have to be subject to strict conditions. That, in turn, required a clearer distinction among the various forms of medical intervention in the end-of-life phase. The broad definition of euthanasia also made it more difficult to achieve statutory regulation on the ending of life on request. That resulted in a movement seeking to achieve two objectives.

The first objective was to limit the scope of the term *euthanasia* to intervention that actively terminated life. Those in favor of this limitation sought to stop the use of the term *passive euthanasia*; in their view, passive euthanasia referred to activities that constituted a form of normal medical intervention that were governed by the physician's professional standards. In the words of the eminent professor of health law Henk Leenen, these cases did not involve euthanasia but, instead, "apparitions of euthanasia."[4] Leenen and his supporters recognized considerable normative differences between the active termination of life, on the one hand, and the withdrawing or withholding of treatment and pain relief, on the other hand. From an ethical and legal perspective, they attached great importance to the distinction between "killing" and "letting die."

The second objective was to restrict the term *euthanasia* to situations involving the active ending of life at the *explicit request* of the patient. The background to this was the sharp legal distinction perceived to exist between actively ending life at the patient's request and actively ending life without such request. The latter form of intervention was regarded as highly problematic, not least because of the provisions of the European Convention on Human Rights (ECHR). The belief was that statutorily regulating the active ending of life on request was compatible with provisions of the ECHR, whereas actively ending life without such request certainly would not be. This development came to a provisional end in 1985, when the Dutch State Commission on Euthanasia published its final report. This commission defined euthanasia as "actively terminating life at the patient's request." Since then, the patient's request has constituted an explicit element of the definition.[1]

Intermezzo I: Relationship Between the Netherlands and Other Countries

It would be no exaggeration to state that the developments occurring in the Netherlands between approximately 1975 and 1985 caused considerable linguistic confusion in the nation's relationships with other countries. Primarily for reasons of domestic politics, the Netherlands was now using a definition of euthanasia that was more restrictive than the interpretation attributed by many other countries to this term. This resulted in considerable confusion in discussions not only between Dutch and foreign parties but also within domestic parties being reproached for incorrectly distinguishing – from a perspective of ethical and legal acceptability – between killing and letting die. Although some of the sharpness of this contrast between the Netherlands and other countries has faded over the past 25 years, it has not yet completely disappeared. Recent examples show that many countries still do not recognize and acknowledge the Dutch definition of euthanasia.[5] In discussions on ending the life of newborn infants with serious disorders (the Groningen Protocol) or withdrawing treatment in the case of comatose patients, "euthanasia" is still in very common use in many countries.

HISTORY: PHASE 3

The classifications and definitions that started being used in the Netherlands in the 1970s and 1980s made a significant contribution to the input used by the researchers commissioned in the years from 1990 onward to conduct empirical studies of day-to-day Dutch practice.[6,7,8,9] For the purposes of this research, they devised a set of terms that, with a few minor changes, is still being used today. This terminology framework recognizes four different categories of medical intervention in the end-of-life phase:

1. Euthanasia and assisted suicide;
2. Life-ending treatment without the patient's explicit request;
3. Pain and symptom relief;
4. Withdrawing or withholding of treatment.

In addition to these four categories, the issue of palliative sedation was also considered in the two most recent empirical studies, published in 2003[8] and 2007.[9]

The classification used in the empirical research since the early 1990s has gained a distinction far exceeding the significance of this research. This system of classification has now developed dynamics of its own and has increasingly formed a framework for the ethical, medical, and social debate. Indeed, it has become common practice, at least in policy discussions, to classify medical decisions in the end-of-life phase in this way. Within the Netherlands, this classification, over time, has come to include widely accepted but usually implicit views on the acceptability of medical intervention in the end-of-life phase. The forms of intervention "above the line" are pain and symptom relief and the withdrawing or withholding of treatment, which are regarded in the Netherlands as "normal medical intervention."[1,10] Patients meeting the indications are entitled to such intervention; the issue of whether they comply with the indications is determined by professional standards and the general legislative rules on patients' rights (in other words, the professional expertise of the physician, the rules on information and consent, and the way in which the interests of patients unable to make their wishes known are represented). "Below the line" are euthanasia and assisted suicide, as well as the ending of life without a patient's explicit request. These latter forms of intervention, which are regarded as "exceptional medical intervention," are those permitted under certain circumstances, but to which the patient has no enforceable right.

Not only must these forms of intervention conform with the relevant professional standards, but they also have to meet the specific, strict conditions stipulated in law (in the cases of euthanasia and assisted suicide) or in case law (in the case of life-ending intervention without the patient's explicit request). In this way, the issue of medical decisions in the end-of-life phase in day-to-day practice in the Netherlands and in the Dutch legal system has been classified and systematized to a high degree, along with broadly supported views on the acceptability (in a general sense) of the various forms of intervention. The discussion is, however, anything but over, as the recent debate on palliative sedation clearly shows. Indeed, there is a range of opinion on where best to place this form of intervention in the classification model, and I will come back to this topic later.

Intermezzo II: Policy and Practice

The developments referred to with respect to the definition of euthanasia and the classification of medical interventions in the end-of-life phase have had a substantial impact on the level of Dutch policy, and I intend to discuss the significance of this for Dutch legislation. At this point, however, I would like to consider how the said definitions and classifications are dealt with in practice. Certainly not everyone regards the definitions as clear and unambiguous, specifically in situations relating to care provided in the end-of-life phase. People can interpret definitions differently, depending, for example, on their moral or other views concerning the acceptability of terminating life. Research has shown that those providing care are influenced not only by objective (in other words, medical) considerations but also by personal views on dying and death.[11] And these views color the way the person views classifications and definitions. A definition that is perfectly clear and unambiguous to one person may be very misleading to someone else.

It is important for a wide variety of reasons that we understand this aspect, not least because the classification of medical interventions in the end-of-life phase (in other words, the four categories, together with palliative sedation), while having proved its value conceptually, is not always of optimal use in day-to-day practice. Empirical research published between 1991 and 2007 on the Dutch practice of medical intervention in the end-of-life phase consistently emphasizes the overlap among the various categories in the classification model. To give two examples:

- In the research published in 1991, 2% of the cases involved situations in which no clear distinction was able to be made between euthanasia and assisted suicide, on the one hand, and pain and symptom relief, on the other hand.[6]
- In the research published in 2007, 3.1% of the cases of continuous deep sedation were classified as euthanasia or assisted suicide, while 2% were regarded as the ending of life without request.[9]

Over the years, it became increasingly easier to make a clear distinction among the various categories in the classification system, partly because the empirical studies have devoted far more attention to the specific means used by the doctor. Nevertheless, the terms used to classify medical intervention by doctors in the end-of-life phase continue to be confused.

To a large extent, this confusion has to be attributed to the significance that the successive empirical studies have attached to the doctor's intention. The question of what a doctor was intending to achieve by intervening has been and continues to be considered when the most appropriate category in which to classify a specific intervention is decided. There has been increasing criticism of that approach in recent years, based on the argument that a doctor's claim that the intention of intervening was to shorten the life or suffering of the patient is certainly not always a good basis for classifying the action as active termination of life (whether on request or otherwise).[5,12] What matters, according to these critics, is what the doctor has actually done (in other words, which method or which dose) and what has actually happened (in terms of accelerating the moment of death). In this context, account must always be taken of the life-shortening effect of interventions that are not (or are not primarily) designed to terminate life. It is widely known, for example, that morphine administered in a dose appropriate for pain or symptom relief can have the side effect of shortening a patient's life. It is perfectly conceivable that a doctor may state in such a situation that the intention was to relieve the patient's suffering, but that does not mean that the doctor's action can or should be classified as actively ending life. That would apply only if the dose administered by the doctor for the purposes of pain or symptom relief was too high or even excessively high. In such cases, describing the intervention as actively ending life could certainly be correct.

All of this means, incidentally, that the empirical data from the independent studies performed in the Netherlands since 1991 may be somewhat "polluted." It is possible, for example, that interventions were classified on the basis of the doctor's stated intentions as "active termination of life," but in retrospect should not have been assigned to that category.

Other sources, too, show that differences of interpretation may exist with respect to the classification of medical interventions at the end of life, both among those providing care, on the one hand, and lawyers, on the other.[11] Literature on the subject contains examples of medical intervention that are characterized differently by the various parties involved in providing the care (doctors, nurses, and so on). Whereas one party regards the intervention as pain relief, another views it as euthanasia and yet another as palliative sedation. As part of his doctoral research, D. van Tol submitted a number of cases to both doctors and lawyers for consideration. While a majority of the doctors classified most of these cases as "normal medical intervention," the lawyers, by contrast, viewed most of the cases as examples of active ending of life.[13] From this we can conclude that the developments in the Netherlands with respect to classifying and defining medical interventions in the end-of-life phase have resulted in only limited clarity and a limited lack of ambiguity. Differences of opinion continue to exist, both among those providing care and between doctors and lawyers, and classifications and definitions either have failed or have managed to alter this situation to only a limited degree.

Intermezzo III: Distinctions Between Medical and Legal Conceptualizations

The differences in interpretation between doctors and lawyers just mentioned highlight a specific aspect of classifying and defining medical interventions at the end of life: in other words, the difference between the medical reality as perceived and experienced by doctors and the way in which lawyers conceptualize medical interventions. It is precisely in those sorts of situations that the relationship between classification and definition, on the one hand, and acceptance and regulation, on the other, become so clearly evident.

It has been proposed on several occasions in the Dutch debate that the concepts of accelerating death and ending life should be distinguished from each other, and that this distinction should also be reflected in terms of liability for punishment, how the action is assessed, and so on.[1,2,5,10] The most widely known proposal was made in 1991 by the Remmelink Committee, which reported on the results of the first empirical research into medical decisions around the end of life. The committee recommended that the "active ending of life at a moment at which vital functions are beginning to fail" be regarded as assistance to the dying and as a normal medical intervention because a doctor's active intervention in such cases is "often inevitable as a result of a patient being terminally ill and close to death." Many doctors (and possibly other people, too) will support the committee's reasoning. Indeed, Govert den Hartogh described the committee's views in this respect as being "widely shared."[12]

Although the Remmelink Committee's proposal has never become generally accepted policy, subsequent committees have expressed support for its approach: It is not considered reasonable for a relatively minor difference between two situations to result in such far-reaching differences in legal consequences. Compare, for example, the following two situations:

- *Situation 1*: At 15:00 on a certain day a dying patient is no longer able to communicate. All those around the patient (doctors and the patient's family) believe that the patient is experiencing severe suffering. Palliative treatment is provided and the sedated patient dies at 22:45 (a natural death).
- *Situation 2*: At 15:00 on a certain day a dying patient is no longer able to communicate. All those around the patient (doctors and the patient's family) believe that the patient is experiencing severe suffering. The doctor decides to administer medication that will end the patient's life. As a result, the patient dies at 16:30 (an unnatural death).

Describing the second situation as "life ending" does not accord with doctors' perception of the position.

That feeling was also discussed in the report presented by the consultative group charged by the ministers of justice and of health, welfare, and sport with formulating review proposals for monitoring the observance of due care in medical procedures relating to newborn infants in the end-of-life phase.[14] As the report stated (pp. 11–12):

> The consultative group is aware of situations in which a doctor administers medication in order to accelerate the death that, owing to the nature of the condition, is expected in the very near future.... According to the letter of the law and the definitions used by the consultative group, decisions such as these are covered by the regulations on the deliberate ending of life and so are required to be reported and reviewed.... The consultative group can imagine that doctors do not regard such decisions as the deliberate ending of life, but instead view them as good terminal care.

A committee of the Royal Dutch Medical Association concluded in a similar context in 1997 (p. 67):

A majority on the committee believe that administering medication after it has been decided to withdraw or withhold treatment, such that [the patient] will die, can constitute part of proper terminal care.... The committee is also aware, however, of the tension between this view and the legal conceptualization of such situations: The primary question in this respect is whether medication has been administered that directly resulted in death. Although the legal assessment of the situation is based on this aspect, there are a number of cases in which medication has been administered in this way that should actually be regarded as the provision of proper terminal care after a decision to withdraw or withhold treatment, and that this decision was in fact sufficient in itself to allow [the patient] to die.[15]

Although the views expressed here have never resulted in any change in policy or regulations, the distinction between medical and legal conceptualizations continues to play an important role, both in day-to-day practice and in discussions of policy and legislation.

HISTORY: PHASE 4

The debate over classifying and defining medical interventions in the end-of-life phase was given a new impulse in the Netherlands in 2003, when more information became available on palliative sedation. In an empirical study into the practice of medical intervention in the end-of-life phase published in 2003, the researchers stated that it was not always possible to make a clear distinction between euthanasia and palliative sedation in all situations.[8] This conclusion led the then-chairman of the Board of Prosecutors General (a group of government prosecutors, chaired by the "attorney general" of the Netherlands, who meet regularly to discuss policy issues) to state that sedating a terminal patient experiencing unbearable suffering to the extent that the patient becomes unconscious could be justified from a medical perspective, but from a legal perspective this could still be regarded as the ending of life. As the chairman said:

It might not be the intention of a doctor who induces a coma in a patient and then stops providing food and water that the patient should ultimately die, but from a criminal law perspective there is a relevant connection. If the patient's death is very likely to be the result of the doctor's action, this can be sufficient to prove intent. It is not required for the doctor also to have wanted the patient's death.[16]

This statement was seen by the medical profession as a barely disguised threat to move action regarded as normal medical intervention into the sphere of criminal law and to subject the issue to legal rules. The public prosecutor seemed then to put words into action by deciding to prosecute a doctor who was accused of ending life without request, but who personally regarded his action as normal medical intervention (in the form of pain relief and sedation).

The expert witness report was one of the reasons why the Breda court decided in November 2004 to accept the doctor's explanation. The court made a clear distinction in this respect between normal medical intervention, on the one hand, and the requirement in criminal proceedings for conditional intent (in terms of the significant likelihood of death), on the other hand. In the case in question, the court ruled that the likelihood of an earlier death (as a result of a sedative and – usually – morphine) was not sufficient in itself to assume a conditional intent to kill a patient. This ruling was upheld by the Hertogenbosch court on July 19, 2005. The Regional Medical Disciplinary Board in Zwolle dismissed the charge of termination of life that had been brought against the doctor by the inspectorate. The Disciplinary Board found that both the medication chosen and the dose applied were consistent with a policy of symptom relief and, therefore, with normal medical intervention.

These high-profile legal proceedings were one of the reasons prompting the Royal Dutch Medical Association to take the initiative to issue a guideline on palliative sedation.[17,18] This guideline, which was published in 2005 and updated in 2009, interprets palliative sedation as the "deliberate reducing of a patient's consciousness in the final phase of life." A distinction is made between two forms of palliative sedation: short-term/intermittent sedation and continuous sedation until the moment of death. The latter (continuous sedation until the moment of death) implies the withholding of food and drink (administered artificially). For this reason, the guideline sees continuous sedation until the moment of death as acceptable only if, while in compliance with various other conditions, the patient has a life expectancy of shorter than two weeks. The information on which the guideline is based shows that in some circumstances, withholding food and drink will not, or no longer in and of itself, have any effect on the patient's life expectancy. If continuous sedation until the moment of death were to start earlier, there could (possibly) be such an effect, and this would blur the distinction between palliative sedation and actively terminating life (whether on request or otherwise).

This example shows how the possible implications of classification and definition in terms of medical ethics and/or legal acceptability can have an impact on the definition or formulation of the conditions and requirements to be observed. Under the guideline, palliative sedation in the case of a patient with a life expectancy of shorter than two weeks is seen as "normal medical intervention." In other cases, there may be reasons for viewing palliative sedation as a form of active ending of life. Just like the definition of euthanasia established in the 1980s, this is typical of the way in which the issue is dealt with in the Netherlands, where solutions reached can generally be counted on as enjoying broad support, both within the medical profession and in wider society. This does not mean that these choices and developments are not subject to critical discussion in the country, but these discussions focus primarily on exceptions and individual aspects of the issue, rather than on basic principles and general frameworks.

DUTCH LEGISLATION

Most of the developments outlined in the previous sections occurred prior to the drafting of the Dutch Euthanasia Act, which came into force in 2002.[5,10] It is important to note that "Euthanasia Act" is the name popularly used for the legislation and not its official name. The official name of the legislation is The Termination of Life on Request and Assisted Suicide (Review Procedures) Act (Wet Toetsing Levensbeëindiging op verzoek en hulp bij zelfdoding). In other words, the legislator opted not to use the term *euthanasia* in the name of the act. From the very start, however, it was clear that the legislation would cover the issues and classification of euthanasia and assisted suicide devised in the early 1990s. Obviously, the word was used frequently in the parliamentary discussions of the bill, both by the ministers responsible and by members of parliament, but, as mentioned, the act itself does not use the term.

The Dutch legislation does not provide an explicit definition of euthanasia. The scope of the Euthanasia Act, as I will refer to it here, has to be derived, therefore, from the legal relationship between this legislation and the Dutch Penal Code (Wetboek van Strafrecht). The scope of the act can consequently be described as the deliberate termination of life by (in the case of euthanasia) or by means of (in the case of assisted suicide) the explicit and properly considered request of the patient. This means that the following medical interventions in the end-of-life phase are not covered by the Euthanasia Act:

a. Withdrawing or withholding treatment;
b. Pain and symptom relief;
c. Palliative sedation;
d. Life-ending intervention without the patient's explicit request.

The medical interventions referred to in a to c are governed by the general legislation on patient rights and the prevailing guidelines or protocols of the medical profession.[1,5] In these cases, therefore, there are no special statutory provisions that apply, and no requirement to report the medical intervention or to consult an independent doctor before performing the intervention (although in extreme situations, this is certainly recommended and regularly occurs in practice). The forms of medical intervention referred to in b and c are covered by the Euthanasia Act if they involve higher doses of medication being administered than professional standards would consider normal for the specific intervention (i.e., pain relief or palliative sedation) and if a relationship can be demonstrated between the administering of this medication and the acceleration of the patient's death.

For other reasons, the termination of life without the patient's explicit request is not covered by the scope of the Euthanasia Act. In the eyes of the legislator, such action is not permitted. Moreover, statutory acceptance of such action would contravene Article 3 of the ECHR (on the right to life). This is notwithstanding the fact, however, that a court may regard the termination of life without the patient's explicit request as legally justified in an individual case. In recent years, courts have accepted such justification in a few cases, and the Groningen Protocol is based on this (albeit limited) legal practice.

To determine the exact scope of the Dutch Euthanasia Act, it is important to consider the statutory requirements and conditions in more detail.[5,10] The primary issue in this respect is the patient's request, one of the key aspects of the statutory provisions. The Dutch Euthanasia Act does not require the patient to be able to express an oral request for his or her life to be terminated right up until the moment of the intervention. Instead of an oral request, a written request is also possible, provided the patient made this request while still able to express his or her will. The other statutory provisions and conditions will then continue to apply, including the crucial requirement for the suffering to be unbearable and with no prospect of improvement. The statutory provision regarding the patient's written request offers a solution in situations where the patient is no longer conscious at the time of the intended euthanasia, but where there are still sufficient grounds and indications for regarding the suffering as unbearable and with no prospect of improvement. If the suffering cannot be described in this way, or cannot continue to be, it is not possible by law to perform euthanasia.

This latter factor means that euthanasia is not possible in the case of a comatose patient. In such cases, it is normally assumed that the suffering cannot or can no longer be regarded as unbearable and with no prospect of improvement, given that a condition for the existence of suffering is that the patient must actually experience it. In the case of a comatose patient, there is still the possibility that treatment (including food and/or liquids) will at some point be withheld or that new complications will no longer be treated, in both cases because providing or continuing to provide treatment is considered medically pointless. As outlined earlier, such situations are not covered by the Dutch Euthanasia Act.

CONCLUSION

Developments in the classification and definitions of the various medical interventions in the end-of-life phase have had a substantial impact on both policy and day-to-day practice in the Netherlands. Initially, the background to these developments was a wish to establish standards and to make a distinction between "normal" and "exceptional" medical interventions, and also to enable "exceptional medical intervention" (i.e., the active ending of life, whether on request or otherwise) to be subjected to specific, strict rules. In this way, a distinction in terms of acceptance and legitimacy was established that has generally been well received within the Dutch legal community and society, but that has not always accorded with foreigners' views on which medical interventions in the end-of-life phase are acceptable and which are not. This has caused considerable confusion and lack of clarity abroad on how exactly to interpret developments in the Netherlands.

Has there been a gradual clarification of day-to-day practice, and are the standards that apply with respect to the duty of care being made more explicit, or are definitions being used to argue away questions on acceptance and legitimacy? Developments in the Netherlands have frequently attracted criticism in this respect. Whether this criticism is justified is largely a question of judgment. The prevailing opinion in the Netherlands, as I see it, is that the developments in classification and definition have helped us to achieve progress, both in setting standards for medical intervention in the end-of-life phase and in improving the quality of medical intervention. That does not mean, however, that there are no longer any problems in this area. As mentioned earlier, the recent developments with respect to palliative sedation triggered a fresh dispute on terms and definitions. Research also shows that providers of care and lawyers continue to label certain cases differently. Classifications and definitions are tools that not only can be used to describe reality but can also specifically influence our view of that reality. As M. A. M. de Wachter has said, "They select, they emphasize, they embody biases."[19] The example of the Netherlands shows both sides of the issue.

References

1. Griffiths, John, Alex Bood, and Heleen Weyers. 1998. *Euthanasia and Law in the Netherlands*. Amsterdam: Amsterdam University Press.
2. Legemaate, Johan. 1998. Twenty-five years of Dutch experience and policy on euthanasia and assisted suicide: An overview. In *Asking to Die – Inside the Dutch Debate about Euthanasia*, ed. David C. Thomasma, Thomasine Kimbrough Kushner, G. L. Kimsma, C. Ciesielski-Carlucci, 19–34. Dordrecht: Kluwer Academic.
3. Leenen, H. J. J. 1990. Euthanasia in the Netherlands. In *Medicine, Medical Ethics and the Value of Life*, ed. Peter Byrne, 1–14. Chicester: John Wiley & Sons.
4. Leenen, H. J. J. 1984. The definition of euthanasia. *Medicine & Law* 3: 333–338.
5. Griffiths, John, Heleen Weyers, and Maurice Adams. 2008. *Euthanasia and Law in Europe*. Oxford: Hart.
6. Maas, Paul J. van der, Johannes J. M. van Delden, L. Pijnenborg, and C. W. N. Looman. 1991. Euthanasia and other medical decisions concerning the end of life. *The Lancet* 338: 669–674.
7. Maas, Paul J. van der, Gerrit van der Wal, Ilinka Haverkate, Carmen de Graaff, John G. C. Kester, Bregje Onwuteaka-Philipsen, Agnes van der Heide, Jacqueline M. Bosma, and Dick L. Willems. 1996. Euthanasia, physician-assisted suicide, and other medical practices involving the end of life in the Netherlands, 1990–1995. *New England Journal of Medicine* 335: 1699–1705.
8. Ontuweaka-Philipsen, Bregje D., Agnes van der Heide, Dirk Koper, Ingeborg Keij-Deerenberg, Judith A. C. Rietjens, Mette L. Rurup, Astrid M. Vrakking, JeanJacques Georges, Martien T. Muller, Gerrit van der Wal, and Paul J. van der Maas. 2003. Euthanasia and other end-of-life decisions in the Netherlands in 1990, 1995, and 2001. *The Lancet*; 362: 395–399.

9. Heide, Agnes van der, Bregje D. Ontuweaka-Philipsen, Mette L. Rurup, Hilde M. Buiting, Johannes E. Hanssen-de Wolf, Anke Janssen, H. Roeline W. Pasman, Judith A. C. Rietjens, Cornelis Prins, Ingeborg M. Deerenberg, Joseph K. M. Gevers, Paul J. van der Maas, and Gerrit van der Wal. 2007. End-of-life practices in the Netherlands under the Euthanasia Act. *New England Journal of Medicine* 356: 1957–1965.
10. Legemaate, Johan. 2004. The Dutch Euthanasia Act and related issues. *Journal Of Law and Medicine* 11: 312–323.
11. Legemaate, Johan. 2005. *De zorgverlening rond het levenseinde – Een literatuurstudie naar begripsomschrijvingen en zorgvuldigheideisen* [Medical care at the end of life – A review of classifications, definitions and requirements]. Utrecht: Royal Dutch Medical Association (in Dutch).
12. Hartogh, Govert A. den. 2003. Mysterieuze cijfers [Mysterious data]. *Medisch Contact* 58: 1063–1066 (in Dutch).
13. Tol, D. van. 2005. *Grensgeschillen* [Boundary disputes]. Groningen: Rijksuniversiteit Groningen (in Dutch).
14. Overleggroep medisch handelen rond het levenseinde bij pasgeborenen. Toetsing als spiegel van de medische praktijk [Monitoring as a mirror of medical practice]. 1997. Ministerie van Volksgezondheid, Rijswijk (in Dutch).
15. Royal Dutch Medical Association. 1997. *Medisch handelen rond het levenseinde bij wilsonbekwame patiënten* [Medical decisions at the end of life and incompetent patients]. Houten: Bohn Stafleu Van Loghum (in Dutch).
16. Wijkerslooth, J. de. 2003. Twee lacunes in de euthanasieregeling [Two gaps in the euthanasia law]. *Opportuun* (June): 10.
17. Legemaate, Johan, Marian Verkerk, Eric van Wijlick, and Alexander de Graeff. 2007. Palliative sedation in the Netherlands: Starting-points and contents of a national guideline. *European Journal of Health Law* 14: 61–73.
18. Verkerk, Marian, Eric van Wijlick, Johan Legemaate, and Alexander de Graeff. 2007. A national guideline for palliative sedation in the Netherlands. *Journal of Pain and Symptom Management* 34: 666–670.
19. Wachter, M. A. M. de, 1992. Euthanasia in the Netherlands. *Hastings Center Report* 22: 23–30.

3

The Legalization of Euthanasia in the Netherlands

Revolutionary Normality

Heleen Weyers

INTRODUCTION

In 2002, the Netherlands became the first country in the world to adopt a law allowing a doctor to terminate a patient's life on the patient's request. For many outside the Netherlands this was shocking. In the Netherlands, however, almost everybody knew that the only thing that really happened was codification of a situation that had existed since the end of the 1980s. Many non-Dutch also mistakenly think that Dutch euthanasia policy is an example of a policy of forbearance (like the Dutch policy on soft drugs) or that the Dutch now have a right to termination of life on request. In this chapter,[a,1,2,3] I try to clear up such misunderstandings by tracing the political, legal, and social practices that shaped the current Dutch law and practice of euthanasia.[b,4]

DUTCH POLITICAL SYSTEM AND CULTURE

The Netherlands is a constitutional monarchy whose parliamentary system emerged in the latter part of the nineteenth century. Characteristic of this system is that the government is responsible to the Second Chamber of Parliament (Lower House) and requires the support of the members of that House. After passing the Second Chamber, a law requires the approval of the First Chamber (the Senate).

[a] This chapter is partly new and partly a compilation of parts of chapters of *Euthanasia and Law in the Netherlands* (1. Griffiths, Bood, and Weyers 1998) and *Euthanasia and Law in Europe* (2. Griffiths, Weyers, and Adams 2008). For a comprehensive history (in Dutch) see 3. Weyers 2004. See these three books for sources of many assertions.

[b] In 1985, the State Commission on Euthanasia defined euthanasia as "intentionally terminating another person's life at that person's request" (see 4. Staatscommissie Euthanasie 1985). If I use the word euthanasia in this sense I write it without quotation marks. Where the meaning of the word is less clear I use "euthanasia."

Dutch elections are held on the basis of proportional representation, so that a party's share of the national vote determines its share of seats in Parliament. Voters can choose among a large number of parties, ranging across the political spectrum from strict religious (Christian) conservatives to populists to left-wing liberals.

By the beginning of the twentieth century, denominational lines divided Dutch society into Protestant, Catholic, and secular (socialist and liberal) segments, each with many of its own societal institutions, including schools and hospitals. Despite its religiously segmented character, the Netherlands has been a stable democracy. The reason for this lies in the pragmatic tolerance adopted by the elites of each segment, who have been businesslike in their dealings with one another and have tended to solve differences concerning the distribution of scarce goods on the basis of proportionality.[5] When an issue could not be resolved by applying the principle of proportionality – for example, in the case of ideologically yes-or-no questions like abortion – avoidance of a definitive resolution was the solution generally sought. Such avoidance took three forms: postponing consideration of the issue (e.g., by referring it to a prestigious committee), redefining it in such a way that the state was no longer responsible for dealing with it, or "depoliticizing" it by making it appear to be a procedural or technical matter and therefore politically neutral.[6] As we will see, although religious differences are less important nowadays in the Netherlands, the political culture of avoiding head-on conflict is still very much alive.

LEGAL BACKGROUND

The Dutch Criminal Code was adopted at the end of the nineteenth century, and its provisions relevant to termination of life on request and assisted suicide – Articles 293 and 294 – were not changed until 2002. Article 293 reads: "A person who takes the life of another person at that other person's express and earnest request is liable to a term of imprisonment of not more than twelve years or a fine of the fifth category." Article 294 reads: "A person who intentionally incites another to commit suicide, assists in the suicide of another, or procures for that other person the means to commit suicide, is liable to a term of imprisonment of not more than three years or a fine of the fourth category, where the suicide ensues."[7]

When the prosecutorial authorities charge someone with a criminal offense, such as terminating a life on request, the case is tried before one of the 19 District Courts. In a District Court, three judges together decide a case. Both the accused and the prosecutor can appeal. The appeal is decided by one of the five Courts of Appeals. In a Court of Appeals, three judges together judge the case anew, dealing with both the facts and the law. Either party can appeal the judgment to the Supreme Court, the highest court in the Netherlands. Five members of the criminal chamber of the Supreme Court decide whether an appeal is justified. The Supreme Court reviews only questions of law. If the Supreme Court decides that an error of law has been made, the case is referred to another Court of Appeals.

At the time that the process of legal change regarding euthanasia began, a number of doctrinal approaches were in theory available for legitimizing the behavior of doctors that seemingly violated Articles 293 and 294 of the Criminal Code. A first possible defense was the "medical exception," which holds that like other offenses against the person, the two articles are implicitly not applicable to doctors. A second defense could have been based on the doctrine of "absence of substantial violation of the law": the idea that behavior that violates the letter but not the purpose of the law does not constitute an offense. A third possible defense offered by Article 40 of the Criminal Code is the excuse of duress and the justification of necessity. The excuse of duress holds that the accused was subject to pressures that he or she could not be expected to resist; it has never been accepted with respect to euthanasia because doctors are expected to withstand pressure by patients or their families. The justification of necessity applies to a person who, in a situation of conflict of duties, prefers to choose the value that, from an objective standpoint, is more important, even if this means doing something that in itself is forbidden.

Finally, the system of legal control over termination of life on request is covered by the Law on the Disposal of Corpses, which requires the city clerk's permission for a funeral or cremation. Such permission is granted if the doctor responsible for treatment files a death certificate on which the doctor certifies that the patient died from a natural cause. If the doctor is not convinced that the death was a natural one, the coroner must be notified. The coroner inspects the body of the deceased, and he or she makes a judgment about the cause of death. If the coroner is convinced that the death was a natural one, he or she files a death certificate; otherwise, the case is to be reported to the local prosecutor, who must decide whether to notify the city clerk that there is no objection to burial or cremation. A doctor who files a false death certificate violates Article 228(1) of the Criminal Code.[c]

HEALTH AND THE HEALTH-CARE SYSTEM

The Dutch are relatively healthy compared with the inhabitants of other countries. Most will live to an advanced age. Further, the Dutch tend to have a high opinion of their health-care system. More than three-quarters of the

[c] Article 228(1) reads: "A physician ... who intentionally issues a false certificate of ... a cause of death ... is liable to a term of imprisonment of not more than three years or a fine of the fourth category." What exactly amounts to a natural cause is a matter of some confusion and disagreement.

population consider the quality of medical care good to excellent, and doctors enjoy a high level of societal trust.[8]

Health-care policy in the Netherlands reflects the country's cultural commitment to social equity and solidarity. In 2006, after 30 years of discussion, a new system of health-care insurance was introduced that requires every resident to take out private insurance, the terms of which are highly regulated. There is a fixed monthly premium for every adult of about €90 and an additional income-dependent premium. The mandatory coverage includes basic care (general practitioner [GP], prescription drugs, hospital care). Coverage can be broadened (e.g., for dental expenses, "alternative" therapies, etc.) if one opts to pay extra. Exceptional costs (such as those for rehabilitation, home care, and a stay in a nursing home or a residential facility) are covered by a universal, compulsory, national health insurance scheme.

General practitioners play major roles in the listing, gatekeeping, and family orientation that characterize Dutch primary medical care.[9] "Listing" means that, in principle, every Dutch inhabitant is registered with a GP. This guarantees patients continuity of care. The gatekeeping function refers to the fact that patients generally do not have direct access to specialists or hospital care but must be referred by their GPs. The impact of gatekeeping is reflected in the low referral rate: More than 90% of all complaints are treated by GPs. As a "family-oriented" practitioner, a Dutch GP generally serves as the personal physician for a patient's entire family. Moreover, GPs make home visits: 4% of all contacts are visits to the patient's home, especially in the case of elderly or very sick persons. GPs are responsible for most cases of termination of life on request (87%).[d,10]

THE BEGINNING OF THE DEBATE ON EUTHANASIA

The 1960s and 1970s were a watershed for Dutch society. From a conservative, tradition-bound country, the Netherlands transformed itself into a hotbed of social and cultural experimentation. The Netherlands took a prominent place in the sexual revolution, the legalization of abortion, the acceptance of drugs, the democratization of educational institutions, the questioning of religious authority (in particular that of the Catholic Church), and so forth. Societal relationships became far more egalitarian and far less authoritarian. Ordinary Dutch people (workers, students, patients, etc.) now generally expect to have their views listened to on issues that affect them.

Before 1970, there was a general lack of interest in euthanasia and very little had been written on the issue in Dutch. This did not change much even when, in 1952, a doctor stood trial for killing his brother at the latter's request. However, at the beginning of the 1970s, the situation radically changed and "euthanasia"

[d] GPs are the responsible doctors in about 44% of all deaths.

became very much a public topic. "Euthanasia" stood for a variety of choices: "voluntary euthanasia" (ending of life on request), "involuntary euthanasia" (ending of life without a request), "indirect euthanasia" (ending of life as an unintended side effect of justified pain relief), "direct euthanasia" (intentionally ending of life), "passive euthanasia" (stopping or withholding treatment), and "active euthanasia" (performing a lethal act). Well-known scholars such as Jan Hendrik van den Berg[e] and Paul Sporken[f] stated their positions[11,12] and soon the topic of euthanasia reached Parliament. The government decided to ask for advice from the Health Council.[g] The Health Council had not yet completed its report when in 1972 a criminal prosecution for euthanasia was brought: the *Postma* case.

The *Postma* Case

Dr. Truus Postma-van Boven was a GP who ended the life of her mother – a widow of 78, who had been in a nursing home since a cerebral hemorrhage left her paralyzed on one side a few months earlier – at the latter's request with an injection of morphine.

In 1973, Dr. Postma stood trial. At the trial, a medical inspector testified (on the basis, he said, of an informal survey of Dutch doctors) that the average doctor in the Netherlands no longer considered it necessary to prolong a patient's life endlessly. In his opinion, it had become widely accepted in medical circles that under certain conditions, when a patient is given pain relief the risk of the patient dying sooner because of this treatment can be accepted. The conditions mentioned by the inspector were that the patient is incurably ill, finds his or her suffering mentally or physically unbearable, has expressed the wish to die, and is, medically speaking, in the terminal phase of illness. The person who accedes to the request must be a doctor, preferably the patient's treating doctor.[13]

The District Court largely agreed with the views reported by the inspector. The only condition it did not accept was that the patient must be in the terminal phase of his or her illness.[h] The court ruled that even though the other conditions had been met, it was wrong of Dr. Postma to have used an injection

[e] A professor in psychiatry and neurology who wrote one of the first Dutch books on medical ethics.

[f] A Roman Catholic priest who was the first Dutch professor in medical ethics.

[g] The Health Council is a scientific advisory organization that informs and advises government and Parliament on issues of public health.

[h] The court rejected this condition because it knew of the existence "of many cases of incurable illness or accident-caused disability, combined with serious physical and/or mental suffering, where the patient is otherwise healthy and can continue living in this state for years. It is not the court's view that such suffering should be denied the relief described by the expert witness" (see 13. *Nederlandse Jurisprudentie* 1973).

that was immediately lethal.[i] In the court's opinion, this was not a reasonable way to achieve the goal of putting an end to the patient's suffering. Dr. Postma was given a conditional jail sentence of one week with one year's probation.[j] Neither Dr. Postma nor the prosecution appealed.

Reactions to the *Postma* Case

The *Postma* case put "euthanasia" definitively on the Dutch societal agenda. The Royal Dutch Medical Association (KNMG)[k] and the Health Council took the position that "active euthanasia" should not be made legal.[14,15] The Health Council's opinion was that in a case in which a doctor feels an obligation to accede to the patient's request, the doctrine of the conflict of duties could be important. Both organizations considered "passive euthanasia" – refraining from or stopping treatment because it is futile or because the patient asked to do so – permissible. Neither organization mentioned "indirect euthanasia." Apparently they considered it normal medical practice. The recently founded right-to-die associations SVE and NVVE[l] and the first Dutch "pro-life organization" NAV (Dutch Association of Physicians)[m] felt the need to take positions.[n] The NVVE and SVE considered both "voluntary active" and "passive euthanasia" permissible. They provided their members with forms in which they could indicate their wishes regarding treatment. The NAV pled for the utmost respect for life and therefore rejected every form of "euthanasia."

In the 1970s, right-to-die societies did not agitate for legalization of "direct euthanasia on request," and most members of the NAV were also members of the KNMG. Beneficence seems to have been a more central concern than self-determination. At the end of the 1970s, however, this quiet climate started to change.

[i] Although the court does not specifically mention the point, its ruling seems to be based on the difference between "indirect euthanasia" (which is what the inspector had in mind) and "direct euthanasia" (what Dr. Postma actually did).

[j] The prosecution had asked for a one-month conditional jail sentence with two years of probation.

[k] The KNMG was founded in 1849 and includes the majority of Dutch doctors.

[l] The first organization, the Stichting Vrijwillige Euthanasie – Foundation for Voluntary Euthanasia (SVE), was founded in January 1973, the second, Nederlandse Vereniging voor Vrijwillige Euthanasie – Dutch Association for Voluntary Euthanasia (NVVE), a few months later.

[m] The Nederlands Artsenverbond (NAV) was founded in reaction to the (liberal) stance of the Dutch Medical Association on abortion in 1972. In the 1980s, the pro-life patients' organization Nederlandse Patiënten Vereniging – Dutch Patients Organization (NPV) and an organization of lawyers who put utmost respect for life first, Nederlandse Juristen Vereniging Pro Vita (NJV), were founded. Aside from these pro-life organizations, a number of religious groups, in particular the strict Calvinist Churches and the Roman Catholic Church, opposed "euthanasia."

[n] Other organizations that took positions are the General Synod of the Dutch Reformed Church and the Humanistic Society (an organization of humanists).

One sign of change was the negative reaction to the government's decision to seek advice from the Health Council before carrying out research into the legality of euthanasia called for in Recommendation 799 of the Assembly of Europe.[o] Asking for this advice was seen as unnecessary postponement.[p] There was also disappointment about the people chosen to join the State Commission on Euthanasia, which was established to advise on the desirability of a change in euthanasia law, most of whom the NVVE did not consider to be experts in the field. Another sign of change was a new case that came to court: the *Wertheim* case, in which more weight was put on self-determination, at least by the defendant.

The *Wertheim* Case

In the spring of 1981, a voluntary euthanasia activist, Ms. Corry Wertheim-Elink Schuurman, was arrested for having assisted in the suicide of a 67-year-old woman. The District Court observed that suicide is not necessarily unacceptable in all situations and that the assistance of others can sometimes be indispensable. However, in light of the prohibition of assistance with suicide in Article 294 of the Criminal Code, such assistance can only be justifiable if certain criteria are met. In the court's view, to justify assistance with suicide it must be evident that the physical or mental suffering of the person was such that he or she experienced it as unbearable; that this suffering as well as the desire to die were enduring; that the decision to die was made voluntarily; that the person was well informed about his or her situation and the available alternatives, was capable of weighing the relevant considerations, and had actually done so; that there were no alternative means for improving the situation; and that the person's death did not cause others any unnecessary suffering. The decision must not have been taken solely by the individual who provided assistance, and a doctor had to be involved.[16]

The District Court held that Ms. Wertheim had not met these criteria and found her guilty of the offense of assisting suicide.

A Prosecution Policy

Following this case, the national Committee of Procurators General decided that every case of euthanasia (Article 293) or assistance with suicide (Article 294) that came to the attention of a prosecutor was to be referred to the committee for a decision on whether to prosecute. The object was to achieve

[o] Recommendation nr. 779 "On the subject of sick and dying patients" asked for national interdisciplinary research commissions to examine the legal boundaries of "euthanasia" carried out by doctors.

[p] With hindsight, we know that the request for this report of the Health Council (1982) offered an excellent starting point for debate.

national uniformity in prosecutorial policy. The conditions as formulated in the *Postma* and *Wertheim* cases were to serve as guidelines for the decisions of the Committee of Procurators General.[17]

REFLECTIONS

In the 1970s, euthanasia was not a political issue, the attempt to get the theme on the political agenda having been deflected by the government, both in 1970 and in 1979, by asking the Health Council for advice.

During the 1970s, however, euthanasia became the subject of social discussion and a few criminal cases. Public discussion seemed to exhibit a trend toward reducing the number of meanings of the term "euthanasia," with the result that behavior that was not problematic from a moral and legal standpoint (refraining from or stopping life-prolonging treatment because it was deemed futile or because the patient had refused it, and death as a side effect of medically indicated pain relief) was increasingly no longer called so.

By the late 1970s, self-determination was beginning to be seen as the most important moral value with respect to euthanasia, at least among some proponents. Until the 1980s, however, beneficence continued to be the most important principle in most people's view, with some holding that the duty to act in the best interests of the patient could lead to a conflict of duties.

The criteria that the person giving assistance must meet in order to avoid being guilty of the crimes covered by Articles 293 and 294 were broadly discussed. It was generally thought that the suffering of the person requesting assistance must be permanent and irreversible and that the euthanasia request must be durable, voluntary, and well considered. Although according to many commentators it was a prerequisite for permissible euthanasia that the patient be in the terminal phase of illness, this view was not shared by the courts. There was consensus that only doctors could perform euthanasia or give assistance with suicide, and that in principle the person rendering assistance must consult with other doctors.

ACCEPTANCE OF EUTHANASIA: LEGAL CHANGE THROUGH CASE LAW

The new prosecutorial policy formulated after the *Wertheim* case led to a number of law cases in the 1980s. Some of them were ultimately decided by the Supreme Court and determined the contours of Dutch euthanasia law. Yet even before the first case was decided by the Supreme Court, other important developments took place with respect to legal change: a parliamentary bill to legalize euthanasia and physician-assisted suicide, and a change in the position on euthanasia by the Royal Dutch Medical Association. Shortly after the Supreme Court's first decision, a second major impulse for change came in the form of the majority report of the State Commission on Euthanasia that was established in 1982.

The Wessel-Tuinstra Bill

Before the State Commission had finished its work, a member of the Second Chamber of Parliament, Ms. Elida Wessel-Tuinstra of the left-liberal party D66, decided that awaiting the commission's report would mean putting off legislative change that she considered urgent. In her opinion, both the person who requests euthanasia and the doctor who agrees to carry it out were exposed to a degree of legal insecurity that was no longer acceptable. She also found it unacceptable that the whole issue of euthanasia had been left to judges and prosecutors. Regulation of euthanasia, in her view, was a responsibility of the legislature. In April 1984, she submitted a bill proposing changes in Articles 293 and 294 of the Criminal Code.[18]

Her bill proposed to make euthanasia and physician-assisted suicide legal if the assistance was given in a responsible fashion "to a patient whose condition is terminal or to a patient whose physical or mental suffering is unbearable" and who had made a voluntary and well-considered request. A number of procedural conditions, such as consultation with a second doctor, were also provided for. Parliamentary action on the bill was postponed until after the State Commission's report.

The Report of the Medical Association

In 1984 the Executive Board of the KNMG published a position paper on euthanasia.[q] The board explicitly stated that its intention was not to address the question of the permissibility of euthanasia.[r] It considered euthanasia to be a fact of life. Euthanasia was defined by the board as "conduct that is intended to terminate another person's life at his or her explicit request."[19] In line with this definition, the board was inclined to drop the distinction between euthanasia and assistance with suicide and to use the same terminology and criteria for both. The board emphasized that only doctors should be allowed to engage in actions that terminate life. The question of euthanasia was seen by the board as one that should be dealt with in the context of the doctor–patient relationship. It recognized that the medical profession has a collective obligation to make a "socially acceptable solution" of the euthanasia issue possible.

The board considered euthanasia performed by a doctor acceptable only if the doctor has taken adequate steps to meet five criteria for due care:

[q] One of the reasons the KNMG took this position was the fact that the State Commission organized hearings in which interested persons and organizations could state their views on euthanasia.

[r] During the discussion in the general membership meeting on the new policy, the chairman stated that the board did not want to take a stand for or against euthanasia. The purpose of the guidelines it had formulated was to assist those doctors who consider performing euthanasia. Debate was closed, with the observation that the new policy was that of the board, not necessarily of all Dutch doctors.

1. The request for euthanasia must be voluntary.
2. The request must be well-considered.
3. The patient's desire to die must be a lasting one.
4. The patient must experience his or her suffering as unacceptable.
5. The doctor concerned must consult a colleague.[19,s,20]

In this report, the KNMG did not propose a change in law, although it did take this step a year later in 1985. To date, the KNMG is still the only national medical association that has taken a positive stance toward euthanasia and its legalization.

The *Schoonheim* Case

The first time the Supreme Court ruled on a case of euthanasia was on November 27, 1984. The case concerned the GP Piet Schoonheim, who in July 1982 had performed euthanasia on a 95-year-old bedridden patient who on several occasions had asked him in a serious and insistent way to do so. After a series of conversations with her, Schoonheid decided to accede to her request.

At the trial in the District Court[t] Schoonheim's lawyer argued that there was an "absence of substantial violation of the law" – because of a change in societal opinion on self-determination – and that Schoonheim had acted in a situation of conflict of duties. The first defense was accepted by the court and Schoonheim was acquitted.[21] The prosecution appealed. The Court of Appeals, Amsterdam, rejected all of Schoonheim's defenses and found him guilty but used its discretion not to impose any punishment.[22] Schoonheim appealed.

The Supreme Court affirmed the holding of the Court of Appeals that the doctrine of absence of substantial violation of the law was not available as a defense. However, the court concluded that the Court of Appeals had not properly considered the appeal to *overmacht*, in the sense of the justification of necessity, and referred the case to another Court of Appeals.[u,23] The Supreme Court explained its decision as follows:

> [O]ne would have expected the Court of Appeals to have considered ... whether, according to responsible medical opinion, subject to the applicable norms of medical ethics, this was, as claimed by the defendant, a situation of necessity.[24]

[s] In 1992, the criterion of a fully documented written record was added (see 20. KNMG 1992). The KNMG criteria reflect the criteria formulated in court cases.

[t] Following the new policy, the Procurators General had decided that prosecution was indicated because Schoonheim had consulted only his assistant.

[u] Half a year passed before the Supreme Court issued its judgment. J. Remmelink (the procurator general who submitted the brief to the Supreme Court, arguing that the court should reject Schoonheim's appeal) later explained the difference between the conclusion of his brief and the court's decision by referring to the fact that in the interim, the Executive Board of the KNMG had adopted a new policy in which it recognized for the first time the legitimacy of euthanasia performed by a doctor (see 23. Remmelink 1992).

The Supreme Court specifically referred to the patient's "unbearable suffering," including, as relevant considerations, the prospect of increasing "loss of personal dignity," the risk that it might become impossible for the patient to "die in a dignified manner," and the existence of alternative ways to relieve her suffering. Not having consulted an independent doctor was not a sufficient reason for rejecting the defense of necessity. The Supreme Court concluded that the approach of the Court of Appeals had not excluded "the possibility that the euthanasia performed by defendant, according to objective medical opinion, must be considered justified, as having been performed in a situation of necessity."[24]

Everyone was surprised that the "Catholic" chamber of the Supreme Court[v] came to this verdict. Proponents of legal euthanasia – such as the NVVE and SVE – received it with delight.[w] Opponents stressed the vulnerability of the accepted defense because of its dependence on the way medical experts understand "responsible medical opinion" and "applicable norms of medical ethics." Lawyers and ethicists discussed the meaning of self-determination as reflected in the court's decision. Opponents and proponents were united in the opinion that the Supreme Court had not accepted a "right" to self-determination with respect to euthanasia.

The Report of the State Commission on Euthanasia

In the summer of 1985, the State Commission on Euthanasia published its report.[x] The commission defined euthanasia as "intentionally terminating another person's life at the person's request."[y,25] For the commission, the patient's request was thus essential to the very concept of euthanasia. This definition makes the term "euthanasia" congruent with the behavior prohibited in Article 293 (killing a person at his or her request).

The commission urged the government and Parliament to clarify the legal situation concerning euthanasia. In its opinion, legislation was essential in order to accomplish such clarification. As far as the justification of necessity was concerned,[z] the commission sought to define criteria to determine when a patient's situation is such that it would be reasonable and acceptable for a doctor, faced with a patient's request to terminate the patient's life, to

[v] The case was decided by five judges, three of whom were Roman Catholic.

[w] The SVE decided to disband since its aim – securing recognition for legal euthanasia within the context of existing law – had been achieved.

[x] The report consisted of a majority report and a minority report in which two members rejected any legalization of euthanasia. The majority report included minority views on some subjects, such as the criterion for the dying process to have commenced.

[y] This definition is much like the one that Henk Leenen, a member of the State Commission, had already formulated in 1977 (see 25. Leenen 1977).

[z] Like the Supreme Court, the commission considered the "medical exception" and the doctrine of "absence of substantial violation of the law" not applicable to the case of euthanasia.

claim that he or she was confronted with a conflict of duties.[aa] The commission emphasized that "the termination of life must be performed by a doctor in the context of careful medical practice, and sufficient procedural control must be guaranteed."[4]

The State Commission proposed a legislative revision of Article 293. The revised article would have provided that euthanasia is legal when performed by a doctor in a medically responsible way, at the request of a patient who is in a situation of "hopeless necessity," and when certain criteria of due care have been met. The commission formulated criteria that very much resemble those of the court cases and of the KNMG.

The State Commission also proposed the addition of a new section to Article 293 that would distinguish euthanasia proper from other medical behavior that leads to the death of the patient but does not constitute euthanasia. Four of these possible treatments were specified in the State Commission's proposal: not initiating or stopping treatment 1) either at the request of a patient, or 2) in a situation in which the treatment is medically futile, 3) not treating an additional illness or disorder for a patient who has permanently lost consciousness, and 4) hastening the moment of death as a subsidiary effect of treatment that is necessary to relieve suffering.

Neither friends nor enemies of legalization of euthanasia had expected that a majority of the State Commission would advise a change in law. Only one member – Henk Leenen[bb] – was known to be in favor of legalization, and during the preceding years two members – Wim Klijn[cc] and Nieboer[dd] – had published articles against legalization. Although proponents of legalization were generally happy with the report, they also raised objections: Some pleaded for the "medical exception," some stressed the need for more control, and some argued that relying on criminal prosecutions is not a good way to regulate medical practice. Opponents, of course, were very upset by the idea of a change in the law.[ee,26]

In early 1986, the government, a coalition of the Christian Democrats (CDA) and the conservative/liberal party VVD, reported to Parliament its tentative conclusions in light of the State Commission's report. The government was

[aa] The commission was unable to reach complete consensus on what the nature of the patient's situation must be. A majority agreed on the criterion that the patient must be suffering "hopelessly" (*uitzichtloos*, without prospect of improvement, senseless), accepting that this suffering could be either physical or mental. A minority wanted to add the criterion that "the dying process must irreversibly have set in" (see 4. Staatscommissie Euthanasie 1985).

[bb] The first Dutch professor in health law. As the founder of Dutch health law, Leenen put much emphasis on patients' self-determination.

[cc] A Roman Catholic moral theologist, professor in medical ethics.

[dd] A professor in criminal law and forensic psychiatry.

[ee] In 1985, an opinion poll on the question "Should a doctor give a lethal injection at the request of a patient to put an end to his suffering?" resulted in 55% positive answers ("yes") and 12% negative ("no") (see 26. SCP 1992).

inclined to view the time as not yet ripe for legislation concerning euthanasia. Nevertheless, should Parliament be of a different view, the government indicated in a "tentative draft of a bill" what sort of legislation would be acceptable to it. In effect, the government proposed to add to the Wessel-Tuinstra bill the additional limitation that euthanasia be legal only in a situation in which there was "a concrete expectation of death."[ff,27] The government also proposed to add a new section to Article 293 specifying, as the State Commission had advised, those forms of life-shortening medical behavior that do not fall under the section.

Confronted with the Wessel-Tuinstra bill, the government's alternative, and a number of more or less fundamental proposed amendments, Parliament took the path of avoidance and referred the matter to the Council of State[gg] for advice.

The Council of State took the position that the public discussion on euthanasia had not yet reached the point at which it was desirable to try to specify in the Criminal Code when euthanasia is permissible. The council nevertheless did advise adding to the Criminal Code a provision making explicit that withholding or withdrawing treatment and pain relief are not covered by Articles 293 and 294, and, in separate legislation outside the code, specifying criteria of due care that a doctor would have to meet before being allowed to invoke the defense of necessity.[28]

Three New Cases

The second case to reach the Supreme Court[hh] concerned Ms. Anna Hendrina Pols, a psychiatrist, who in August 1983 ended the life of a friend at the latter's request. In its ruling in the *Pols* case, the Supreme Court rejected the medical exception as an available defense for euthanasia. The court held that it did not appear that the prohibition concerning euthanasia in Article 293 had been intended as subject to an exception for doctors. Furthermore, contrary to the defendant's claim, there was no settled social consensus that euthanasia is a form of "normal medical practice" that can be considered to fall within the medical exception.[29,ii,30]

[ff] The government thereby adopted the position of the minority within the majority of the State Commission.

[gg] The Council of State belongs to the highest constitutional bodies in the Netherlands. At that time, government was obliged to ask for the advice of the Council of State before presenting a bill to Parliament, and members of Parliament who wanted to submit a bill were allowed to do so. Nowadays, every bill has to pass the Council of State.

[hh] During the 1980s and 1990s, a number of doctors stood trial. Almost all had reported what they had done, and none had been unconditionally sentenced to jail.

[ii] Ultimately, Dr. Pols was sentenced to a conditional jail sentence of two months subject to two years' probation (see 30. *Tijdschriftvoor Gezondheidszorg* 1987).

In June 1985, the anesthetist Pieter Admiraal stood trial for a case in which he had carefully followed the substantive criteria formulated by the KNMG. One of the questions raised at the trial was whether Admiraal should have consulted more experts (in particular, a neurologist and a psychiatrist). The District Court ruled that Admiraal had been confronted by a situation of necessity, that he had carefully weighed the conflicting duties and interests, and that in doing so he had made a justifiable choice. He was acquitted. Neither the prosecutor nor Admiraal appealed, and so the latter became the first Dutch doctor who carried out euthanasia and was acquitted.[31,jj,32]

From the *Admiraal* case it became clear that a doctor who complies with the criteria of due care would not be convicted for carrying out euthanasia. This was confirmed by the minister of justice, who notified the KNMG in September 1985 that doctors who comply with the due care criteria published by the association's Executive Board would not be prosecuted.

A prosecution in 1987 settled beyond doubt that a doctor can count on not being prosecuted so long as he or she has met the criteria of due care, and that a failure to consult another doctor is not in itself sufficient ground for a criminal prosecution. The case concerned a GP who had given lethal injections to a cancer patient at her explicit request. When criminal charges were brought, the doctor moved to quash the indictment. The court did so. In its view, the undisputed facts required the conclusion that prosecution of the doctor for euthanasia could not succeed, since if there were a trial it would soon become evident that the defendant had acted in a situation of necessity. The Supreme Court let the decision stand.[33]

Euthanasia Is Not a "Natural" Cause of Death

The reports of the Health Council (1982) and of the State Commission (1985) called attention to the need to create an adequate system of control over euthanasia practice. This problem was first addressed in the form of the question as to whether a doctor can properly file a certificate of natural death after performing euthanasia. The general view was that euthanasia cannot be considered a "natural" cause of death.

In 1985, a criminal case was brought that definitively settled this issue. The case concerned a doctor who in December 1983 had ended a patient's life in a nursing home at her explicit request. He filed a death certificate stating that the cause of the patient's death had been natural. The doctor was tried for euthanasia and for submitting a false certificate (Article 228[1] of the Criminal Code). The doctor's defense to the euthanasia charge was based on the justification of necessity. The District Court agreed and found him not guilty

jj The final acquittal of the doctor in the *Schoonheim* case took place in 1986 (see 32. *Nederlandse Jurisprudentie* 1987).

of euthanasia. The doctor's lawyer also invoked the justification of necessity as a defense to the second charge. The court did not agree, and the Court of Appeals and the Supreme Court upheld its decision: Allowing doctors to file false death certificates would undermine legal control of termination of life, and the defendant's reliance on his oath of secrecy was rejected with the argument that this oath gives a doctor the right to remain silent, but not to give false information.[33]

REFLECTIONS

In the period 1970–1982 there had been considerable discussion about how to define "euthanasia." This question was given a definitive answer by the State Commission on Euthanasia in 1985. The definitional criterion for euthanasia is to be found in the voluntary and well-considered request.

The exact meaning of the second substantive criterion of lawful euthanasia – that the patient's suffering be unbearable – was not settled in the 1980s (and, to some extent, still is not). Some members of the State Commission thought a necessary condition to be that the patient must be in the "terminal phase" of illness, but the courts have always rejected this condition. The majority of the State Commission thought that the patient must be in a situation of "hopeless necessity," while the KNMG spoke of "unacceptable suffering." Over the course of its legislative history in Parliament, the Wessel-Tuinstra bill changed several times in this respect. The Supreme Court seems to take the most expansive view by indirectly rejecting the criterion that a patient be in the terminal phase of illness and referring to the threat of "loss of personal dignity" as sufficient.

The procedural criteria have been much less a subject of debate. Consulting a colleague, reporting to the authorities, and record keeping are all seen as important. However, the exact legal status of the criteria of due care has not always been clear. In themselves, neither not reporting nor not consulting stands in the way of successfully invoking the justification of necessity with respect to euthanasia.

The majority of the State Commission advised legalizing euthanasia, a proposal that had already been given form in the Wessel-Tuinstra bill. Such a bill could, in principle, count on a majority in Parliament. At that time, however, such a majority was blocked by the presence of Christian Democrats in the government. But even the government, though very reserved, did not totally reject legalization. It postponed the question by asking the Council of State for advice. The content of the advice it received – not to change euthanasia law substantially – suited the government's purpose.

In this period, it was the courts that were responsible for legalizing euthanasia under specific conditions. It became established in a series of court decisions that when a patient who is suffering unbearably and hopelessly makes a voluntary and well-considered request, and a doctor accedes to the request, the doctor is not guilty of a crime under Articles 293 or 294 of the Criminal Code. In short, in the 1980s Dutch law on euthanasia did effectively change.

Can the judicial policy in relation to euthanasia properly be called one of "forbearance" (*gedogen*) like the Dutch policy on soft drugs? Forbearance is an accepted legal practice in the Netherlands. It is one of the several possible official reactions to a violation of the law and consists of refraining, on policy grounds, from initiating a prosecution. In this sense, the policy formulated in 1982 by the Committee of Procurators General can be seen as one of forbearance.

The ruling of the Supreme Court in the *Schoonheim*case (1984), however, made euthanasia in conformity with the criteria of due care legal. In 1985, the minister of justice confirmed that the public prosecutors would not prosecute a doctor who in carrying out euthanasia has complied with the criteria of due care formulated by the KNMG, and in 1987, the Supreme Court stated that a doctor could count on not being prosecuted as long as he or she had met the due care criteria. These developments fundamentally changed the position of the public prosecutors. The minister's statement made prosecution unlikely, but the verdict of the Supreme Court gave prosecution no prospect of success. Since the prosecutorial authorities were no longer confronted with a violation of the law, decisions not to prosecute were henceforth based on legal rather than policy considerations, and it became impossible to describe the nonprosecution of doctors any longer as due to a policy of forbearance.[34]

As far as the process of legal change is concerned, the most obvious differences between the Netherlands and other countries seem to lie in the fact that Dutch authorities were willing to prosecute (in other countries, prosecutions are rare), that the Dutch courts did not decline to take the lead (elsewhere, such as in the UK, Canada, and the United States, the courts seem often to prefer to avoid controversy and refer the issue to the legislatures), and that the KNMG considered it the responsibility of the medical profession to take the lead in finding a socially acceptable solution to the euthanasia issue.

The legal solution of "conflict of duties" ties the legalization of euthanasia to the doctor rather than to the patient. It is the doctor who is confronted by conflicting duties – relieving suffering and not violating the prohibition of killing – and this implies that self-determination is not the basic principle on which the legalization is based. Self-determination is a necessary condition of legal euthanasia, but no "right" of the patient is involved. The limited role of self-determination in the Dutch situation is often overlooked because the well-heard voices of scholars like Leenen put so much emphasis on self-determination. The duty that conflicts with the duty of respect for life is the professional ethical duty to prevent suffering. It is thus beneficence, not self-determination, that is the leading principle underlying the legalization of euthanasia.

Put another way, self-determination in and of itself could never be a sufficient justifying principle for euthanasia, since it is the involvement of *another* person – the doctor – that requires justification. Self-determination underlies the patient's right to suicide, but beneficence is required to justify the involvement of a doctor.

INTEGRATING EUTHANASIA LAW IN LEGISLATION

From the 1980s on, pressure increased for legislative codification of the change that case law had brought about. But such codification was difficult to realize so long as Christian Democrats were in government, as they had been since 1917. Avoidance is the usual strategy of Dutch politicians when confronted with a fundamentally controversial issue and – as we will see – it was used in the 1990s even after the Christian Democrats were no longer represented in government. The time gained by avoidance, however, was well used. The criterion of unbearable and hopeless suffering was further developed – for example in the *Chabot* case – and research on medical practice at the end of life was carried out, providing a wealth of unique data.

In 1998, the final stage of the process of statutory legalization got under way, resulting finally in legislation in 2002. Two new prosecutions also redefined the significance of self-determination in Dutch law.

Government in Action

In January 1987, the government notified Parliament that it would look into the possibility of a bill (as advised by the Council of State) to make explicit that withholding and withdrawing treatment and pain relief were not covered by Articles 293 and 294 and to specify criteria of due care, without, however, legalizing euthanasia as such. In practice, this was an opportunity for further delay, since the government proposed first to ask the Health Council for advice concerning the criteria of due care. But the council answered very quickly. In March 1987, it reemphasized the importance of fully informing the patient; of ensuring that his or her request is voluntary, well considered, and durable; of consultation; and of full record keeping.[35] The government also asked the Committee of Prosecutors General for its views concerning the advice of the Council of State. The Prosecutors General reacted very negatively to the advice of the Council of State and the government's draft bill.[kk,36] At the very end of 1987, the government submitted a bill by which essentially nothing in the Criminal Code would be changed,[ll,37] a bill that was considered not

[kk] They objected to the device of a "negative definition of an offense" (the specification of behavior not included in Article 293) and to specifying criteria for the defense of necessity outside the Criminal Code.

[ll] Instead of changing Articles 293 and 294, the bill would have added two provisions to the Law on Medical Practice: 1) the exclusion of death due to termination or noninitiation of treatment and to pain relief from the scope of Articles 293 and 294, and 2) minimum criteria that a doctor who performs euthanasia would have to meet. It would be up to the prosecutors and the courts to determine to what extent these provisions outside the Criminal Code were relevant to the defense of necessity.

recommendable by almost everybody. The government's bill had to compete with the (three-times-revised) initiative of Wessel-Tuinstra still pending in Parliament.

In May of 1989, before parliamentary consideration of the Wessel-Tuinstra bill and the government's alternative were complete, the center-right government fell and was replaced by a center-left government. During the formation of the new government, the parties agreed that further legislative initiatives regarding euthanasia should await the findings of a commission appointed to conduct research into the extent of current euthanasia practice.[38]

The Remmelink Commission

The Commission Appointed to Carry Out Research Concerning Medical Practice in Connection with Euthanasia (referred to as the "Remmelink Commission" after its chairman)[mm] was established in January 1990. Its research was supposed to provide insight into "the state of affairs with respect to the practice of acts or omissions by doctors which shorten the life of a patient, with or without an explicit and serious request."[39] To carry out the research, the support of doctors was necessary. In return for its cooperation, the KNMG insisted on a reporting procedure for doctors who had carried out euthanasia. In November of 1990, the minister of justice announced such a procedure.[40] In broad terms, the new reporting procedure was based on the assumption that a doctor who has performed euthanasia may not file a certificate of natural death but must notify the coroner of what he or she has done. At the same time, the procurators general issued instructions governing police investigation of reported cases, the gist of which was that the whole investigation should be as discreet as possible.[41]

The Remmelink Commission delivered its report in September 1991.[42] The research put an end to more or less wild speculations concerning the extent of euthanasia. The findings indicated that about 1.7% of all deaths per year were due to euthanasia and 0.2% to assistance with suicide. The research also revealed that in 0.8% of all deaths, the life of a patient was ended without the patient having made an explicit request.[nn]

The general reception of the report can best be characterized as a collective sigh of relief that there was apparently no real problem. The Labor Party – long supporters of the Wessel-Tuinstra bill – was promptly able to agree with the Christian Democrats that no substantial legislative change was required. The government proposed to withdraw its 1987 bill and to substitute a new one, which did no more than put a legal foundation under the new reporting procedure.[43] As the Remmelink Commission had advised, this procedure

[mm] Remmelink was a professor in criminal law and procurator general of the Chamber of Criminal Law of the Dutch Supreme Court.

[nn] Death due to pain relief and due to forgoing treatment was far more frequent – 17.5% of all deaths in both categories.

would now also be applicable to cases of termination of life without an explicit request. The criteria for due care would be incorporated in the reporting procedure. This proposal – an amendment to the Law on the Disposal of Corpses – was quickly enacted (1994).

In the same year, the government fell and a new so-called Purple Government was formed. The new government consisted of three parties – the social-democratic PvdA, the right-wing liberal VVD, and the left-wing liberal D66 – all of which had been in favor of the Wessel-Tuinstra bill of 1984. It came as a great disappointment to many[oo] when this government announced that it did not intend to introduce legislation to delete euthanasia from the Criminal Code but instead to initiate a second round of research into the practice of euthanasia.[44,pp,45,46]

Termination of Life and Incompetent Patients

While familiar procedures to postpone statutory codification of changes that in practice had already taken place in euthanasia law played out in the political arena, developments in the courts did not stop. A theme that again attracted attention was that of medical practices at the end of life for patients who lack decision-making capacity. In 1985, the KNMG had established a commission Commissie Aanvaardbaarheid Levensbeëindigend handelen (CAL) to advise it on the acceptability of life-ending acts with respect to these patients. In 1990, the CAL issued the first of a series of position papers that ultimately dealt with newborns, patients in permanent coma, demented patients, and patients suffering from psychiatric diseases.[qq,47] However, probably the most influential report on the topic was published not by the KNMG but by the Dutch Association for Pediatrics (NVK): *To Act or to Abstain? The Limits of Medical Practice in Neonatology.*[48] The gist of these reports is that what requires justification is not *stopping* treatment but *prolonging* treatment.

With respect to compromised babies, the NVK took the position that initiating or continuing treatment is justifiable only if one has good grounds for

[oo] Since 1991, less than 10% of the population answered "no" to the question "Should a doctor give a lethal injection at the request of a patient to put an end to his suffering?" (see 1. Griffiths, Bood and Weyers 1998).

[pp] In light of the government's position, the NVVE decided that it was necessary to keep up the pressure for legislative reform. In April 1996, it published a new proposed bill on euthanasia (see 45. NVVE 1996). The gist of the proposed revisions of Articles 293 and 294 of the Criminal Code was that euthanasia and assistance with suicide by a doctor would not be illegal when performed in accordance with the criteria for due care, which the bill included. The NVVE bill would also have added a new article making it legal to supply a person not currently suffering, but who does not want to undergo physical or mental deterioration, with the means for a "gentle death." This idea had first been advanced by a prominent Dutch lawyer and former Supreme Court judge, Huib Drion (see 46. Drion 1991).

[qq] Collected and edited in 1997 (see 47. KNMG 1997).

supposing it benefits the patient. The consequences of this position for most severely compromised newborns are clear: If the patient cannot benefit, there is no justification for prolonging life; thus, physicians should refrain from providing (further) treatment (in particular, artificial respiration but also, for example, artificial administration of food and drink), and doing so will inevitably lead to the baby's death. When justifiable withholding or withdrawing of treatment leads to unacceptable suffering, the report maintains that actively terminating the life of the baby is appropriate. Two prosecutions (*Prins* and *Kadijk*) have made clear that Dutch judges accept this argument. Both doctors were acquitted on the basis of justification of necessity.[49,50] In 2002, these developments were completed by the formulation of guidelines for active termination of life in severely compromised newborns (the Groningen Protocol).[rr]

For patients in a persistent vegetative state, the CAL argued that there are two legitimate reasons for stopping treatment: an advance directive in which treatment is refused and the futility of further treatment.[ss,51]

For deeply demented patients, the same argument as for babies and patients in an irreversible coma can be made. Most discussions in the Netherlands on demented patients concern whether a patient who in advance considers being deeply demented unacceptable can receive euthanasia. This is seen as highly problematic. Patients with dementia in an early stage can be competent enough to make a voluntary and well-considered request for euthanasia or assistance with suicide. There are a handful of examples of patients whose requests are complied with by doctors who report what they have done. So far, the prosecutorial authorities have accepted all of these cases as legitimate.

Patients suffering from psychiatric disorders may be competent to request physician-assisted suicide, and their suffering may meet the criteria of being unbearable and hopeless. Beginning in the mid-1980s, the courts were confronted with a number of cases involving such patients. The judgments in these cases seemed to allow room for assistance with suicide for psychiatric patients.

The *Chabot* Case

A famous case in which psychiatric disorder played a role is the *Chabot* case. In September 1991, the psychiatrist Boudewijn Chabot supplied a 50-year-old woman with lethal drugs at the woman's request. Over a period of several years, the woman had undergone a series of extremely traumatic experiences

[rr] In July 2005, the Groningen Protocol was adopted for use throughout the country by the NVK.

[ss] In 1989, a District Court ruled in a case of a patient in an irreversible coma that artificial feeding constitutes medical treatment and, therefore, falls within the authority of a doctor to terminate "medically futile" treatment. The decision was upheld by the Court of Appeals (see 51. *Nederlandse Jurisprudentie* 1989).

that had deprived her of all desire to continue living. Her psychic traumas were in principle susceptible to psychiatric treatment (which would, however, have been long term and with limited chance of success), but she consistently declined therapy. Chabot found her request well considered and that for her, suffering was unbearable and hopeless.

The District Court and the Court of Appeals found Chabot's defense of necessity well founded. On appeal, the Supreme Court reaffirmed its earlier judgments that euthanasia and assistance with suicide can be justified if the doctor acted in a situation of necessity.[52] The court rejected the argument of the prosecution that this justification is not available in the case of assistance with suicide given to a patient whose suffering is nonsomatic and who is not in the terminal phase of an illness. It agreed with the holding of the Court of Appeals that "the wish to die of a person whose suffering is psychic can be based on an autonomous judgment."

The Supreme Court, however, concluded that in the circumstances of this case, there was insufficient evidence to support the defense of necessity, since there was no statement from an "independent medical expert who has at least seen and examined the patient himself." (Chabot had consulted seven experts, none of whom considered it necessary to examine the woman.) The court added that although failure to consult a colleague – whether or not the latter examines the patient – does not in an ordinary case foreclose the defense of necessity, in the case of suffering that is not somatically based, evidence of consultation including actual examination of the patient is essential. Chabot was found guilty of the offense of assistance with suicide (however, no punishment was imposed).

The *Chabot* case thus put an end to the idea that being in the terminal phase of illness is a necessary condition for legal euthanasia or physician-assisted suicide. It also makes clear that the suffering of the patient does not necessarily have to be physical. But the exact nature of the patient's suffering was not yet completely settled. It returned again in another famous case, the *Brongersma* case, to be discussed later.

The *Chabot* case provoked much debate. One of the central questions was why a *doctor* has to be involved in such a case. At the time, Chabot answered that question by pointing to the fact that doctors are the only ones who have access to the necessary drugs. Others objected to the ever-increasing "medicalization" of death[53] or argued against a tendency toward acceptance of unconditional self-determination.[54]

The Second National Study

The results of the research promised by the government in 1994 became available at the end of 1996.[55] They generally confirm the picture presented by the research for the Remmelink Commission in 1991, and the political message – that with regard to medical practice in connection with euthanasia and assistance with suicide there is not much reason for great public concern – was essentially the same. But the new research also directly addressed the question of the effectiveness of the reporting procedure, and here the findings were more problematic. The rate of reporting, while improved (from 18% to 38%), was still rather low, and it seemed that the more dubious cases (and, in particular, cases of termination of life without an explicit request) were hardly being reported at all. The problem of effective enforcement of the legal rules concerning euthanasia thereby became a central concern in the public debate.

The KNMG and the NVVE argued that legal insecurity resulting from the failure to adopt legislation was the root of the problem. The government, on the other hand, argued that the problem lay in the distaste of doctors for having their behavior assessed by lawyers, and that doctors might be more inclined to report if the criminal character of the reporting procedure were reduced. It was therefore decided to put a buffer between doctors and prosecutors by creating Regional Review Committees to review reported cases.[56] Each committee, composed of a lawyer, a doctor, and an ethicist, would judge whether a doctor had complied with the criteria for due care. If a committee found that this was the case, it would advise the prosecutorial authorities not to prosecute. In principle, the prosecutorial authorities would follow the advice of the committee. The Regional Review Committees commenced work at the end of 1998. In their first period of work (1998–2002, when the new law changed their position) the Regional Review Committees assessed about 6,750 cases, and almost all of them were judged to have met those criteria. The majority of the "not careful" cases involved problems concerning consultation. Prosecutorial authorities decided not to prosecute any of the cases.[tt]

For cases regarding termination of life of incompetent patients, another committee was to be installed. But although plans for this committee languished for many years in the filing cabinets of government officials, the committee (limited to newborns) finally came into being in 2006.[uu]

In 1998, another new facility was created: a service for GPs to consult if they are considering carrying out euthanasia. This service (known under the acronym SCEN, for Support and Consultation Euthanasia in the Netherlands) informs GPs about the criteria for due care and provides a trained, independent consultant. The consultant functions as a check on whether the criteria have been met in a specific case.[57] In their annual reports, the Regional Review

[tt] Since the enactment of the euthanasia law in 2002, this is still the case. Between 1998 and 2008, 28 cases were judged as being "not careful." As of August 2008, none of the doctors involved had been prosecuted.

[uu] The letter announcing the committee states the assumption that active termination of life will be preceded by a decision to withhold or withdraw treatment because the baby is not expected to survive or because the prognosis for its later health is extremely poor. The influence of both the NVK report and the CAL report with respect to the criteria that must be taken into account, as well as criteria for due care, is obvious. To date (2008), the committee has not received any reported cases to review.

Committees have commented that cases in which a SCEN doctor was involved as consultant rarely gave rise to any problem. (In 2005, the facility was extended to specialists in hospitals and nursing homes.)

Legislative Codification of Legalization

In 1998, elections were in the offing. The "Purple Government" had not seized the opportunity to legalize euthanasia. D66, the political party that had introduced the first euthanasia bill in 1984, took the coming elections as an opportunity to put euthanasia back onto the legislative agenda. Together with individual parliamentarians of the other parties constituting the coalition government (PvdA and VVD), D66 introduced a bill to legalize euthanasia.[vv,58]

The elections resulted in a second coalition government of the same three parties, and the new government adopted the legislative proposal as a government bill, which became The Termination of Life on Request and Assisted Suicide (Review Procedures) Act of 2002. The bill set out a number of criteria for due care, amended Articles 293 and 294 to provide that a doctor who meets the criteria and reports the death of his or her patient to the coroner on the appropriate form is not guilty of an offense, and put the Regional Review Committees on a statutory foundation, making final their determination that a doctor has met the criteria.

The statutory criteria are that the doctor must

- be satisfied that the patient's request was voluntary and well considered;
- be satisfied that the patient's suffering was unbearable and that there was no prospect of improvement;
- have informed the patient concerning his or her situation and prospects;
- have discussed the situation with the patient and, together with the patient, be convinced that there was no reasonable alternative in the light of the patient's situation;
- have consulted at least one other, independent, doctor who must have seen the patient and given a written opinion on the due care criteria listed in the four previous points; and
- have terminated the patient's life or provided assistance with suicide with due medical care and attention.

The preamble to the bill emphasized its central objectives: transparency of euthanasia practice and legal certainty. The value of patient self-determination was not very prominent in the bill.[ww] The situation to be codified was the

[vv] In that year, the number of positive responses to the question "Should a doctor give lethal injections at the request of a patient to put an end to his suffering?" fell from 58% to 50%, but not because opposition grew (only 9% answered "no"). Five years later, and two years after enactment of the law, the results were almost the same (51% and 9%) (see 2. Griffiths, Weyers, and Adams 2008).

[ww] Nevertheless, opponents of the bill expressed the opinion that self-determination was the hidden, underlying principle of the bill.

conflict of duties that forms the basis of the justification of necessity. Self-determination is not a part of this conflict, and lawmakers emphasized that the bill does not provide for a right of self-determination; the new defense is only available to a doctor who complies with the criteria for due care, and a doctor has no duty to perform euthanasia.[59, 60]

As far as the legality of euthanasia is concerned, the law of 2002 does little more than ratify what the State Commission, the KNMG, the courts, and the prosecutors had already accomplished. The only genuinely new provisions concern a) the legality of euthanasia pursuant to a prior written request by a person who has become incompetent, and b) the position of minors. Formally, the law puts more emphasis on the criteria of consultation and reporting by making these prerequisites to legal euthanasia (something the courts had not done). However, during the parliamentary debates, the minister of justice assured Parliament that prosecution policy with respect to these criteria would not change. Therefore, as in the 1980s and 1990s, neither not reporting nor not consulting a second doctor stands in the way of legal euthanasia.

Parliament discussed the bill between February 2000 and April 2001. Recurring themes were the central values underlying the bill, the significance of the advanced written request provided for in the bill,[xx] the position of minors who ask for euthanasia,[yy] and the legality of assisted suicide for patients whose suffering is not due to a medical complaint but is "existential" in nature.[zz,59,60]

Despite the many questions that arose during the debates, the Second Chamber of Parliament accepted the bill in November 2000 without many changes. Forty members (of the Christian parties and the socialist party SP) voted against the bill and 104 in favor of it. In April 2001, the First Chamber likewise accepted the bill, with 46 senators in favor and 28 against. The law became effective on April 1, 2002.

The new law was heavily criticized from abroad, but there was not much reaction to this criticism in the Netherlands. The Dutch apparently knew that in principle nothing had changed, and a majority approved of the law.

Legal security and effective control are seen as the most important goals of euthanasia legislation. Whether these goals are being achieved has been evaluated in new research into the medical practices at the end of life, in 2001[61] and

xx A doctor whose patient is suffering unbearably but is no longer competent can honor the earlier written request. The patients referred to most often in the parliamentary debates are those in a late stage of dementia. The advance request of a patient with severe dementia was supposed to be important only for those patients who, besides dementia, also suffer from other conditions.

yy The provision that a request for euthanasia by a minor between 12 and 16 could be honored by a doctor even if one of his or her parents objected provoked a storm of criticism. When it became clear that in the opinion of the doctors concerned the provision was superfluous, it was withdrawn.

zz Many questions were raised, in particular about the *Brongersma* case. The minister of justice asserted that the bill was not intended to cover such a case (see 60. *Second Chamber of Parliament 2000–2001*).

2005.[62] The results show that the reporting rate rose from 18% (1990) to 41% (1995), then to 54% (2001) and 80% (2005). Although there is discussion on differences in the classification of particular practices as euthanasia between doctors and researchers.[63,64] The conclusion must be that doctors' willingness to report has grown during the 15 years of policy formulation regarding reporting procedures.

Perhaps surprisingly, the number of euthanasia cases fell after the enactment of the law. In 1990 there were an estimated 2,700 cases of euthanasia, in 1995 there were 3,600 cases, in 2001 3,800 cases, and in 2005 only 2,425.[aaa] One reason that may account for the decline in the number of euthanasia cases is the apparent increase in the frequency of terminal sedation (from 5.6% in 2001 to 8.2%, or 7.1% of all deaths).[bbb,61,65,66]

The *Brongersma* Case

In April 1998, the GP Philip Sutorius assisted one of his patients – a well-known former senator named Edward Brongersma – in committing suicide. Brongersma, 86 years old at the time of his death, had had a very active, politically and socially engaged life, but his physical condition had deteriorated to the point that he found his situation unbearable and sought his GP's help to end his life.

In reporting what he had done, Sutorius characterized the reasons for Brongersma's request as "lonely, feelings of senselessness, physical deterioration, and a long-standing wish to die not associated with depression." To a

aaa Reporting to the Regional Review Committees grew during the parliamentary debates and decreased thereafter (1998: 2,209; 1999: 2,216; 2000: 2,123; 2001: 2,054; 2002: 1,883; 2003: 1,815; 2004: 1,886; 2005: 1,933; and 2006: 1,923 (see 2. Griffiths, Weyers, and Adams 2008). The frequency of termination of life without a request has also declined (from 0.8% of all deaths in 1990 and 0.7% in 1995 and 2001 to 0.4% in 2005). As far as we know, the reporting rate of termination of life without a request is almost zero.

bbb The researchers of the 2001 study concluded that in about 10% of all deaths, terminal sedation had been applied. They noted that they themselves had classified some cases of terminal sedation as euthanasia. There were cases in which administration of sedatives was with the express purpose of hastening death, usually at the explicit request of the patient (see 61. Van der Wal et al., 2003). The head of the prosecutorial authorities reacted publicly to these results in a way that challenged one of the pillars of Dutch euthanasia policy over the preceding 15 years. He argued that if terminal sedation is so similar to euthanasia, there ought to be some external control. His position led to questions in Parliament. The minister and state secretary of health took the position that the medical profession should formulate a guideline regarding terminal sedation (see 65. *Second Chamber of Parliament 2003–2004*). The KNMG appointed a committee to do this and approved the committee's proposed guideline in December 2005 (see 66. KNMG 2005). In the meantime, there had been a court case and a disciplinary case on terminal sedation. Both abandoned the earlier double-effect line of argument, as did the KNMG committee – that it is not the intention of the doctor that determines the proper categorization of his or her behavior but, rather, the question of whether the drugs as administered were "medically indicated."

question concerning Brongersma's suffering Sutorius replied, "The person in question experienced life as unbearable." And to a question whether there were treatment alternatives, he answered, "No, the person in question 'weighed the pros and cons,' and there was no disease [to treat]." The prosecutorial authorities decided to prosecute.[ccc]

The first trial took place in October 2000, on the same day as initial parliamentary deliberation on the government's bill. Many members of Parliament asked whether the bill sought to legalize behavior such as that of the doctor in the Brongersma case, making clear that they were opposed to this. But the District Court, relying heavily on one of the expert witnesses, accepted the view that Brongersma's suffering was unbearable and hopeless (in the sense of there being no reasonable prospect of improvement) and acquitted Sutorius.[67]

The judgment of the District Court provoked strong reaction. Through its chairman, the KNMG publicly distanced itself from the judgment. The association decided to appoint a committee to advise it with respect to the boundaries of legitimate assistance in dying and whether the existing framework of norms and rules regarding assistance with suicide should be changed.[ddd,68]

The Court of Appeals reversed the judgment of the District Court. Although the court regarded it as good that doctors are concerned about the suffering of their patients and seek to relieve even purely existential suffering, it nevertheless ruled that relieving suffering that does not have a medical cause is not a part of the professional duty of a doctor. The court rejected Sutorius's appeal to the justification of necessity – based on the conflict of duties to which a doctor in his professional capacity can be exposed – and the case was appealed to the Supreme Court.

In December 2002, the Supreme Court ruled on the *Brongersma* case. The Supreme Court rejected all of Sutorius's defenses, its most important conclusion being that the reasons given by the Court of Appeals for rejecting the justification of necessity were legally correct. A doctor who assists suicide in a case in which the patient's suffering is not predominantly due to a "medically classified disease or disorder," that is, a clinically diagnosed disease/condition, but stems from the fact that life has become meaningless for the patient, acts outside the scope of a physician's professional competence.[69]

ccc Since the case antedated the Regional Review Committees, Sutorius's report went straight to the prosecutorial authorities.

ddd The committee issued a report in 2004. In its opinion, further development of the criteria used by doctors to assess the suffering of a patient is a more promising way to deal with the limits of medical authority than trying to distinguish between "medically based" suffering and other suffering. Doctors, especially GPs and nursing home doctors, can be experts with regard to existential suffering at the end of life; the committee argued that this expertise should be further developed (see 68. KNMG 2004). The KNMG has yet to react to the report.

The *Brongersma* case is unique in the development of Dutch euthanasia law in that judicial decision making and parliamentary debate were closely interwoven. The questions raised and statements made in Parliament about the coverage of the new law figured prominently in the decision of the Supreme Court as arguments for rejecting Sutorius's appeal.

The ruling of the Supreme Court is widely seen as an attempt to limit the possibility of euthanasia by bringing in (or putting more stress on) the idea of a medically classifiable disease. It is not clear that the approach taken will hold in practice. The trials in the District Court and the Court of Appeals made clear that the concept of "disease" is open to more than one interpretation. Further, doctors can use the concept of disease in a strategic way: stressing the patient's disease or disorder as a cause of suffering.

The core subject of the *Brongersma* case – widely referred to as being "weary of life" – is closely related to a debate that has been going on in the Netherlands since 1991, when the former Supreme Court judge, Huib Drion, argued that very old single persons who are "finished with life" should have the right to receive lethal drugs from their physician.[eee] The NVVE and another smaller right-to-die society (Foundation for Voluntary Life) have embraced variations on this idea and are seeking permission to carry out an experiment to establish whether a "last will pill" can safely be made available.[fff,70]

Legal Resistance to Patient Self-Determination

In the early years of the public discussion about euthanasia, it was already clear that people who suffer from a (terminal) illness are not the only ones who ask for assistance in dying. Others who seek such assistance are old people who are "weary of life," people with chronic diseases who cannot endure the prospect of many more years to come, and people in psychic distress. Because doctors are reluctant to assist them with suicide, even when the legality of doing so is clear, these patients must look elsewhere for help.

Some of those who do not get help from their doctor approach right-to-die societies. Since the 1980s, the NVVE has given personal advice to its members about effective means for ending one's life,[ggg] and since 1996 its members have been able to buy a booklet with information about ways to do so. Questions have been asked in Parliament about the permissibility of giving information about ways to commit suicide. The general opinion is that giving information

[eee] The NVVE had tried to give the idea a legal status in 1996 (see 45. NVVE 1996).

[fff] In the spring of 2008, 74% of the Dutch population appeared to be in favor of a controlled distribution of the "last will pill." Almost 50% think that the facility should be legalized (see 70. NVVE 2008).

[ggg] In the early 1990s, a doctor closely linked to the NVVE was prosecuted for assistance with suicide. In this case, the Supreme Court observed that giving information about how to end one's life does not amount to "assistance" under Article 294 of the Penal Code, but "steering" the suicide does.

ought not to be prohibited.[71] During the 1990s, another organization began offering assistance: Stichting De Einder (The Horizon Foundation). De Einder not only offers information and the opportunity to talk about one's desire to die but is also willing to be present at the time of the suicide.

Since 1999, four persons working for the NVVE or De Einder have been prosecuted for involvement in a suicide. Two prosecutions were initiated when family members of the deceased complained to the prosecutorial authorities; in the other two cases, the "suicide consultant" either alerted the police himself or attracted attention by publishing about the case. In the first case, which involved a psychologist of the NVVE, the District Court ruled that an obligation to prevent the suicide of a competent person does not exist. The court held that the psychologist acted carefully and acquitted her.[72]

The other three cases involved volunteers of De Einder. In one case, the suicide consultant was sentenced to 12 months' imprisonment, of which 8 were conditional. The Court of Appeals took the position that the consultant had overstepped many boundaries and that there was reason to fear repetition.[hhh,72] The consultant appealed, arguing that preparatory acts are different from assistance with suicide. The Supreme Court, however, affirmed the ruling of the Court of Appeals that the moment at which the assistance takes place is not decisive in answering the question of whether Article 294 of the Criminal Code has been violated.[iii,73] Another case involved the founder of De Einder.[jjj] He had made the suicide possible by exchanging drugs with a 25-year-old woman who wanted to die. The District Court gave him an unconditional jail sentence of one year, but the Court of Appeals reduced the penalty[kkk] because the defendant showed remorse and stated that he was ceasing his work as a suicide consultant.[74] In both cases, the courts made very clear that self-determination is not an "ultimate value" and accountability is very important. The last case in which a lay person stood trial for assistance with suicide ended with an acquittal. The District Court observed that talking and giving information and moral support do not amount to assistance with suicide.[lll]

In 2007, Chabot published a study on "self-directed deaths in consultation with proxies" in the Netherlands. From this study, it appears that it is not only suicide consultants but also people in a person's immediate social surroundings who give their support. Chabot distinguishes two methods: "voluntary refusal of food and fluid" and "taking lethal medication attended by a confidant."[75]

[hhh] The assistance consisted of opening a jam jar and a bottle of liquor; putting things such as water, yogurt, bowls, liquor, and a plastic bag near the woman; and helping her to consume the medicines and alcohol and to put a rubber band around her neck (see 72. *Tijdschrift voor Gezondheidsrecht* 2004).

[iii] The defendant stopped his work as a suicide consultant.

[jjj] The man was well known as a suicide consultant both from the annual reports of the foundation and from his publications.

[kkk] To 12 months, of which 8 were conditional, with two years' probation.

[lll] In the spring of 2007, the prosecutor withdrew his appeal (*Relevant* 2007/2: 14).

The support given by others varies, from direct assistance (e.g., collecting lethal drugs) to being present so that the person does not have to die alone. According to Chabot, the number of life-ending cases of this sort exceeds substantially the number of cases of euthanasia carried out by doctors. He estimates that there are 1,600 cases per year of using drugs and 2,800 cases of refraining from eating and drinking.[76]

REFLECTIONS

Between 1987 and 2002, a variety of efforts were made to codify the results that the courts had reached earlier. Most of them were left stranded, not for want of majority support from the population[mmm,77] and in Parliament but as a result of the exigencies of forming coalition governments. In the end, after a government took power for the second time without participation by Christian Democrats, the statutory codification of what the courts had recognized was finally realized.

During the same period, and as a direct consequence of the legislative stalemate, two major national studies were made of euthanasia and other medical practices that shorten life. Stimulated in part by the findings of this research, the public debate – having in an earlier period been narrowed down to euthanasia and assistance with suicide – was widened again to include other medical practices that shorten life. First in reports of several medical professional bodies and shortly thereafter in case law, the problems of assistance with suicide in the case of psychiatric patients and of shortening the life of severely compromised newborns began to receive serious attention. Toward the end of this period, public discussion focused increasingly on the problem of effective regulation.

The most recent evaluation of the law on euthanasia shows that 30 years of debate and legal policy have produced considerable transparency in the form of a high reporting rate. From the work of the Regional Review Committees we can conclude that reported cases almost always comply with the criteria of due care. From this perspective, Dutch euthanasia policy can be considered successful.

Enactment in 2002 of the law on Termination of Life on Request and Assisted Suicide (Review Procedures) did not put an end to Dutch developments regarding medical practice at the end of life. With the new criterion in the *Brongerma* ruling that a patient have a medically classifiable disease, the Supreme Court tried to halt developments that reduced the emphasis on suffering as a criterion for due care. At the same time, however, suicide consultants (who do not consider their acts to be assistance with suicide) and right-to-die

[mmm] See 77. Weyers 2005, and 2. Griffiths, Weyers, and Adams 2008, for a full account of the changes in value orientations in the Dutch population and its meaning for a change of law.

societies looking for possibilities to help their members put more emphasis on self-determination (and less on the nature of suffering).

In the coming years we can expect developments regarding patients with diminished capacity. Because of the increasing number of older persons, it is to be expected that the problem of persons who want euthanasia if they become seriously demented and of elderly persons who are weary of life will receive increasing attention.

CONCLUSION

The Netherlands is the first country in the world that legalized termination of life on request. Although in principle revolutionary, this legalization can be seen as quite common for the way the Dutch treat societal and political problems.

The overwhelming majority of the Dutch population is at least not against legal euthanasia, and a major part of the population favors the possibility. An explanation can be found in the tendency of the Dutch to trust their doctors, especially their GPs, and their health-care system. Although the idea that euthanasia is a danger for vulnerable patients certainly exists, it is not very widespread in the Netherlands.

The most characteristic example of the Dutch method of dealing with societal problems is the way the KNMG operated. Triggered by law cases and the invitation of the State Commission to give its opinion on euthanasia, the board of the association accepted the responsibility of the medical profession for euthanasia. The way it sought not to take a stand in the debate but to provide willing doctors with guidelines exhibited a talent for strategic maneuvering. The KNMG's position can also be considered an example of a Dutch characteristic that James Kennedy calls *bespreekbaarheid*, "discussibility," the idea that problems can best been handled by discussing them openly.[78]

Although euthanasia is a controversial topic even in the Netherlands, societal discussion on it has been restrained. The common coloring of the debate, as of many other Dutch debates, is that both parties have a right to their opinion. Such an attitude causes more problems for those who resist change than for those who champion it. The problem for the former is that they are expected to give room to others to do as they like. (The fact that opponents of euthanasia did not receive much attention in this chapter reflects the rather limited voice they had in the debate.) The justification of necessity, and thereby the central position of doctors in euthanasia practice, contributed to this keeping of pressure low in the public debate.

This chapter has shown that Dutch euthanasia law changed long before the criminal code was formally amended. That a fundamental legal change takes place in the courts is not unusual in the Netherlands (the right to strike and to abortion are other examples where the courts pioneered).

The legislative process concerning euthanasia is an example of the fact that fundamental change in the Netherlands is seldom abrupt. One of the reasons the process took as long as it did is the politics of avoidance. Postponement by appointing advisory committees (for example, the Health Council) and postponing consideration until more information becomes available (here, by multiple national studies) are good examples of this characteristic approach. Dutch political processes generally exhibit an effort to achieve as much consensus as possible. In the case of euthanasia, postponement led to vastly increased insight into its actual practice. Many Dutch citizens and politicians interpreted the findings of these studies as a relief. In this way, the data helped to "depoliticize" the issue of euthanasia. The Regional Review Committees have also contributed to the high level of public confidence in euthanasia practice. As a result, the whole matter has virtually disappeared from the political agenda.

To conclude this chapter, it is good to stress the differences that may exist between the Netherlands and other countries as far as the regulation of euthanasia is concerned: trust in the medical profession, acceptance of responsibility by the leading professional medical organization (the KNMG), prosecutors willing to bring cases against doctors, judges not afraid to lead legal change, politicians looking for broad consensus, and an orientation toward openness in the search for control.

References

1. Griffiths, John, Alex Bood, and Heleen Weyers. 1998. *Euthanasia and Law in the Netherlands*. Amsterdam: Amsterdam University Press.
2. Griffiths, John, Heleen Weyers, and Maurice Adams. 2008. *Euthanasia and Law in Europe*. Oxford and Portland: Hart Publishing.
3. Weyers, Heleen. 2004. *Euthanasie: Het proces van rechtsverandering* [Euthanasia: The process of legal change]. Amsterdam: Amsterdam University Press.
4. Staatscommissie Euthanasie. 1985. *Rapport van de Staatscommissie Euthanasie* [Report of the State Commission on Euthanasia]. The Hague: Staatsuitgeverij.
5. Lijphart, Arend. 1968. *The Politics of Accommodation: Pluralism and Democracy in the Netherlands*. Berkeley: University of California Press.
6. Andeweg, Rudy, and Galen Irwin. 1993. *Dutch Government and Politics*. London: Macmillan.
7. Rayar, Louise, and Stafford Wadsworth. 1997. *The Dutch Penal Code*. Littleton, CO: Fred B. Rothman & Co.
8. Van der Schee, E., and D. Delnoij. 2005 Dokter geniet nog steeds aanzien: Onderzoek consumentenvertrouwen in zorg [Dutch still trust their doctors: Results of survey research among health-care consumers]. *ZorgVisie* 35: 28–29.
9. Van Rooij, Elise, et al. 2002. *Health and Health Care in the Netherlands: A Critical Self-assessment of Dutch Experts in the Medical and Health Sciences*. Maarsen: Elsevier Gezondheiszorg.

10. Onwuteaka-Philipsen, Bregje, et al. 2007. *Evaluatie Wet toetsing levensbeëindiging op verzoek en hulp bij zelfdoding* [Evaluation of the Termination of Life on Request and Assisted Suicide (Review Procedures) Act of 2002]. The Hague: ZonMw.
11. van den Berg, J. H. 1969. *Medische macht en medische ethiek* [Medical power and medical ethics]. Nijkerk: Callenbach. Translated as *Medical Power and Medical Ethics*. 1978. New York: W. W. Norton.
12. Sporken, Paul. 1969. *Voorlopige diagnose. Inleiding tot een medische ethiek* [Diagnosis for the time being: Introduction to medical ethics]. Utrecht: Ambo.
13. *Nederlandse Jurisprudentie* 1973, nr. 183: 558.
14. KNMG (Koninklijke Nederlandse Maatschappij tot bevordering der Geneeskunst). 1973. Voorlopig standpunt van het hoofdbestuur inzake het euthanasievraagstuk [Provisional position of the governing board with respect to the question of euthanasia]. *Medisch Contact* 19: 587–588.
15. Gezondheidsraad. 1972. *Interim-advies inzake euthanasia* [Interim advice concerning euthanasia]. The Hague: Ministerie van Volksgezondheid en Milieuhygiëne.
16. *Nederlandse Jurisprudentie* 1982, nr. 63: 223.
17. *Second Chamber of Parliament, Appendix, 1981–1982*, 1757.
18. *Second Chamber of Parliament 1983–1984*, 18 331, nr. 2 and 3.
19. KNMG (Koninklijke Nederlandse Maatschappij tot bevordering der Geneeskunst). 1984. Standpunt inzake euthanasie [Position on euthanasia]. *Medisch Contact* 30: 990–997.
20. KNMG (Koninklijke Nederlandse Maatschappij ter bevordering van de Geneeskunst). 1992. Richtlijnen KNMG en Nieuwe Unie '91 [Guidelines of the KNMG and Nieuwe Unie '91]. *Medisch Contact* 47: 29–32.
21. *Nederlandse Jurisprudentie* 1983, nr. 407.
22. *Nederlandse Jurisprudentie* 1984, nr. 43.
23. Remmelink, J. 1992. *Spanningen tussen recht en strafwet. Rede gehouden door prof. mr J. Remmelink ter gelegenheid van zijn afscheid als procureur-generaal bij de Hoge Raad der Nederlanden op de buitengewone zitting van het college op woensdag 29 april 1992* [Tension between law and the Criminal Code: Valedictory lecture of Professor J. Remmelink as Procurator General of the Supreme Court of the Netherlands, delivered at the extraordinary session of the court on Wednesday, April 29, 1992]. The Hague: Ministry of Justice.
24. *Nederlandse Jurisprudentie* 1985, nr. 106.
25. Leenen, H. 1977. Euthanasie in het gezondheidsrecht [Euthanasia in health law]. In *Euthanasie* [Euthanasia], ed. P. Muntendam, 72–147. Leiden: Stafleu's Wetenschappelijke Uitgeverij.
26. SCP (Sociaal Cultureel Planbureau). 1992. *Sociaal en cultureel rapport 1992* [Social and cultural report 1992]. The Hague: VUGA.
27. *Second Chamber of Parliament 1985–1986,* 19 359, nr. 2.
28. Second Chamber of Parliament 1985–1986, 18331, nr. 43.
29. *Nederlandse Jurisprudentie* 1987, nr. 607.
30. *Tijdschriftvoor Gezondheidszorg* 1987, nr 35.
31. *Nederlandse Jurisprudentie* 1985, nr. 709.

32. *Nederlandse Jurisprudentie* 1987, nr. 608.
33. *Nederlandse Jurisprudentie* 1988, nr. 157.
34. Weyers, Heleen. 2001. Euthanasia: The process of legal change in the Netherlands. In *Regulating Physician-Negotiated Death: Recht der Werkelijkheid* [Journal of the Dutch/Flemish Association for Socio-Legal Studies], ed. Albert Klijn, Margaret Otlowski, and Margo Trappenburg, 3: 11–27.
35. Gezondheidsraad. 1987. *Advies inzake zorgvuldigheidseisen euthanasie* [Advice concerning the due care criteria for euthanasia]. The Hague: Ministerie van Volksgezondheid en Milieuhygiëne.
36. *Second Chamber of Parliament 1986–1987*, 19 359, nr. 8.
37. *Second Chamber of Parliament 1987–1988*, 20 383, nr. 2 and 3.
38. *Second Chamber of Parliament 1988–1989*, 21 132, nr. 8 (coalition agreement): 47.
39. *Second Chamber of Parliament 1989–1990*, 20 383, nr. 13: 2.
40. *Second Chamber of Parliament 1990–1991*, 21 800, nr. 23: 2.
41. Richtlijnen meldingsprocedure euthanasie en hulp bij zelfdoding: Jarenlange onduidelijkheid voorbij [Guidelines reporting procedure on euthanasia and assistance with suicide: Many years of uncertainty coming to an end]. 1990. *Medisch Contact* 45: 1303–1304.
42. Maas, Paul van der, J. J. van Delden, and L. Pijnenborg. 1992. *Euthanasia and Other Medical Decisions Concerning the End of Life.* Amsterdam: Elsevier.
43. *Second Chamber of Parliament 1991–1992,* 22 572, nr. 2 and 3.
44. *Second Chamber of Parliament 1993–1994*, 23 715 nr. 11 (coalition agreement): 32.
45. NVVE (Nederlandse Vereniging voor Vrijwillige Euthanasie). 1996. *Voorontwerp euthanasiewet* [Draft euthanasia bill]. Amsterdam: NVVE.
46. Drion, H. 1991. Het zelfgewilde einde van oude mensen [The choice for ending life by elderly people]. *NRC-Handelsblad* 19, October 19.
47. KNMG (Koninklijke Nederlandse Maatschappij ter bevordering van de Geneeskunst). 1997. *Medisch handelen rond het levenseinde bij wilsonbekwame patiënten* [Medical practice at the end of life in the case of noncompetent patients]. Houten/Diegem: Bohn Stafleu van Loghum.
48. NVK (Nederlandse Vereniging voor Kindergeneeskunde). 1992. *Doen of laten? Grenzen van het medisch handelen in de neonatologie* [To act or to abstain? The limits of medical practice in neonatology]. Utrecht: NVK.
49. (Henk Prins) *Nederlandse Jurisprudentie* 1996, nr. 113.
50. (Gerard Kadijk) *Tijdschrift voor Gezondheidsrecht* 1996, nr. 35.
51. *Nederlandse Jurisprudentie* 1989, nr. 909.
52. *Nederlandse Jurisprudentie* 1994, nr. 656: 3154.
53. Trappenburg, Margo. 1995. Het belang van medische bescheidenheid [The importance of medical modesty]. *Socialisme en Democratie* 52: 263–273.
54. Achterhuis, Hans, et al. 1995. *Als de dood voor het leven. Over professionele hulp bij zelfmoord* [Scared to death: On professional assistance to suicide]. Amsterdam: Van Oorschot.
55. Van der Wal, Gerrit, and Paul van der Maas. 1996. *Euthanasie en andere medische beslissingen rond het levenseinde* [Euthanasia and other medical decisions on connection with the end of life]. The Hague: SDU.
56. *Second Chamber of Parliament 1996–1997*, 23 977, nr. 13.
57. Onwuteaka-Philipsen, Bregje, and Gerrit van der Wal. 1998. *Rapport steun en consultatie bij euthanasie in Amsterdam* [Report on support and consultation in

Amsterdam]. Amsterdam; Instituut voor extramuraal geneeskundig onderzoek/ Afdeling sociale geneeskunde Vrije Universiteit Amsterdam.
58. *Second Chamber of Parliament 1997–1998*, 26 000.
59. *Second Chamber of Parliament 1999–2000*, 26 691, nr. 6: 16–17, 24.
60. *Second Chamber of Parliament 2000–2001*, nr. 9: 17–18.
61. Van der Wal, Gerrit, Agnes van der Heide, Bregje Onwuteaka-Philipsen, and Paul J. van der Maas. 2003. *Medische besluitvorming aan het einde van het leven: De praktijk en de toetsingsprocedure euthanasie* [Medical decision making at the end of life: Medical practice and the assessment procedure for euthanasia]. Utrecht: De Tijdstroom.
62. Onwuteaka-Philipsen, Bregje, et al. 2007. *Evaluatie Wet toetsing levensbeëindiging op verzoek en hulp bij zelfdoding* [Evaluation of the Termination of Life on Request and Assisted Suicide (Review Procedures) Act of 2002]. The Hague: ZonMw.
63. Den Hartogh, Govert. 2003. Mysterieuze cijfers: Meldingspercentage van euthanasie kan niet meer stijgen [Mysterious numbers: Further increase in the reporting rate is not possible]. *Medisch Contact* 58: 1063–1066.
64. Van Tol, Donald. 2005. *Grensgeschillen: Een rechtssociologisch onderzoek naar het classificeren van euthanasie en ander medisch handelen rond het levenseinde* [Boundary disputes: A legal-sociological study of the classification of euthanasia and other medical behavior at the end of life]. Ph.D. diss., University of Groningen.
65. *Second Chamber of Parliament 2003–2004*, 29 200 XVI, nr. 268: 9.
66. KNMG (Koninklijke Nederlandse Maatschappij tot bevordering der Geneeskunde). 2005. *KNMG-richtlijn palliatieve sedatie* [KNMG guideline on palliative sedation]. Utrecht: KNMG.
67. *Tijdschrift voor Gezondheidsrecht* 2001, nr. 21.
68. KNMG (Koninklijke Nederlandse Maatschappij tot bevordering der Geneeskunst). 2004. *Op zoek naar normen voor het handelen van artsen bij vragen om hulp bij levensbeëindiging in geval van lijden aan het leven: Verslag van de werkzaamheden van een commissie onder voorzitterschap van prof. J. Dijkhuis* [Norms for behavior of doctors in the case of requests for assistance in suicide due to suffering from continued life: Report of the Dijkuis Committee]. Utrecht: KNMG.
69. *Nederlandse Jurisprudentie* 2003, nr. 167.
70. NVVE (Nederlandse Vereniging voor Vrijwillige Euthanasie). 2008. Driekwart Nederlanders voor laatstewilpil: 74% van de Nederlanders voor de laatstewilpil. http://www.nvve.nl/nvve2/pagina.asp?pagkey=99569&metkey=375 (accessed October 31, 2010).
71. *Second Chamber of Parliament, 2002–2003, Appendix:* 1143.
72. *Tijdschrift voor Gezondheidsrecht* 2004: 178–179.
73. LJN: AR 8225, Supreme Court, 01853/04.
74. LNJ: AY7270, Court of Appeals Amsterdam, 23–006489–05.
75. Chabot, Boudewijn, and Arnold Goedhart. 2009. A survey of self-directed dying attended by proxies in the Dutch population. *Social Science & Medicine* 30: 1–7.
76. Chabot, Boudewijn. 2007. *Auto-euthanasie: Verborgen stervenswegen in gesprek met naasten* [Self-euthanasia: Low-visibility ways to die while in contact with those to whom one is close]. Amsterdam: Bert Bakker.

77. Weyers, Heleen. 2005. Legal recognition of the right to die. In *Contemporary Issues in Healthcare Law and Ethics*, ed. A. Garwood-Gowers, J. Tingle, and K. Wheat, 253–267. Edinburg and other cities: Elsevier Butterworth Heineman.
78. Kennedy, James. 2002. *Een weloverwogen dood. Euthanasie in Nederland* [A well-considered death: Euthanasia in the Netherlands]. Amsterdam: Bert Bakker.

4

The Normative Context of the Dutch Euthanasia Law

Esther Pans

This chapter focuses on the normative considerations and choices underlying The Termination of Life on Request and Assisted Suicide (Review Procedures) Act (Wet Toetsing Levensbeëindiging op verzoek en hulp bij zelfdoding, or WTL), also known as the Dutch Euthanasia Act.[1]

Under the WTL, physician-assisted death[a] is still a criminal offense, but the Criminal Code has been amended to exempt physicians from criminal liability if they report their actions and meet the so called "criteria of due care" as formulated in the WTL. According to these requirements, the attending physician must:

- be satisfied that the patient had made a voluntary and carefully considered request;
- be satisfied that the patient's suffering was unbearable and that there was no prospect of improvement;
- have informed the patient about his or her situation and prospects;
- be satisfied that it is their mutual opinion that there is no reasonable alternative, given the patient's situation;
- have consulted at least one other independent physician, who must have seen the patient and given a written opinion that the case met the criteria for due care; and
- have terminated the patient's life with due medical care and attention.

[a] "Physician-assisted death" encompasses both euthanasia and physician-assisted suicide. In the Netherlands, these two forms of intentionally ending the life of a patient by a doctor on the patient's explicit request are often taken together because they are subject to the same legal criteria. Besides, in the Dutch context, the role of the physician in assisted suicide is just as central as in euthanasia, the only difference being that in the first case the patient drinks a potion (in the physician's presence) while in the second case the physician performs the life-ending intervention, usually by means of a lethal injection.

This chapter summarizes 1. Pans.2006.

Our interest in the normative background to these rules is twofold. First, the reasoning behind a rule is simply always of interest from a scholarly point of view – especially so in our case, in which the subject matter is essentially ethical. If the legislator tells us that under certain circumstances a doctor is allowed to kill or assist in the killing of his patient, we naturally wonder on what moral basis such a rule was drafted. But our interest goes further. The law itself may be a fait accompli, but its wording hardly is self-explanatory. Among other criteria, what constitutes a "carefully considered request" or, even more so, what "unbearable suffering" means requires interpretation. Understanding the normative background of the WTL is key in that process.

This chapter focuses on the four principles that underlie the WTL: compassion, autonomy, dignity, and the protection of life. It explores the social and medical context of Dutch euthanasia practice, the history of the law and the "open" nature of the norms in the WTL, and the key features of the WTL, as well as the philosophical understandings and legal implications of the four core principles that lie behind it.

SOCIETAL AND LEGAL CONTEXT

The Dutch Sociomedical Environment

The law governing euthanasia is closely tied to its Dutch sociomedical environment. This notion can hardly be overstated. Among the numerous factors that shape this environment, two are particularly noteworthy: universal access to care and the centrality of family physicians.

In the Netherlands, health care of high quality is equally available to all – the poor receive the same medical treatment as the rich. Virtually every citizen is insured against costs for health care. The cost of care is not on the patient's mind, and so financial considerations are unlikely to affect patients' decisions whether or not to seek further treatment.

The pivotal figure in the Dutch medical system is the family physician/general practitioner (*huisarts*). In 2007, 88% of physician-assisted death was performed by family physicians, comparable to numbers in preceding years.[2] The relationship between family physician and patient is one of trust and personal attention. Typically, it spans a considerable period of time. In the treatment of life-threatening illnesses, medical specialists will report back to the family physician, who will then discuss these reports with his or her patient. The family physician's position of being well informed regarding the patient's history, person, and medical condition is important in judging the seriousness of the patient's suffering and whether his or her request for euthanasia or assisted suicide is voluntary and carefully considered. These two aspects, as will be discussed further, form the basis of the physician's judgment about the patient's request.

The law rests on these social and medical preconditions and cannot simply be "translated" to other contexts or other countries. The Dutch "lesson" about euthanasia must be thoroughly reconsidered before it can be applied elsewhere.

Developments Preceding the WTL

When the WTL came into force on April 1, 2002, it no doubt marked a milestone in the Dutch debate. But it can hardly be said to have substantially *changed* Dutch law. The goal – as legislators repeatedly stressed – was not to set new rules but, on the contrary, merely to codify developments in case law that had been taking place since as early as 1973. The WTL does not establish new practices or legal requirements. Indeed, all of the "criteria of due care" can be found, literally or in substantially the same form, in the preceding case law.

Two articles of the Dutch Criminal Code, Articles 293 and 294, provide criminal penalties for physicians who performed euthanasia or assisted a patient to commit suicide. Article 293 states: "A person who takes the life of another person at that other person's express and earnest request is liable to a term of imprisonment of not more than twelve years." Article 294 provides that "[a] person who intentionally incites another to commit suicide, assists in the suicide of another, or procures for another person the means to commit suicide, is liable to a term of imprisonment of not more than three years ... where the suicide ensues."

However, physicians could plead immunity from criminal liability on the basis of the concept of *overmacht,* "necessity" (Criminal Code, Article 40).[b] With respect to physician-assisted death, the necessity in question is the physician's "conflict of duties." According to a 1984 decision by the Dutch Supreme Court (the *Schoonheim* case),[3] "conflict of duties" refers to a situation in which, in accordance with accepted scientific norms in medicine and the norms of medical ethics, the physician faces two or more incompatible obligations between which he or she is forced to choose. To fall within the defense of "necessity," the physician's decision must be one that can reasonably be justified when considered objectively and in view of all the circumstances of the case.

The Supreme Court held the following factors to be particularly relevant, although they are not the only considerations: 1) the unbearableness of the patient's suffering, including the prospect of increasing "loss of personal dignity," 2) the risk that it might become impossible for the patient to die in a dignified way, and 3) the absence of alternative ways to relieve the patient's suffering. Depending on the specific case at hand, there may be other relevant facts to be taken into account. The Supreme Court thus formulated the basic rules we now find in the 2002 law.

[b] This concept is also referred to in the literature as *force majeur*.

Moreover, from the beginning, the courts made clear that it is not always required that the patient be terminally ill or imminently dying. In 1994 (the *Chabot* case),[4] the Supreme Court explicitly stated that when the cause of suffering is psychological and the patient is not in the terminal phase, his or her expressed wish to die can be granted, provided that the attending physician concurs and an independent medical expert has visited and examined the patient as well. The Supreme Court emphasized that such cases call for extreme care and demand a "reluctant," cautious approach by the attending physician. In 2002 (the *Brongersma* case),[5] the court formulated a general restriction: The patient's suffering must (mainly) be based on a psychological or somatic medical diagnosis.

Although Articles 293 and 294 of the Criminal Code are still applicable, under the WTL criminal law has lost its central role. Rather than public prosecutors being the ones to evaluate alleged cases of euthanasia, five Regional Review Committees now carry out that role. Where previously the criminal courts confronted just a few – often pioneering, atypical – cases, these committees assess each and every reported case of euthanasia. The committees have three members: a legal expert, a physician, and an expert on ethical issues. When a review committee finds that the doctor has acted with due care, the Public Prosecution Service will not be informed and no further action will be taken. The public prosecutor still has the authority to prosecute every case, whether or not it has been approved by a committee, but in practice this rarely happens.

KEY FEATURES OF THE WET TOETSING LEVENSBEËINDIGING

Casuistry and "Open" Norms

One of the striking features of the 2002 law on euthanasia is the open, abstract wording of its central requirements. A "carefully considered request" and, even more so, "unbearable suffering" require interpretation. The legislature's decision to frame requirements in this way was deliberate.

By demanding interpretation, these open norms enable the review committees to judge each reported case of euthanasia in terms of its own unique circumstances. This approach is known as casuistry. Casuistry takes as its starting point the conviction that the solution to complex, subtle, multilayered moral problems is not to be found in general, universal principles. A direct, uniform translation of a general principle to a specific case is not possible because complex moral issues involve multiple relevant points of view, unique situations, and distinctions, for which there is no single correct solution. The aim should be to analyse cases one by one and to do justice in each particular case. This opens the possibility of reaching agreement on a case-by-case basis about the meaning of abstract norms in complex and difficult ethical problems, while consensus on an abstract, general level is not required.

The method of casuistry implies a gradual arranging of cases, from the transparent to the contested. The process of decision making then comes down to applying basic moral rules (maxims, principles) and articulating and classifying the circumstances that are relevant in a particular case. The different arguments that apply in each case are viewed in their mutual cohesion; assessment leads to a variety of results, each with a certain degree of probability.

In the context of assessing cases of euthanasia, physicians and review committees adopt an attitude of interpretation. That means that they include in their decision making the meaning and intention of the criteria for due care set out in the law. They refine the application of the norms in light of the goals of the WTL; the interests of the physician, patient, and society that are protected by these norms; and the values and principles that are realized in the law, especially the principles of compassion, autonomy, dignity, and the protection of life.

From an international perspective, the downside of building this casuistic assessment of cases into the law is that Dutch euthanasia practice may seem arbitrary to outsiders. The policy may be especially hard to defend in the international context, where concerns about protecting patients tend to favor clear, strict, uniformly applicable norms to safeguard the valuable legal good of human life. From the Dutch perspective, especially from physicians' perspective, another problem with casuistry is that general rules are difficult to provide. This causes uncertainty with respect to potential prosecution, especially with respect to nonparadigmatic cases. A paradigmatic case is that of a terminally ill patient who has a very short life expectancy (hours to days). In particular, for a physician who is being prosecuted because of the lack of clarity as to whether his or her particular case satisfied the legal norm (Schoonheim, Chabot, Brongersma), the "open" nature of the norm is quite burdensome. Furthermore, physicians, and sometimes review committees, do not always clearly articulate the norms behind their decisions, and their deliberations are difficult to reconstruct.

Notwithstanding these objections, in the Netherlands this casuistic method may well have been the only possible way to regulate the complex and sensitive problem of euthanasia. If the legislature had attempted to formulate concrete, detailed provisions, there probably would have been no provisions at all.

Medical Ethics

The legislature was also reserved in explicating the normative background to the WTL. The approach might be termed "theory modest" insofar as no need was perceived to justify the law in terms of moral principles, or to argue for priority among such principles. The parliamentary history (*parlementaire geschiedenis*) – the written account of discussions between the government as initiator in the lawmaking process and the Dutch Parliament – states that after decades of intensive public debate, in the Netherlands there is a broad consensus that in paradigmatic cases, physician-assisted death should not be criminally prosecuted. This mere fact is the overriding justification for the WTL.

True as this may be from a democratic point of view, it appears to leave little to work with for those who must interpret the WTL in actual cases. Euthanasia and assisted suicide are fundamentally ethical matters. If the law gives only general directions for determining whether a given case does or does not adhere to the law, should or should not be subject to prosecution, the review committees are left to look elsewhere for the wisdom they need to make that determination. In other words, in following the casuistic method embodied in the law, where do committees find the basic moral rules (maxims, principles) that, in combination with all relevant circumstances of the case, lead to the "right" conclusion?

Just as it provided the blueprint for the wording of the WTL, preceding case law also provides the moral frame of reference for interpreting it. In judging whether there is a "conflict of duties" that would support a defense of necessity, the Supreme Court has referred to scientific and ethical norms accepted in the medical profession; the parliamentary history explicitly states that this continues to be the case under the WTL. This brings us to our next question: What are those norms and how are they understood in regard to euthanasia and assisted suicide?

Ethics and the Normative Framework of WTL

Judges were the ones who "decriminalized" euthanasia and physician-assisted suicide, yet they were not, and did not want to be, the ones who determined the content of the norms governing practice. The courts focused on procedural aspects – "if there is a 'conflict of duties,' the doctor is not punished if he makes the 'right' choice"; and for the content of the norms – "which is the 'right' choice" – they relied on the authority of medical and ethical experts. Although everything now in the WTL is ruled by the Supreme Court, it originates from medical and ethical sources.

In the ongoing interpretation of the WTL, medical and ethical standards will be as vital as they were in the earlier stages of the debate. But what can we expect from medicine and ethics?

We cannot expect these disciplines to offer absolute guidelines of proven validity or even conceptual definitions on which there is complete consensus. Ethics is not hard science. While there may be no universal consensus about euthanasia and assisted suicide, however, as I discussed earlier, certain fundamental ideas are widely accepted. Thus, for example, there is a broad, common understanding of the physician's duty to relieve suffering, of patient autonomy, of dignity, and of the duty to protect life (to be discussed in more detail).

The review committees will follow approaches that are authoritative in medicine or for which they find a high degree of support within the profession. But many debated questions remain, of course. In areas in which there is no consensus, a physician should be aware that he or she ventures into an area within which the legitimacy of the interventions is debatable. There is a considerable chance that a review committee will decide that the physician's action was not in conformity with the norms of medical ethics.

The absence of clear, universally agreed-upon principles in medical ethics poses challenges for physicians and review committees. Medical ethics regularly encourages reflection; it is valuable in offering tools for thought or providing a context in which to understand the case at hand; it can be especially helpful when the understandings it yields are directly applicable in practice, as is often the case. By promoting close consideration of concepts such as autonomy, suffering, empathy, voluntariness in decision making, hopelessness, the protection of life, compassion, beneficence, dignity, right to life, value of life, and quality of life, medical ethics can lead to a deeper understanding of individual cases. So, too, can it provide valuable insight into the nature of suffering, the experience of pain, and the grounds for *informed consent* that can help clarify issues. At the same time, however, in medical ethics nuances and further reflections create new questions. Thus, even coupled with medicine's scientific standards, the norms of medical ethics do not always offer a generally accepted, undisputed direction for fleshing out the meaning of the legal standards for euthanasia.

Where cases are recognized as similar to paradigm cases in morally relevant ways, we can say that there indeed do appear to be clear, authoritative rules because the paradigm cases themselves embody consensus among participants (physicians and review committees) – even when the underlying moral justification for euthanasia or assisted suicide is not made explicit. In paradigm cases and those that "fit" the model they set out, most Dutch people think the facts speak for themselves, as it were. In the hard cases at the margins, however, the conceptual justification carries much weight. These cases at the margin are also the domain in which new juridical understandings are developed, drawing on – but not necessarily exclusively guided by – the insights that medical ethics can offer.

CORE MORAL PRINCIPLES

Despite the lack of unambiguous agreement on universal guiding principles with respect to euthanasia and physician-assisted suicide, one can detect a common thread in medical ethical approaches to the duty to relieve suffering, to autonomy, to dignity, and to the protection of life. Approaches to these four core issues provide some solid ground for interpreting the criteria of due care for euthanasia. For each principle I shall present a short exposition of the fundamental moral principles of the WTL, both theoretically and practically.

Duty to Relieve Suffering

Medical ethics recognizes that suffering, and the physician's duty to relieve suffering, pose significant challenges. On the one hand, suffering is multicausal, multidimensional, and unique to the individual. Why does one person suffer unbearably with lung cancer in a certain stage but not another person in a comparable situation? Suffering is highly determined by the individual because it can relate to any aspect of a person. Even more so, suffering is mostly of a mixed nature: part psychological, part somatic, part social, part spiritual, and so on. The causes and the nature of suffering are only partly open to analysis, both for the suffering individual and for others.

On the other hand, we are convinced that we are able to empathize, relate to, experience, and feel the suffering of another human being. Significant literature on suffering – for example, the work of the Dutch philosopher Henri Wijsbek – builds on empirical studies of pain to differentiate forms of suffering and to identify the characteristics of specific types of suffering and the factors that can magnify or minimize the possibility of feeling, and of observing, suffering.

Some forms of suffering are, in general, less open to be shared and felt, but for the individual experiencing them they can certainly be unbearable and hopeless. This is particularly true of forms of chronic psychological suffering, with which it may be very difficult to empathize, even though the physician's duty of compassion rests on the ability to perceive and in some measure share the patient's experience of suffering. The more difficult it is to understand the patient's suffering empathically, the harder it can be to identify appropriate treatment options. As a result, patients whose suffering is psychological may be disadvantaged in comparison to patients whose suffering has a somatic cause. The unbearable and hopeless nature of psychological suffering is less likely to find acceptance than is suffering that has primarily somatic roots. To the extent that psychological suffering often concerns relatively young patients with a long life expectancy, the matter becomes even more problematic, as, of course, does the issue of free will – that is, the question of whether the patient's request for euthanasia in such circumstances is truly voluntary or colored by a psychiatric disorder.

Identifying and assessing suffering can be challenging in other ways as well, for example, when physician and patient are from different cultural backgrounds or when the physician has had little or no previous contact with the patient. Just as important, the obligation to recognize and appropriately relieve suffering demands of the physician not only medical knowledge but also general insight about human beings and sensitivity to the existential meanings that illness and suffering may carry for patients. Physicians who lack knowledge or skill in any of these areas will be less able to address suffering effectively.

Autonomy and Self-Determination

The second core principle is the principle of (respect for) autonomy. In criminal law the significance of autonomy is limited: to prevent coercion. That is one of the reasons why autonomy in euthanasia may be a necessary but not sufficient condition and is not the foundational principle. Because the legal framework of euthanasia and assisted suicide resides in criminal law, without a patient's request we are speaking not of euthanasia but of murder. That also explains why, among other factors, assisted dying is neither a patient's nor a physician's duty. A patient must request it of a physician.

Furthermore, from a philosophical point of view, the autonomy of a human being is not unproblematic. Concepts such as "freedom," "voluntariness," and "autonomy" are rife for discussion in both ethics and philosophy. This is even more so where euthanasia and physician-assisted suicide are concerned because these involve situations of *overmacht* (necessity, or *force majeure*). Uncertainty is often the rule in such situations, where degree of voluntariness or suffering, feelings of depression that come and go, fear, pain, stress, and pressure of time all threaten to confound decision making. Add to which the fact that the patient occupies a vulnerable position in the (hierarchical) system of health care, as individual against the health-care "apparatus" that may mistakenly presume – or be presumed – to be in control, and whose "informed" consent rests on the ultimately insurmountable gap in knowledge between physician and patient.

In the WTL, the notion of autonomy becomes visible in the first legal criterion of due care, the requirement that there be a "voluntary and well-considered request of a patient to end life." From a philosophical perspective, this requirement is somewhat problematic, as noted, even more so in the light of the specific problem of the voluntariness of the wish to die. From a practical perspective, however, as a condition that should apply for the legally acceptable practice of euthanasia, the voluntariness and well-considered nature of a patient's request are reasonably susceptible to assessment and evaluation.

The significant limitations imposed on patient autonomy by decision making in the context of the system of health care were important considerations behind the legislative decision not to ground Dutch euthanasia policy primarily on autonomy. There are always very pressing, forceful circumstances that determine the request for euthanasia or physician-assisted suicide, and the ultimate question is always how free a "voluntary" request to die can be in the face of serious suffering. There are unavoidable tensions between the requirement that the patient's request be "well considered" and the requirement that at the same time his or her suffering be "unbearable" and "hopeless."

One of the key choices made by the legislature was that euthanasia or physician-assisted suicide remain an intervention of last resort. While a patient's autonomy is sharply limited in scope, the physician is allowed to reject a request for any reason and is not required to explain his or her reasoning. When a physician declines a request there is no duty to consult, and the rejection of a request is not regulated in any particular way. But neither is any restriction placed on the patient's withdrawal of a request. Thus, as a positive right – that is, a right to make a claim on another's behavior – autonomy is strictly regulated, while as a negative right – that is, a right to reject – it has strong significance. This is in keeping with the way that patients' autonomy is seen generally in health law: Patients' right to refuse medical treatment is strongly protected, whereas the right to request or to receive specific medical treatment always demands more than just the will of the patient (i.e., a medical indication).

That said, however, patient autonomy does play a very important, if somewhat indirect, role in the assessment of unbearable suffering. How someone experiences his or her suffering depends to a large measure on personal perception. A physician may take into account all the different circumstances of a case. He or she does not personally have to find the suffering unbearable but must identify with the fact that this particular suffering is unbearable *for this particular patient.* To this extent, there remains an essential role for autonomy in the process of decision making with respect to euthanasia or assisted suicide.

If it has been established that a patient wishes to realize his or her capacity for self-determination through a voluntary, well-considered, and explicit request to die, that the patient no longer chooses to continue to live, then a physician is authorized – never obliged – to enter into the complex medical-ethical process of weighing the pros and cons in decision making for euthanasia. For the physician, that means balancing the duty to alleviate suffering, on the one hand, with the duty to protect life, on the other.

Dignity

Thirdly, there is the principle of (respect for) human dignity. The loss of dignity was recognized as a relevant factor in suffering in the 1984 *Schoonheim* case, in which dignity was directly related to dying. The parliamentary discussion of the WTL focused specifically on the strong relationship between dignity and the problem of euthanasia in regard to dementia, coma, and being "weary of life." However, empirical research carried out throughout the Netherlands suggests that loss of dignity plays an essential role in practically all cases in which euthanasia is performed and reported.

The research shows that loss of dignity often plays an important role in all types of suffering. Interviews with physicians in 2001 and 2002[6] made clear that the reason mentioned most frequently for requesting euthanasia is meaningless suffering (65%), followed by deterioration/loss of dignity (44%), general feelings of weakness/fatigue (43%), the prevention of worse/ongoing suffering (36%), the prevention of deterioration (35%), dependence (33%), and pain (29%). The prominence of deterioration/loss of dignity, prevention of worse or ongoing suffering, and dependence among the reasons for euthanasia requests indicate the role that dignity plays in patients' suffering. We are left to conclude that requests originate in large part from patients' need to experience a dignified death, in which suffering is neither prolonged unnecessarily nor intolerable to endure.

This also means that in the paradigmatic cases of euthanasia (especially cancer, lung disorders, and neuro-muscular diseases), the experience of loss of dignity is often a significant component of the patient's suffering. Judges and legislators decided that loss of dignity can play a role solely *as a factor in suffering* but cannot independently justify euthanasia or physician-assisted suicide.

Yet what dignity means is not very clear. Although "dignity" figures prominently in treaties on human rights and has inspired reflection from the earliest philosophical essays to our current deliberations, it is by no means a clear and concise concept. In medical-ethical literature, loss of dignity is associated with many different issues: loss of mental and physical abilities, inability to live in ways consistent with one's values, dependence, irrationality, and the absence of choices. That there is no broadly supported definition of dignity seems understandable because dignity may relate to every single aspect of a person.

The Dutch system of law takes the notion of the intrinsic dignity of every human being as the starting point, or "basic norm," with respect to every individual, regardless of gender, age, decision-making capacity or other characteristic. On this foundation, the WTL offers the competent person an additional possibility – carefully regulated and limited – to give his or her own moral direction to the personal meaning of dignity. That does not mean that a physician must follow this personal view of a patient, but that at least the physician should take the patient's view into serious consideration when deciding whether to accept a request for euthanasia, especially a request that is grounded in the patient's perception (or fear) of loss of dignity.

The decision to recognize dignity only in the context of suffering and not as an independent rationale for euthanasia can be defended on good grounds: that broader interpretations of dignity might pose a danger. The explicit restriction articulated by the Supreme Court in the *Van Oijen* case (2004), that only the person involved is in a position to and allowed to determine whether his or her life still has dignity, fits well with this normative decision. The case involved a patient whose situation could be described as "ultimate degeneration" when the physician, Wilfred Van Oijen, performed euthanasia on her. The patient's life was shortened by only a few hours, but because she was not observably suffering and had not requested that her life be ended, Van Oijen was not in a position to perform euthanasia, irrespective of how "undignified" he felt the patient's situation was. Thus, the principle of autonomy and the duty to relieve suffering restrict the significance of dignity in decisions for euthanasia.

So far the review committees have given dignity the most far-reaching recognition as a factor of suffering in early dementia. That is striking because these cases do not concern dying with dignity but living with dignity, in a social or spiritual sense.

In 2008 the Dutch Association for Voluntary Euthanasia (NVVE) issued a position statement on dignity in which it advocated a more central role for dignity in life-ending interventions than is presently permitted.[7] Time will tell if this position will find support with Dutch physicians, politicians, and the general public.

All said, then, the role of dignity is not unimportant. As a factor of suffering it clearly can have a large impact on the assessment of a request for euthanasia. That is legitimate because if one supports the position that the alleviation of suffering is decisive for allowing euthanasia and then acknowledges that suffering may emerge from the many facets of a person, one should also acknowledge that loss of dignity might be a justification for euthanasia.

Duty to Protect Life

The fourth core principle governing euthanasia and physician-assisted suicide under the WTL is the duty to protect human life. Although it is the hardest to define and most elusive of all the principles relating to euthanasia, the duty to protect life nevertheless forms the basis of legislation. The protection of life entails two elements of law: the right to life and the value of life. The first element concerns the interest in being alive; the second concerns the more abstract notion that every human life is owed respect.

The right to life is founded on human rights and fixed in international treaties; it has an explicit place in the requirement that the patient him- or herself must make a voluntary, well-considered, and persistent request for euthanasia. The value of life is more or less related to what is designated as the intrinsic dignity of human beings, and finds its most explicit support in religious and philosophical traditions. A physician must incorporate both aspects in the assessment of a request for euthanasia and to balance his or her duty to protect life against the duty to alleviate the suffering of the patient.

That protecting life is *the* core principle and normative foundation in euthanasia is seen in the substantive and procedural criteria of due care – conditions for prudential practice – all of which aim at ensuring that practice is as restricted and careful as possible. The criteria of due care focus on *avoiding* euthanasia. The decision to continue to frame euthanasia as an offense against life in criminal law also reflects the focus on protecting human life.

If the traditional approach in the Netherlands focused on the *sanctity* of life approach, however – on the intrinsic value and absolute inviolability of human life – the present approach focuses on the *quality* of life. The 2002 law recognizes that human life can be evaluated – but *only* by the person whose life it is – and can be judged to be below the standard at which that individual believes continuing to live is meaningful. On this reasoning, protecting life can include resisting degeneration and endlessly prolonging life by medical interventions. Protecting life thus extends to the chance for people to die.

This is a remarkable step. To include the notion that life may be protected best by ending it designates a totally new view of the protection of life. As long as autonomy plays a crucial role – in the sense that only a (competent) patient may ground a request for euthanasia on the loss of dignity or other aspect of quality of life – there is a guarantee that the process follows the patient's wishes. Significant risks might emerge were autonomy not maintained as a strict condition and loss of dignity allowed to play a role in a physician's decision making about euthanasia without a patient's request to end life. Difficult problems would be posed if euthanasia were carried out for patients who lack decision-making capacity – for example, those in a coma or those who have late-stage Alzheimer's disease, presenting confrontations within the present system of law.

The desirability of protecting life finds expression in the legal regulation of euthanasia and physician-assisted suicide and in the criteria of due care. Essentially, these focus on preventing euthanasia and guaranteeing a restrictive and careful practice. We cannot stress too strongly that euthanasia is not considered to be normal medical practice, but is seen as exceptional intervention, an intervention of last resort. It may be that since the introduction of the WTL, the role of criminal law has become more peripheral, but if physicians do not comply with the criteria for due care, then a case can be made that euthanasia remains a serious crime, to be answered by imprisonment of up to 12 years. The key role of the duty to protect life is translated directly into maintaining the potential criminal nature of euthanasia. Although from time to time some advocate that euthanasia and physician-assisted suicide be truly "decriminalized," this does not seem very likely to happen for the foreseeable future.

References

1. Pans, Esther. 2006. *De normatieve grondslagen van het Nederlandse euthanasierecht* [The normative foundations of the Dutch euthanasia law]. PhD diss., VU Amsterdam. Nijmegen: Wolf Legal Publishers.
2. Review Commitees. 2009. "Annual Report." http://www.euthanasiecommissie.nl/en/review-committees/annualreport/ (in Dutch and in English).
3. Hoge Raad (Supreme Court of the Netherlands), November 27, 1984, NJ 1985, 106 (the *Schoonheim* case).
4. Hoge Raad (Supreme Court of the Netherlands), June 21, 1994, NJ 1994, 656 (the *Chabot* case).
5. Hoge Raad (Supreme Court of the Netherlands), December 24, 2002, NJ 2003, 167 (the *Brongersma* case).
6. Wal, Gerrit van der, et al. 2003. *Medische besluitvorming aan het einde van het leven. De praktijk en de toetsingsprocedure euthanasie* [Medical decisions at the end of life: The practice and the evaluation procedure]. Utrecht: De Tijdstroom.
7. NVVE (Nederlandse Vereniging voor Vrijwillige Euthanasie). 2008. Perspectieven op waardig sterven [Perspectives on dying with dignity]. Discussion paper. http//www.nvve.nl/nieuws/Perspectievennota.pdf (accessed February 2008).

5

Dutch Social Groups on "Euthanasia"

The Political Spectrum on Ending Life on Request

Heleen Weyers

The Dutch debate about "euthanasia"[a,1] started in the late 1960s and ended for the time being in 2002 with a change in the statutory law. Social groups as well as political and legal actors played important roles. This chapter focuses on the voices of social groups that figured prominently in the debate and how those voices changed over the course of debate.

It is not possible here to present the full history of the debate over its more than 30 years. Instead, this chapter explores four critical moments in the public conversation: the release of the first report on euthanasia by the Health Council and the case of Dr. Truus Postma-van Boven,[b] both in 1973; the hearings of the State Commission on Euthanasia in 1984; the publication in 1991 of the Remmelink Report, the first nationwide research into medical practice at the end of life; and the submission in 1998 of the euthanasia bill that ultimately became law.

The analysis that follows examines the positions taken by organizations representing physicians, patients, and religious denominations. Physicians' perspectives are represented in the views expressed by the Royal Dutch Medical Association (KNMG),[c] which since 1984 has supported doctors who comply with patients' requests to end their lives, and the Dutch Association of Physicians (NAV),[d] which opposes ending life on request. Patients' perspectives are represented here by the Dutch Association for Voluntary

[a] The word *euthanasia* has many meanings. In the Netherlands, since 1985 euthanasia is defined as "intentionally terminating another person's life at that person's request" (see 1. Staatscommissie Euthanasie 1985). When I use the word in this sense I write it without quotation marks. Where the meaning of the word is less clear I use "euthanasia."

[b] A general practitioner who was prosecuted for ending life on request.

[c] Koninklijke Nederlandse Maatschappij tot Bevordering der Geneeskunst, founded in 1849. The KNMG is a federation of doctors' organizations, with a membership of 40,000 members in 2008.

[d] Nederlands Artsen Verbond, founded in 1973, with 400 members as of 2007.

Euthanasia (NVVE),[e] the Foundation for Voluntary Euthanasia (SVE),[f] and the Foundation for Voluntary Life (SVL)[g] – all three of which support ending life on request – and the Dutch Patients Organization (NPV),[h] which opposes it. Finally, we include the perspectives of spokesmen of three churches that contributed prominently to the debate: the Dutch Reformed Church (NHV), the Calvinist Churches (GK),[i,2] and the Roman Catholic Church (RKK).[j,2,3]

THE HEALTH COUNCIL REPORT ON EUTHANASIA AND THE *POSTMA* CASE (1973)

The Dutch debate was sparked in the late 1960s when a physician proposed to withdraw life support from a young woman, Mia Versluis, who had been in a coma for several months as the result of an operation. Her father, outraged at what he considered "euthanasia," filed a complaint against the physician who had been the responsible anesthetist during the operation.[k,4] With this case, the Dutch were for the first time publicly confronted with medical behavior that potentially shortens life. In 1969, the issues involved in the case of Mia Versluis were formulated in an unusually provocative way by a well-known Dutch scholar, Jan Hendrik van den Berg.[5] His booklet led to questions in Parliament that resulted in the founding of the Committee on Medical Ethics within the national Health Council, which in turn began developing a position paper on "euthanasia" in 1970. Before the committee had completed its work, another law case came to public attention. In 1972, it became clear that a doctor would come to trial for ending her mother's life at the mother's request

[e] Nederlandse Vereniging voor Vrijwillige Euthanasie, founded in 1973, which had more than 100,000 members as of 2007.

[f] Stichting Vrijwillige Euthanasie, founded in 1973. The SVE was a small but vocal discussion group with some 15 members. It closed down in 1985.

[g] Stichting Vrijwillig Leven, founded in 1996 by some members of the NVVE who thought this organization did not stand up enough for self-determination. As a foundation, the SVL does not have members. An indication of its size is its approximate 2,500 donors.

[h] Nederlandse Patiënten Vereniging, founded in 1982. In 2007 the NPV had 75,000 members.

[i] The Dutch Reformed Church and the Calvinist Churches, together with the Lutheran Church, were united in 2000. At that time about 17% of the Dutch were members of one of these churches (see 2. Becker 2005).

[j] Despite its strong Calvinist history, Roman Catholicism remains the leading faith community in the Netherlands. In 2000 almost 32% of the Dutch were members of this church (see 2. Becker 2005). With respect to ending life on request, it should be noted that the churches do not necessarily represent the views of believers. For example, a majority of Catholics were opposed in 1966 (55% answered "no" to the question "Should a doctor give a lethal injection at the request of a patient to put an end to his suffering?"), but by 1991 Catholics were indistinguishable from the rest of the population (58% "yes"). Dutch Reformed are only slightly less supportive than the general population (16% "no") and the Calvinists are least supportive of all (34% "no") (see 3. Griffiths, Bood, and Weyers 1998).

[k] Ultimately, the action led to a decision by the Court of Appeals in Amsterdam that put forward procedural criteria for decisions to terminate life-sustaining treatment.

(the *Postma* case).[l] The Health Council postponed publication of the ethics committee report until the case concluded.

In the report published in 1973, the ethics committee defined "euthanasia" as "deliberately acting or deliberately refraining from acting so as to shorten the patient's life when that is in the best interest of a patient whose condition is incurable."[6] The report distinguished several types of "euthanasia": "voluntary euthanasia," carried out with the express consent of the patient; "nonvoluntary euthanasia," carried out without the consent of the patient; "passive euthanasia," that is, hastening death by withholding or withdrawing life-sustaining treatment; and "active euthanasia," the use of life-shortening measures. With regard to "passive euthanasia," the committee took the view that under certain circumstances, a doctor can refrain from employing life-prolonging measures. The committee had two specific situations in mind: "voluntary euthanasia," when it is the patient who refuses treatment, and "nonvoluntary euthanasia," when the doctor considers it a medical-ethical duty to refrain from further treatment. The ethics committee held that "active euthanasia" should not be permitted and did not find it necessary or desirable that the law concerning "euthanasia" be amended.

Pending the publication of the Health Council report and the ruling in the *Postma* case, several social groups had already started to formulate their positions on "euthanasia." Like the Health Council, physicians, patients, and churches were also grappling with the challenge of defining euthanasia at this early stage of the debate.

One of the first organizations to take a public stance on the issue was the General Synod of the Dutch Reformed Church, which published its report, *Euthanasia, Meaning and Boundaries of Medical Behavior*, in 1972.[7] In contrast to the Health Council, the synod distinguished "indirect euthanasia," that is, hastening death as an unintended side effect of pain relief,[m,8,9] from "passive euthanasia," hastening death by stopping or not starting treatment, and from "active euthanasia," the deliberate ending of a patient's life by medical means.

The synod's report held both "indirect" and "passive euthanasia" to be permissible. With respect to "indirect euthanasia," the authors doubted whether pain relief shortens life. Even if this is the case, they reasoned, being free from pain is a necessary condition if one is to experience the end of life as an integral part of life. With respect to "passive euthanasia," the authors took the position that the wish of a competent patient to refuse a life-prolonging treatment at the end of life ought to be taken very seriously. They held that the difference between "passive" and "active euthanasia" was not one of principle but of psychology. Further, they held that the boundaries between "passive" and

[l] See Chapter 3 for more information on the *Postma* case.

[m] What is elsewhere referred to as "double effect" (see 8. Rachels 1986 and 9. Kuhse 1987).

"active euthanasia" are fluid. They did not take a position on the permissibility of "active euthanasia" in consideration of the fact that people hold different views about these matters.

Neither the Calvinist Churches nor the Roman Catholic Church in the Netherlands took specific public positions on the question at this time.[n,10,11]

Among the different views mentioned by the General Synod was the perspective of a group of doctors who organized themselves as the Dutch Association of Physicians. The NAV – formed in opposition to the position taken by the Royal Dutch Medical Association on abortion – took the stand that doctors should be guided in their work by the principle of absolute respect for human life. The NAV spoke out not only against abortion but also against "euthanasia" (without defining different types of it as had the General Synod and the Health Council). The NAV regarded all these practices as contrary to the professional ethos of medicine and, hence, as activities in which doctors should not participate.[12]

For its part, in 1973 the board of the KNMG published a provisional position paper on "euthanasia" in response to the *Postma* case and the report of the Health Council.[13] Like the ethical committee of the Health Council, the board of the KNMG took the position that doctors should respect the decision of a competent patient to refuse treatment and that a doctor should stop treating after such a refusal. The board considered the hastening of death as a side effect of medically indicated pain relief not to be "euthanasia." Like the Health Council's Committee on Medical Ethics, the KNMG board noted that "active euthanasia" was prohibited, and the board unconditionally supported existing law that held physicians accountable for "euthanasia" in the criminal courts.

Meanwhile, the news that Dr. Postma would be prosecuted led a number of her patients to set up a working group to encourage people to voice their support for "voluntary euthanasia." Two days after Dr. Postma's conviction in 1973, the group decided to continue its work as a formal association, the Dutch Association for Voluntary Euthanasia. The NVVE aimed first at ensuring social acceptance for ending life on request and, ultimately, its legalization.[14] At the time, the NVVE argued that legalization was not yet advisable.[15]

A few months before the formation of the NVVE, another patient organization was created to advocate for "voluntary euthanasia": the Foundation for Voluntary Euthanasia. Like the NVVE at that time, the SVE did not strive to change the law but sought only to have "voluntary euthanasia" recognized as

[n] In the 1950s, Pope Pius XII (RKK) had already articulated viewpoints on medical practice at the end of life. In his answers to questions from physicians, he advised that a treatment that is "disproportionate" need not be started, and further that pain relief that has the unintended side effect of hastening death can be justifiable (see 10. Pope Pius XII 1957a and 11. Pope Pius XII 1957b). Elsewhere, the pope clearly indicated that active termination of life was unacceptable.

acceptable within the existing legal framework. In the 1970s, both the SVE and the NVVE spent much of their time designing living wills that allowed patients not only to express their preferences to refuse life-prolonging treatment for a serious disease or after an accident but also to request "active euthanasia" when recovery to an acceptable state would not be expected.

To conclude: The positions taken by these various groups show the boundaries of the debate in the 1970s. With the exception of the NAV, which strongly opposed "euthanasia" – without specifying its meaning – there appeared to be consensus that some medical practices at the end of life that were labeled "euthanasia" were in fact acceptable. In particular, "indirect euthanasia" (hastening death as a side effect of necessary pain relief) and "passive euthanasia" (in the form of refusal of life-sustaining treatment and refraining from futile medical treatment) were seen as ethically and legally justified. The first was accepted on the ground of beneficence, the second on the ground of patient self-determination, the third as being against medical ethics. Although some room was seen, especially by the NVVE and SVE, for actively ending the life of a patient on request ("voluntary active euthanasia"), this was hardly ever considered motivated by referring to self-determination.

THE HEARINGS OF THE STATE COMMISSION ON EUTHANASIA (1982–1985)

In October 1982, the Dutch government established a State Commission on Euthanasia to examine the desirability of changing law with respect to "euthanasia." The commission prepared a discussion paper and a list of questions, and invited interested individuals and organizations to share their views in a series of public hearings held in 1984. In 1985, the commission issued a final report and recommendations that were based partly on analysis of the testimony it had heard. Key testimony focused on such questions as: Should the law on termination of life on request be changed? If the law should be changed, how should termination of life on request be regulated? What criteria of due care should be required? Which medical practices at the end of life do and, importantly, do not fall under the concept of ending life on request?[16]

In its notes for the hearings, the State Commission made reference to the position of the Health Council (1982) that ceasing a treatment that only postpones the moment of death, administering pain relief that has the unintended but foreseeable and accepted side effect of shortening life, and refraining from treatment at the patient's request are "normal medical practice."[17] The commission distinguished this kind of medical behavior at the end of life from ending life on request. All of the organizations that responded to the invitation to comment on the discussion paper concurred with the division between "normal medical practice" and ending life on request. Organizations differed, however, with respect to the idea of the permissibility of intentionally ending a life on request and legalizing the practice.

The spokespersons of the Roman Catholic Church and the Calvinist Churches both offered testimony opposing ending life on request. The Calvinist Churches went on to elaborate their point of view further in a joint report with the Dutch Reformed Church shortly after the publication of the State Commission's report.

The Roman Catholic Church in the Netherlands rejected the ending of life on request as being against "natural medical ethics." In their eyes, ending a life on request rests on the pretension of having life at one's disposal. They rejected it because killing is considered to be an attack on the dignity of the person and because of the doctrine of the sanctity of life. Therefore, ending life on request should be forbidden. For the sake of humanity, a society cannot afford a plurality of opinions on this issue, the RKK stated.

In a similar view, the Calvinist Churches opposed termination of life on request as a violation of the fundamental relationship between God and man: Because God is the owner of life, human beings do not have a right to self-determination. Further, they argued, the duty to preserve life is the absolute condition for the existence of the legal community. The Calvinist Churches also pointed to the danger of the slippery slope on this matter.

In a report published in 1985,[18] the Calvinist Churches, together with the Dutch Reformed Church, broadened the subject. They translated the moral question of "euthanasia" – defined as intentionally ending a life on request or in the best interest of the patient – into a question of whether persons are autonomous creatures. In their answer to this question, autonomy and self-determination were conceptually reformulated as responsibility[o] and stewardship. Besides autonomy, the churches invoked the principle of "quality of life": They took the position that in cases of complete defacement, death can be preferable to life. Therefore, under certain circumstances the decision to end one's life is not "necessarily unjustified."

The initial report did not discuss changing the law governing euthanasia. However, as a result of the reactions to this report, a second, revised edition addressed the question.[19] Although the report recognized a general right to die, it argued that this right did not justify legalizing "euthanasia." The report held that the right to die is more limited than the primary right to life. It contended, further, that it was not possible to define exceptional cases clearly and objectively enough to ensure that such cases would remain the exception.[19]

Like the churches, the Dutch Patients Organization testified in opposition to ending a life on request and to the prospect of any change in the law. The NPV saw the ending of life on request as a violation of fundamental Christian beliefs about the sanctity of life, arguing that all human beings deserve protection, irrespective of their stage or quality of life. In the NPV's view, human life is a seamless continuum from conception to death. They rejected the

[o] In the Dutch discussion, self-determination almost always is coupled with responsibility.

suggestion in the questions of the State Commission that individuals have a right to choose death. Rather, they argued that medicine and law jointly have an unconditional duty to preserve life. The NPV likewise rejected the proposition that societal perspectives or social norms could determine whether termination of life on request is ethically justified or should be legally permitted. Legalizing such acts, in their view, carried the grave danger that as social perspectives changed, vulnerable patients – such as patients with mental illness or severely handicapped newborns – would be put at risk, and trust in doctors would be undermined.

The patient organizations that strove for legal termination of life on request – the SVE and NVVE – also responded to the State Commission. The SVE took the position that ending a life on request should not be punishable in cases in which certain requirements of due care were fulfilled. But although they pleaded for more social control and regulation of ending life on request, the SVE opposed changing the law.[p] The NVVE, in contrast, saw change in the law as necessary in order to make termination of life on request available for patients. In their view, it should not be punishable so long as certain conditions were met.

Dutch physicians' organizations were similarly divided in their responses to the State Commission. The NAV reiterated the position it had taken in 1973: Protecting the intrinsic value of human life is the basis of the *Rechtsstaat*,[q] and ending life on request contradicts the Hippocratic Oath, which is at the heart of medical professionalism. They opposed any change in the law and called for existing law to be applied consistently. They argued that it is not possible to define a category of legally permissible termination of life on request, citing the elasticity of proposed criteria for due care.

By the time the State Commission convened hearings in 1984, the executive board of the KNMG had changed its position on euthanasia to hold that euthanasia should not be illegal under certain defined conditions. The board was looking for greater legal certainty for patients and doctors. It emphasized that only doctors should be allowed to engage in actions that terminate life on request, as they are the only ones who have the knowledge to be able to diagnose and offer prognoses and the only ones qualified to administer the drugs needed. Furthermore, the board argued, doctors can be controlled by disciplinary law. In their response to the State Commission, the KNMG did not ask for a change in law, although they would do so just a year later.

To conclude: As these reactions to the work of the State Commission on Euthanasia show, the opinions of societal groups changed in the 1980s, though

[p] In 1985 after the verdict in the *Schoonheim* case made clear that euthanasia can be lawful, the SVE closed down.

[q] A concept in continental European legal thinking that literally means "state of law." It refers to a state in which the rights of people are protected by the law and the exercise of governmental power is constrained by the law.

mostly on the liberal side of the political spectrum. The most significant of these changes is the shift in the KNMG's position, from opposing the ending of a patient's life by a doctor on the request of a patient to not merely supporting it but seeing it as a fact of life in medical practice. We also see calls emerging for a change in the law, both by the KNMG and by the NVVE, which by the mid-1980s seem to have thought that their first aim – societal acceptance of termination of life on request – had been achieved,[r,20] and thus that the time had come to advance its second goal: a change in the law.

Three other considerations deserve attention. The report of the hearings of the State Commission showed a consensus with respect to medical practices at the end of life that do not fall under the concept of euthanasia. This reflects the general consensus in the Netherlands that while life deserves respect, the duty to respect it is not absolute. It also reflects agreement that patients themselves can decide whether or not they want treatment. This agreement about self-determination did not extend to termination of life on request.

From the hearings, it becomes clear that the line between proponents and opponents to euthanasia is not identical to the line between those who are for and against a change in the law. Some proponents of euthanasia are against the latter.

The report also showed that new arguments were being brought into the debate. In addition to the sanctity of life and absolute respect for life, opponents stressed concerns about a slippery slope and the undermining of societal trust (in doctors). Both opponents and supporters of legal change put forward arguments about the need to control termination of life on request.

THE REMMELINK REPORT ON MEDICAL PRACTICES AT THE END OF LIFE (1991)

In 1990, the Dutch government commissioned a group of researchers to study medical practices at the end of life. The research, which was published in 1991 in what came to be known as the Remmelink Report,[21] showed that in 1990, 38% of all deaths in the Netherlands (some 49,000 cases) was preceded by a decision of a doctor who knew that it would probably shorten the patient's life. In the majority of cases, these decisions concerned withholding or withdrawing life-sustaining treatment (some 22,500 cases, or 17.5% of all deaths) and pain relief (also 17.5% of all deaths). With respect to these two categories, the research distinguished several subcategories, including pain relief with the subsidiary purpose of hastening death (4,500 cases) and stopping treatment with the express purpose of hastening death (11,000 cases). A minority

[r] Opinion polls show that the NVVE was correct in this assessment. To the question "Should a doctor give a lethal injection at the request of a patient to put an end to his suffering?" in 1970, 53% of respondents answered "yes" and 24% "no." In 1985, 55% answered "yes" and 12% "no" (see 20. Sociaal Cultureel Planbureau 1992).

of cases involved decisions to actively intervene to end life at the patient's explicit request (2.3% of all deaths, about 2,700 cases a year). Approximately 1,000 deaths (0.8%) involved decisions to actively end life without an explicit request on the part of the patient. With respect to the criteria of due care, developed in the 1980s, the researchers found that only 18% of all cases in which physicians actively intervened to end a life were reported as such. They found that compliance with other due care criteria – the presence of unbearable and hopeless suffering, a voluntary and well-considered request, and consultation with a second doctor – was generally good.

These results led the government to several conclusions. First, in practice, ending life on request does not lead to wrongs. Second, the reporting rate should be improved. To reach this goal, the government proposed that the reporting procedure implemented in behalf of the research be mandated by law. Third, it was too soon to formally change the legal status of termination of life on request.[22]

Among the many organizations that published responses to the report and the government's decision were the doctors' organizations KNMG and NAV and the patients' organizations NPV and NVVE. In this instance, however, the churches issued no position statement.

The NAV was deeply concerned not only that Dutch practice regarding termination of life on request had gone much too far, but also that the attention paid to the rather small number of these cases was distracting attention from the far larger number of cases in which decisions had the effect of shortening the patient's life. Decisions to forgo life-sustaining treatment or provide pain relief that might hasten death were taken at least partly with the intent of shortening life. The NAV believed that Dutch thinking was unbalanced on this matter to the point that people failed to appreciate the enormity of the report's findings and hardly understood their consequences.[23]

The NAV held that the kind of quality-of-life reasoning that led to decisions that a given treatment was futile or that pain medications could be given despite the possibility of hastening death violated the bedrock ethos of medicine. In the eyes of the NAV, a doctor has no right to make judgments about quality of life. They refer to the European Convention on Human Rights to stress that life deserves absolute respect and that this ethics should govern doctors' practice at all times. The organization feared that if the trend revealed by the report continued, government policy would ultimately abrogate fundamental human rights.

The response of the board of the KNMG was at the opposite end of the spectrum. In their view, the findings of the Remmelink Report showed that there were far fewer cases of termination of life on request than had been thought and that, in general, doctors acted with due care.[24] In the KNMG's view, this supported their argument that doctors who met recognized criteria of due care should not be subject to prosecution. Although the board acknowledged that public oversight and regulation of termination of life on request was important, they were disappointed that the government had not gone farther and removed termination of life on request, properly carried out, from the sphere of criminal justice.

Dutch patients' organizations were equally divided in their responses to the Remmelink Report. The Dutch Patients Organization was alarmed because government had opened the door to legal recognition of termination of life on request.[25] The NPV took the position that in doing so, government would disregard its responsibility to legally protect citizens and would give doctors power of decision, resulting in legal uncertainty for patients and inequalities among patients. The NPV viewed the findings with foreboding, because of what they saw as the alarming prevalence of practices intended to shorten life, because of the low rate of reporting, and because doctors who object to reporting could label their behavior as pain relief or forgo treatment without consequences.

The NPV held that the government had in effect accepted ending life on request. In their view, the proposed policy provided legal protection for doctors, rather than holding them accountable for their practices. Such a policy neglected the primary responsibility of government to protect citizens. The NPV called urgently for a policy that would reaffirm the prohibition in the Criminal Code against doctors terminating life and that would instruct the prosecutorial authorities to actively seek out and prosecute physicians who acted in violation of that prohibition.

In contrast, in an unpublished letter to the Parliamentary Commission on Justice and Health, the board of the patients' organization NVVE called for removal of criminal sanctions against doctors who honored durable, explicit, and earnest requests for euthanasia made by competent persons. They argued further that such requests should be honored not only for terminally ill patients but also for people who suffer from chronic illness or mental rather than physical anguish. The NVVE argued for regulation of the ending of life on request outside of criminal law.[26]

To conclude: Whereas in 1984 there had been general agreement across the political spectrum on the distinction adopted by the State Commission on Euthanasia between controversial and noncontroversial medical practices at the end of life, there was now strong dissent from the conservative groups. Both the NAV and the NPV revisited their earlier acceptance of forgoing treatment and pain relief with the side effect of shortening life as legitimate, and were now shocked by the fact that those acts were sometimes carried out partly or explicitly with that goal in mind. Both groups condemned those practices. To these organizations, it was clear that the Netherlands had stepped onto a slippery slope.

At the other end of the spectrum, the NVVE, by broadening the scope of the patients to include those who were not terminally ill, was stressing patient self-determination more than it had previously. Moreover, now that legal recognition had been won for termination of life on request, the KNMG and NVVE were emphasizing statutory recognition of the practice.

At the beginning of the 1990s, then, we see increasing polarization between those who were "pro-life," opposing all forms of intentional ending of life, and those who argued that termination of life on request should not only be permitted but also gain statutory recognition. This polarization, however, did not lead to a noisy debate in which opponents and proponents execrated each other. Just like before, the debate was rather calm.

STATUTORY CHANGE: LEGALIZATION OF ENDING LIFE ON REQUEST (2002)

The last phase of the legalization of ending life on request started in 1998 as the Dutch Parliament began considering a bill to that effect. Before Parliament opened its discussion of the proposed legislation, societal groups were invited to comment on it. Although the responses were never published in parliamentary proceedings, we have found the reactions of our index groups.

As to be expected, the Dutch conference of Roman Catholic bishops objected to the proposed legislation both in principle and out of concern for its likely consequences.[s,27] They argued that passage of the bill would effectively remove any legal sanction from ending life on request in the Netherlands, which was unacceptable. Legal "justification" – that is, adherence to criteria of due care – should in no way be allowed to override the duty to preserve life. The government, they argued, has a paramount duty to protect citizens in their relationships with one another.

The bishops also pointed to the adverse consequences of the bill, including a decline in public morality, further loss of respect for life, pressure on doctors to terminate life on request, erosion of trust in doctors, a decline in the willingness to help people who are suffering, and the creation of a climate in which patients would feel obligated to spare their intimates the burdens of difficult, long-lasting care. The bishops called on all responsible policymakers not to take the path set out in the legislation.

The United Protestant Churches also called for a halt in efforts to legalize death on request and urged a collective societal moment of reflection to evaluate the consequences of existing policy for respect for life. Already, they held, moral standards had become unstable, life had come to be valued in economic terms, and society had lost concern for those in need. In the churches' view, what was urgently needed was a very different legal framework from the one proposed, a framework for end-of-life care that emphasized the duty to preserve life and addressed the responsibilities of caregivers.

The Protestant churches concluded that to permit physicians to terminate life on request violates a fundamental value and crosses a border that should not be passed. They worried that the legislation would put the Netherlands on

[s] The paper has been published in 27. de Lange and Jans 2000.

a slippery slope, especially because, in their view, the criteria for due care were subjective. They feared that if individual wishes came to be decisive in setting the law, the very basis of society would be undermined and the duty to protect life would be endangered. Finally, they worried that passage of the legislation would have the pernicious effect of promoting a vision of life and health that did not accept handicaps, chronic disease, and deterioration.

The professional medical organizations were, as expected, divided on the bill. The KNMG welcomed the proposal as putting an end to the paradoxical situation in which doctors found themselves with respect to ending life on request. They expected the bill to increase doctors' willingness to report and would, therefore, create greater opportunity to guarantee transparency and ensure the quality of practice for death on request.[28] To the KNMG, the bill represented the fruition of policymaking efforts over the previous several years.

The NAV was against the proposed legislation.[29] In their eyes, the bill damaged constitutional protections of human life and human dignity. The NAV took the position that the law would not be applied uniformly given the subjective nature of the criteria for assessing physicians' actions, particularly the key requirement that the patient's suffering be "unbearable" and "hopeless." Moreover, they were concerned that acceptance of the bill would frustrate good end-of-life care. By permitting termination of life on request, the legislation would normalize these practices. Not only would patients be put under pressure to choose these options at the end of life, but so too would doctors. Accepting the bill would also put doctors back on a pedestal and inappropriately give them the power to decide over life and death. As the NAV saw it, supporting or opposing the bill was nothing less than choosing what kind of society the Netherlands would be: Like abortion, termination of life on request is no good for the patient, the doctor, and society, and it should be rejected.

With respect to patients' organizations, the NPV did not respond directly. However, we can infer its views from the position taken by Care for Life,[f] a platform on which the NPV participated. The proposal deeply concerned Care for Life. If passed, they saw it having far-reaching effects on the medical profession, society as a whole, and the *Rechtsstaat* in the Netherlands. In the view of Care for Life, the legislation would open the door to increasing numbers of cases of termination of life on request. As law, it would encourage a social climate in which the obligation to provide maximum care, irrespective of the individual's condition, would no longer be obvious. The effects on quality of life, and the quality of society, would be grave.

Beyond these general objections, Care for Life objected to specific provisions in the bill. They believed that the draft legislation violated human rights

[f] Care for Life is a gathering of idealistic organizations that speaks up for human life in all phases of life, starting with conception (see http://www.rmu.org/index.php?paginaID=106).

set out in international conventions and noted the difficult position in which the legislation put conscientious objectors: Legalizing death on request would impose moral beliefs on those who did not share them.

For its part, the NVVE welcomed the legislation but at the same time took the position that it should be improved.[30] They were concerned that, as drafted, it would create unnecessary barriers for doctors and patients because the proposed criteria for due care were too onerous.

Response from the Foundation for Voluntary Life in general followed that of the NVVE. The SVL argued that the bill should have taken as its starting point Article 11 of the Dutch Constitution, which guarantees bodily integrity. They also felt that the proposal, as drafted, embodied the perspective of the medical profession rather than of patients. They called on Parliament to change the language of the bill to refer to the "person involved" instead of "patient,"[31] thereby stressing the importance of self-determination.

To sum up: The churches opposed the bill that regulated ending life on request. In their objections, they emphasized the consequences on society and the legal system more than religious arguments.

The diverging positions of the two doctors' organizations did not change substantially between 1991 and 2002. Throughout, the KNMG had supported ending a life on request as responsible medical practice when carried out with due care, and had stressed the need for transparency and for clarity in the law. They saw legalization of death on request as having positive consequences. The NAV, for its part, steadfastly opposed ending a life on request on grounds of respect for life (and the duty to preserve it) and the negative consequences it would have for medicine, law, and society in general. For the NAV, legalization could only have negative consequences.

The perspectives of patients' organizations likewise remained largely unchanged, with the NVVE continuing to support and the NPV continuing to oppose death on request. The one change that did take place was the emergence of the SVL, whose views on self-determination were even more liberal than those of the NVVE.

The divergence that had occurred at the beginning of the 1990s deepened at the beginning of the new millennium.

THE DUTCH SPECTRUM ON "EUTHANASIA"

Not all of the organizations examined in this chapter responded formally at each key moment in the euthanasia debate between 1972 and 2002 (we miss the view of churches especially in 1991). Nor was the organizational landscape entirely constant over that time, at least among patient advocates, whose organizational profile changed with the formation of the NPV in 1982, the dissolution of the SVE in 1985, and the formation of the SVL in 1997. Nor do the positions formally expressed by organizations necessarily represent the views of all of their individual members. Nonetheless, exploring the positions taken by key organizations at crucial moments in the development of Dutch public thinking concerning the ending of life on request gives a good insight into the developments in the spectrum of opinions over the course of the three decades before the practice was formally recognized in legislation.

In the beginning of the Dutch debate on ending life on request, it was not at all clear which medical behavior at the end of life fell under the concept of "euthanasia." Already in the 1970s, some behavior that was so labeled was considered not morally or legally problematic: pain relief with the unintended side effect of hastening death ("indirect euthanasia"), stopping treatment because treatment was medically futile ("nonvoluntary passive euthanasia"), and stopping treatment because the patient refused it ("voluntary passive euthanasia"). This consensus received its formal affirmation by the report of the State Commission on Euthanasia. The State Commission took the position, and all the organizations that let their voices be heard in the hearings agreed, that these practices are part of "normal medical practice" and should not be labeled as euthanasia. From that time on, it was clear that the debate would concentrate on intentional termination of life on request.

Our review of the available position statements of leading organizations shows increasing polarization of perspectives across the political spectrum. As the debate evolved, organizations revised their positions, clarifying their arguments and sometimes developing new arguments. However, the climate in which the various arguments have been uttered has not changed. The discussion has been very peaceable throughout.

In the 1970s, there was not much disagreement. Both medical associations were against the possibility of intentional termination of life on request. Both patients' organizations (the NPV did not yet exist) were in favor of this possibility. But at the time, neither prevailed in seeing the practice legalized. Surprisingly, the only Dutch church that spoke out on ending life on request (NHK) was not totally against this possibility.

From the hearings of the State Commission on Euthanasia it is not only clear that there was consensus on "normal medical practice" but also that participants disagreed on the legalization of intentionally ending life on request. Polarization, however, became more apparent in the reactions to the Remmelink Report.

On the liberal side, right-to-die societies initially put little emphasis on patient self-determination with respect to ending life on request, instead seeing doctors as playing an important role. After 1991, however, the NVVE came to stress autonomy as a fundamental value that would be served by ending life on request. In the late 1990s, the SVL took that argument even further.[u]

Over time, the KNMG became a stronger proponent of the availability of ending life on request, calling for legalization in 1985 and thereafter. The argument on which it based its support, however, is not and has never been patient

[u] After the bill became law, the differences between the two organizations largely disappeared.

self-determination. In its plea for a change in the law, the KNMG was looking for legal clarity for doctors (and patients) and ways to ensure transparency in practice.

On the conservative side, the opposition to medical behavior that potentially shortens life became more entrenched over this period. The NPV and NAV, which agreed with the distinction of the State Commission's classification between euthanasia and normal medical practice, were horrified by the 1991 Remmelink Report – not so much by the extent of the practice of euthanasia revealed by the report but by what they learned about the extent to which deaths occurred as a result of decisions to limit treatment or provide pain relief with the express or subsidiary intention of ending life. To them, it was obvious that the Netherlands was sliding down a slippery slope. It strengthened their position that ending life on request should not be legalized.

A notable change in the public debate during this period was the growing conservatism of Dutch Protestant churches with respect to "euthanasia": Whereas in 1972 the Protestant churches had seen it as "completely justifiable,"[32] by 1985 they had come to see it less positively as "not necessarily unjustified." By the end of the 1990s, their position was that ending a life on request was a "violation of a fundamental value" and completely unacceptable.

It is remarkable that the organizations that opposed euthanasia, though inspired by religion, invoked religious arguments only at the beginning of the debate. During the debate, the religious arguments were replaced by consequentialist ones, obviously due to the little weight given to the former. This characteristic of the Dutch debate on euthanasia – the diminishing of religious arguments – is also to be seen in the reaction of the churches. During the debate, they increasingly invoked arguments relating to good care, societal mistrust, and slippery slopes.

In the near future, one controversy will remain in the debate on medical behavior at the end of life – the role of self-determination. The NVVE and SVL are looking for more room for this value; such room is disputed by the KNMG (ending life of request is defended by the conflict of duties), the churches, the NAV, and the NPV (who all defend respect for life and fear for negative societal consequences).

References

1. Staatscommissie Euthanasie. 1985. *Rapport van de Staatscommisie Euthanasie* [Report of the State Commission on Euthanasia]. Vol. 1: 59. The Hague: Staatsuitgeverij.
2. Becker, T. J. 2005. Church membership investigated (1950–2002). In *The Dutch and Their Gods: Secularization and Transformation of Religion in the Netherlands since 1950*, ed. Erik Senger, 60. Hilversum: Uitgeverij Verloren.
3. Griffiths, John, Alex Bood, and Heleen Weyers. 1998. *Euthanasia and Law in the Netherlands*. Amsterdam: Amsterdam University Press.

4. Beslissing Gerechtshof Amsterdam [Decision Court of Appeals, Amsterdam] 1969. *Nederlandse Staatscourant* 55: 7.
5. Berg, J. H. van den. 1969. *Medische macht en medische ethiek*, Nijkerk: Uitgeverij G. F. Callenbach. Translated as *Medical Power and Medical Ethics*. 1978. New York: W. W. Norton.
6. Gezondheidsraad. 1972. *Advies inzake euthanasie* [Advice concerning euthanasia]. Den Haag: Ministerie van Volksgezondheid en Milieuhygiëne.
7. Generale Synode der Nederlands Hervormde Kerk. 1972 *Euthanasie. Zin en begrenzing van het medisch handelen* [Euthanasia: Meaning and limiting of medical behavior], 's-Gravenhage: Boekencentrum.
8. Rachels, J. 1986. *The End of Life*. Oxford: Oxford University Press.
9. Kuhse, H. 1987. *The Sanctity-of-Life Doctrine in Medicine: A Critique*. Oxford: Claredon Press.
10. Pope Pius XII. 1957a. Trois questions religieuses et morales concernant l'analgésie [Three moral and religious questions about analgesia]. *Acta Apostolicae Sedis* 49: 129–147.
11. Pope Pius XII. 1957b. An answer to a question about 'reanimation.' *Acta Apostolicae Sedis* 49: 1027–1033.
12. Statutes of the NAV (Dutch Association of Physicians).
13. KNMG (Koninklijke Nederlandse Maatschappij tot bevordering der Geneeskunst). 1973. Het euthanasievraagstuk [The euthanasia issue]. *Medisch Contact* 28: 578–589.
14. Statutes of the NVVE (Dutch Association for Voluntary Euthanasia).
15. NVVE (Nederlandse Vereniging voor Vrijwillige Euthanasie). 1978. *Rapport van de Adviescommissie Wetgeving betreffende toelaatbaarheid euthanasie* [Report of the Advice Committee Legislation on the permissibility of euthanasia], Amsterdam: NVVE.
16. Staatscommissie Euthanasie. 1985. *Rapport van de Staatscommissie Euthanasie* [Report of the State Commission on Euthanasia]. Vol 3: 7–11. The Hague: Staatsuitgeverij.
17. Gezondheidsraad. 1982. *Euthanasie. Advies inzake euthanasie uitgebracht door de Gezondheidsraad* [Euthanasia: Advice on euthanasia by the Health Council]. 's- Gravenhage: Staatsuitgeverij.
18. Van den Berg, J. et al. 1985. *Euthanasie en pastoraat* [Euthanasia and pastoral care]. Leusden: Kerkinformatie.
19. *Euthanasie en pastoraat* [Euthanasia and pastoral care]. 1988. 's-Gravenhage: Uitgeverij Boekencentrum B.V., p. 19.
20. Sociaal Cultureel Planbureau. 1992. Sociaal en cultureel rapport 1992 [Social and Cultural Report 1992]. Rijswijk: Sociaal en Cultureel Planbureau.
21. Van der Maas, Paul J., et al. 1992., *Euthanasia and Other Medical Decisions Concerning the End of Life*. Amsterdam: Elsevier.
22. *Second Chamber of Parliament 1991–1992*, 20 383, nr. 14.
23. Commentaar Nederlands Artsenverbond op het kabinetsstandpunt [Comment of the NAV on the viewpoint of the Cabinet]. 1991. *Medisch Contact* 46: 1543–1546.
24. Euthanasie. Reactie hoofdbestuur KNMG op het regeringsstandpunt [Euthanasia: Reaction of the Board of the KNMG on the viewpoint of the Cabinet]. 1991. *Medisch Contact* 46: 1541–1543.

25. Nederlandse Patiënten Vereniging, *Reactie van de Nederlandse Patiënten Vereniging op het Kabinetsstandpunt euthanasie* [Reaction of the NPV on the Cabinet's viewpoint on euthanasia] 1991. Veenendaal: NPV.
26. Euthanasie uit het strafrecht [Remove euthanasia from the Penal Code]. *Euthanavisie* 1992, nr. 1: 10.
27. de Lange, F., and J. Jans, eds. 2000. *De dood in het geding. Euthanasiewetgeving en de kerken* [Death at issue: Law on euthanasia and the churches]. Kampen: Uitgeverij Kok.
28. Hagenouw, R. 1999. Wetsvoorstel Toetsing Levensbeëindiging op verzoek en hulp bij zelfdoding' [The Termination of Life on Request and Assisted Suicide (Review Procedures) Act]. *Medisch Contact* 54: 1452–1453.
29. Hildering, P. 2000. Bezwaarschrift NAV [Petition NAV]. *Pro Vita Humana* 7: 11–13.
30. Standpunt NVVE betreffende wetsvoorstel euthanasie. Amsterdam 16–11–1999 [OpinionoftheNVVEontheeuthanasiabill:Amsterdam,November16,1999].1999. http://www.nvve.nl/nvve2/dossierdetail.asp?pagkey=71802&dossier=72075.
31. Gill. K., and G. Schellekens 1999. Wetsvoorstel euthanasia en hulp bij zelfdoding [Bill on euthanasia and assisted suicide]. *SVL Nieuws*, no. 5: 1–3.
32. de Lange, F. 2000. Verschuivingen in het kerkelijk spreken – Verschuivingen in het debat over euthanasie [Shifts in clerical speaking – Shifts in the debate on euthanasia]. In 26. F. de Lange and J. Jans 2000, pp. 46–58.

6

The Dutch Social Fabric

Health Care, Trust, and Solidarity

Margo Trappenburg and Hans Oversloot

INTRODUCTION

In this chapter, we will discuss the social and political "fabric" of the Dutch euthanasia regime. The Dutch regime – described more extensively in other chapters – can be characterized as both liberal and moderate. It is liberal compared to many other countries where euthanasia is strictly forbidden. It is moderate because of the many safeguards involved: Dutch people are not entitled to euthanasia or physician-assisted suicide, and doctors cannot perform euthanasia as they see fit. Both patient and doctor must adhere to legal criteria and procedural norms.

Three strands that make up the social fabric of this regime come very clearly to the fore in the literature on euthanasia in the Netherlands. They have kept the regime liberal as well as moderate.

The first strand is the consensual character of the Dutch social and political culture. Dutch political elites – adherents of various ideologies, with different opinions on euthanasia – felt that they had to work out a regulatory regime that would suit most of them, rather than a regime that would accommodate liberal preferences while disregarding religious or conservative objections, or vice versa.

The second strand is the Dutch health-care system, in particular the system of general practitioners, who supposedly know their patients much better than most hospital doctors. General practitioners are entrusted with euthanasia decisions because of their knowledge of their patients.

The third strand is the trust that Dutch patients have in their doctors and their willing submission to rules and decisions made by the medical elite. Dutch patients trust their doctors with their lives and deaths, even more literally than patients in countries where euthanasia is forbidden. Dutch patients seem to be willing to accept medical decisions in other areas as well; they tend to accept that "you can't always get what you want" with regard to health care.

Recent social and political changes could begin to fray this tightly woven fabric, however. In the early years of the twenty-first century, new populist parties have challenged traditional political elites, altering the consensual character of Dutch politics. Similarly, as more and more women physicians enter general practice on a part-time basis, fewer general practitioners (GPs) fit the traditional model of the longtime, trusted advisor who knows the patient and family well and can be called at all hours. Finally, the introduction of a more market-based health-care system that – as is emphasized again and again in public and political debate – puts patients in the driver's seat as consumers is undermining patients' willing submission to the rules and decisions of the medical elite.

In what follows we will explore whether and how these changes may – in the long run – also change the Dutch euthanasia regime itself.

THE THREE STRANDS IN FOREIGN EYES

Several foreign commentators have expressed wonder about the reason that euthanasia was first legalized in the Netherlands. What made the country unique or unusual in this respect? Israeli researcher Raphael Cohen-Almagor noticed with alarm the wide consensus among what some have called the "euthanasia elite," the researchers, ethicists, lawyers, politicians, and policy-makers involved in the euthanasia regulations:

> What was striking in my discussions was the prevailing acceptance of the euthanasia procedure. There were only a few dissenters who were willing to oppose the system. My first fourteen interviewees were, on the whole, in favor of the policy, and I felt a growing unease in encountering such unanimity of opinion.[1]

American medical anthropologist Frances Norwood points – with warmth and approval – to the unique relationship between Dutch patients and their general practitioners:

> What I first noticed conducting observations with *huisartsen* [general practitioners] was that their daily practice was quite different from what I had observed ... in the United States. Dutch *huisartsen* tend to work alone in offices situated within neighborhoods, homes converted into office space typically, and they continue to this day a long tradition of conducting home visits, or house calls.... Another important distinction between the Dutch and U.S. general practice is the power differential, the relationship between patients, families and *huisartsen*. In some ways the power differential in terms of physician authority is more equalized between Dutch patients and *huisartsen* than between their US counterparts.[2]

Dutch GPs take time to discuss their patients' personal life. Unlike the majority of contemporary American doctors, they do not restrict themselves to their patients' medical condition. A conversation between patient and *huisarts* tends to become a form of mutual consultation, a kind of conference. Patient and doctor try to reach consensus, although in this process patients generally follow the doctor's lead.

Whereas Norwood was impressed by the easy relationship between GPs and their patients, Herbert Hendin, professor of psychiatry at New York Medical College, was struck by what he perceived as the uncanny amount of trust in physicians that he found in the Netherlands. Apparently, possibly because of their personal acquaintance with their doctors, Dutch patients are willing to grant their physicians the right to end their suffering by putting them to death. Hendin observed:

> The Dutch accept the authority of physicians in ways that would seem foreign in the United States. Malpractice suits are rare in the Netherlands. Even when physicians end the lives of patients who have not requested it, the Dutch are inclined to be forgiving on the grounds that the physicians' intentions were benevolent.[3]

Hendin attributes this leniency to what he considers to be the ambivalent Dutch attitude toward authority. As traditional Protestants, the Dutch defied the authority of the pope and of the Roman Catholic Church, yet they appear to be willing to accept "authority that is less direct and obvious; doctors and judges fall into this category."[3]

These and other foreign observers point to three characteristics of Dutch (political) culture that also have relevance for explaining the way in which the legal framework and the actual practice of euthanasia came about – and have been maintained: 1) the culture of consensus, in which elites of all sorts seem to make complicated decisions together in some fuzzy way; 2) the familiarity between Dutch GPs and their patients; and 3) general willingness to submit to the medical elite. In fact, these observations by "outsiders" and "foreigners" do not differ much from (earlier) observations by "insiders" and "natives," and (the effects of) these findings continue to be discussed by Dutch social scientists, political theorists, and moral philosophers.

A CLOSER LOOK AT THE SOCIAL AND POLITICAL FABRIC OF THE EUTHANASIA REGIME

Dutch political culture has usually been described as pragmatic, consensual, and corporatist. The country's electoral system is based on proportional representation. Broadcasting time, mayoralties, and high-ranking positions in government bureaucracy are also distributed according to various proportionality principles. Coalition governments are a fact of life; no individual political party has ever managed to win a majority of seats in Parliament. Sensitive issues touching on religion or morality are carefully discussed in advisory councils and expert committees. Labor relations are discussed in advisory councils in which employer organizations and trade unions try to agree on cutbacks, wage raises, job security, and so on.[4] Political scientist Rudy Andeweg characterizes the political system as follows:

> "Cosy consensus" is the *Economist*'s pet phrase to describe Dutch politics. Indeed, whatever criterion is used, or whatever aspect of the political system is analysed, the

Netherlands always scores high on cooperation and low on competition. Together with Austria, Belgium and Switzerland, the Netherlands is regarded as one of the classic cases of consociational democracy, in which the destabilizing effects of deep social divisions are neutralized by cooperation among the leaders of the social segments. Neo-corporatism – a combination of non-competitive relations among interest associations with bargaining between interest associations and government – is also characteristic of the Dutch system.[5]

In such a system elites of all kinds learn that they must be moderate and that at one moment or another they will have to agree on important points, or at least do business together. Andeweg stresses that Dutch political elites tend to search for consensus and compromise. A large number of legislative government proposals are approved by both ruling coalition parties and parties in opposition.

Consensus and compromise seeking is also practiced in the arena of interest groups. Once a decision is taken and a compromise has been reached, protest tends to disappear in the Netherlands. The political debate about abortion ended in 1981 when a compromise bill was finally adopted. After that, both the pro-life and the pro-choice movements virtually disappeared, despite the fact that neither had accomplished its goals.[5] One might expect a similar course of events with regard to euthanasia after the introduction of the current law in 2002. Proponents of a more liberal regime as well as opponents of the present law would then accept the chosen compromise. They would not fight either for an extension of the present possibilities or for tighter rules and regulations.

To understand the way in which the practice of euthanasia in the Netherlands originated, and how this practice has been maintained, one must pay special attention to the relationship between patient and doctor, that is, the relationship between patient and GP.[6] Studies of euthanasia in practice have shown time and again that euthanasia is very much a matter between family doctor and patient, rather than a medical procedure confined to hospitals or nursing homes.[7,8,9] It involves a process that was intended to safeguard Dutch patients from unexamined or hasty decisions about ending their lives by compelling them to convince their family doctor that they really want to die. That process of persuasion requires more than a single conversation. The doctor, for his or her part, is legally obligated to seek consultation from another physician in assessing whether a decision to perform euthanasia is appropriate.

American media may portray Dutch citizens as free-spirited individuals preoccupied with drug abuse, abortion, and pornography right up to the time they end their lives prematurely by means of euthanasia, but citizens' willingness to submit to medical authority disproves that caricature. The Dutch acknowledge authority and do accept limits on ethical issues; in most cases, they are willing to forgo the treatments that physicians choose not to employ. For example, for a long time prenatal diagnosis was available only to pregnant women and aspiring parents who were categorized as having a medical "indication," such as maternal age, family history, or a previous child with a genetic condition. One could not receive an amniocentesis without such an acknowledged medical indication, even if one were willing to pay for it. Similarly, the ideology of natural birth is very much alive among the medical elite (especially among midwives), and up till very recently Dutch women could not demand an epidural because of a preference for a less painful birth process than the one nature provides.

New medical technology, such as predictive genetic testing, is not simply thrown on the market following government approval; it is regulated through medical channels, and people have access to it if their doctor thinks that they have a proper medical reason. Former Health Minister Elizabeth Borst-Eilers, who is a member of D66 – generally considered the most liberal political party in the Netherlands with respect to (regulation of) ethical issues – announced in a white paper on new genetic technology:

> In my eyes [the health-care sector and the medical profession] should produce a protocol for predictive genetic diagnostic research. Consensus about indications must decide when and under what conditions the use of this kind of technology could be appropriate.... The fact that professionals will act in accordance with professional standards will guard us against unjustified demands for genetic diagnostic research from patients, and against requests that could lead to an excessive burden on the patient and no compensatory advantages in case of an unfavorable outcome.[10]

Medical professionals must write protocols and uphold professional standards. A mere request should not suffice to get a predictive test, nor should a mere request ever be enough to grant someone a mercy death.

One might say that these three characteristics – the culture of consensus, the special relationship patients have with their GP, and people's submissive attitude toward the medical elite – have made the Dutch euthanasia regime what it is today, a moderately liberal regime: moderately liberal in that it provides individual freedom of choice within a formal, legal framework that sets limits to individual self-determination; moderately liberal because two doctors must classify the patient's suffering as unbearable before they would consider going along with a wish to die.

Its liberal aspects make the regime unacceptable to citizens with strong traditional religious views, who feel that we should not intervene in God's way. But neither does it satisfy hard-core social liberals. For those who think that an individual's life is his or her own for the taking, who are convinced that people fully own their individual lives, and who believe that a request alone should be sufficient to get euthanasia, the present regime is not liberal enough, or perhaps not even liberal at all.

All three seemingly fixed characteristics have recently become more or less unhinged, however, and are perhaps now in a state of flux. In the remainder of this chapter, we discuss what is happening to Dutch political culture, the traditional GP system, and the general populace's acceptance of medical authority. We also explore the implications of these changes for the euthanasia regime and whether it is likely to become more conservative or more liberal in direction, including even, perhaps, a change in the legal status of euthanasia.

FROM CONSENSUS POLITICS TO POPULISM OR POLARIZATION?

From 1918 to 1994, the Dutch were governed by a coalition of one or more Christian Democratic political parties, and most of the time by either a Social Democratic party or a Liberal party. During that time, the Netherlands had center-left coalitions (Christian Democrats plus Social Democrats) or center-right coalitions (Christian Democrats plus Liberals). For those citizens who were interested in changing the law on moral issues (such as abortion, euthanasia, equality between men and women etc.), this state of affairs was often disappointing. The Christian Democratic participation in each and every government was a clear impediment to "progress" – as the Social Democrats and Liberals of different persuasions were inclined to characterize the changes they desired.

The Social Democrats and the Liberals differed widely on socioeconomic issues, but with respect to moral questions they were expected to be able to come to an agreement fairly easily. After all, beginning in the 1970s, the Netherlands had become a highly secularized country, in which traditional, observant Christians (Protestants of different persuasions as well as [Roman] Catholics) had become a minority. Thus, a politically liberal regime with regard to moral issues was regarded as fitting and proper. However, Liberals and Social Democrats were never able to let their potential agreement on ethical issues prevail over their diverging socioeconomic convictions. They always preferred a like-minded Christian Democratic coalition partner on socioeconomic issues. For this reason, a "purple coalition" (of the red Social Democrats and the blue Liberals) was expected to remain merely a dream of the political leaders, member-activists, and voters of D66, a smaller party with strong liberal preferences on moral issues.

In 1994, however, D66 got a chance to realize its dream. The 1994 parliamentary elections had led to a stalemate. There was neither majority support for a coalition of center and right nor a feasible majority for a center-left coalition. Thus, the larger parties would have to cooperate with D66, which had won quite a number of seats. D66 made it clear that they were only willing to talk about their dream: a purple coalition of Liberals, Social Democrats, and, obviously, D66. Four months after the 1994 election, the so-called Purple Government was a fact; it would survive the next elections in 1998 and last until 2001.[a]

During its first years (1994–1998), the purple coalition was extremely popular, but its popularity faded the longer it was in office. The Social Democrats

[a] Factual information about Dutch coalitions at http://www.parlement.com.

signed a coalition agreement dominated by a significantly new perspective on state regulation of the public and private sector, calling for public services to be privatized and market incentives to be introduced into government. Social Democratic Prime Minister Wim Kok announced that his party would have to lose its "ideological feathers" and embrace modern times.[11]

The Liberal Party, traditionally known as tough on crime and more recently as tough on immigrants, was led by Vice Prime Minister Hans Dijkstal, who was generally considered to be soft on both these issues. The purple coalition thus led to substantial convergence between the two traditional opponents in Dutch politics. Political scientists drew attention to the effect that this convergence might have on the electorate in the long run. In effect, the purple coalition put an end to Dutch citizens' traditional expectations that elections would allow for a choice between center right and center left (even if politics meant that their preferred party would always have to give up some of its political preferences). Putting an end to this choice, political scientists pointed out, would make the country susceptible to populism.[12,13,14] If people cannot choose between competing political elites because they have good reason to think that these are all alike, they may decide to vote for someone who challenges the political elite as such and who presents him- or herself as the representative of a totally different *kind* of politics (nonpolitics).

Such was the situation when Pim Fortuyn, a columnist of a widely read weekly, decided to take part in the 2002 parliamentary elections. His platform was a mix of issues that had been neglected during the purple years: He took a tough stance on crime, he promised to be extremely tough on immigrants, and he had no sympathy for the privatization of public services, although he found the Dutch welfare state far too generous in many respects. Fortuyn was highly ideological, though he could hardly be praised for ideological consistency. His "ideology" was quite personal, in some respects idiosyncratic, but not, therefore, unpopular; on the contrary.[b] Opinion polls predicted a very successful election result.

On May 6, 2002, Fortuyn was murdered by an animal rights activist. His list of candidates participated, in Fortuyn's name, in the general election of May 15 and managed to win 26 (of 150) seats in Parliament. But the Pim Fortuyn parliamentary group was soon torn apart. They could not decide who should lead them; they seemed to disagree on many issues, both procedural as well as

[b] Pim Fortuyn, from a lower-middle-class Roman Catholic family, had studied sociology in Groningen, where he was appointed assistant professor when he was a Marxist. Later in life he had, in vain, applied for a leading position in the Christian Democratic Party. Openly homosexual, he perhaps would have fitted better within the Social Democratic Party, but although his career – as a consultant and interim manager – had been fostered by people prominent in that party, he would delight in pestering the Social Democrats in particular – which fitted well with the traditional position of the weekly *Elsevier* (a right-wing nonreligious periodical), for which he worked as a columnist.

substantive; there was a clash of personalities. None of them had any parliamentary experience, which turned out to be a major handicap when the party was asked to participate in the new coalition (Christian Democrats, the Liberal Party [SJY], and the Pim Fortuyn Party). Their May 2002 electoral result would never be equaled again, and the Pim Fortuyn Party formally ended its existence in 2007. In 2003, a traditional center-right cabinet took office, and in 2006, a center-left coalition succeeded it, suggesting that the normal routine in Dutch politics had been restored. However, Dutch politics did not really get back to business as usual.

The populist threat presented by the Pim Fortuyn Party was overtaken, first by the former immigration minister, Rita Verdonk, and then by Geert Wilders, a dissenting member of Parliament who left the Liberal Party in 2004 to start his own Partij voor de Vrijheid (Party for Freedom). This new populist party won 9 seats in Parliament in 2006 and 24 in 2010. The present coalition is a center-right minority Cabinet supported in Parliament by the Party for Freedom.

Compared to members of previous Parliaments, members at present feel much more insecure than their predecessors. When asked what they would do in case differences of opinion come to the fore between themselves and their voters, a high percentage of parliamentarians have indicated that they would follow their voters, rather than their own preferences. Before the Fortuyn upheaval, this percentage was much lower.[15]

The events of September 11, 2001, followed by the rise of populism, contributed to politicians' feeling of insecurity with respect to the Muslim minority in the Netherlands. There are about 850,000 Muslims in the Netherlands at present, out of a total population of 16 million.

The religion of Islam was imported into the Netherlands in the 1960s and 1970s by Turkish and Moroccan "guest workers," and subsequently by the spouses and family members who joined them. A large percentage of the first generation of Turkish and Moroccan immigrants speaks Dutch only poorly. This lack of fluency often persists in later generations. Many of the original immigrants' descendants prefer to marry in their parents' (or grandparents') native country and bring their spouses – few of whom have any Dutch and many of whom are not literate in their own language – to the Netherlands. The result is that their children do not learn Dutch at home, which creates difficulties when they enter the Dutch educational system.[16]

Many of these families live in highly segregated neighborhoods where they associate infrequently with native Dutch-speaking people; for many ethnic minority children, their teacher will be the first Dutch-speaking person they meet on a regular basis, and they do not meet a teacher until they are four years old. School segregation is prevalent in the Netherlands, and immigrant children often spend their school years in classrooms dominated by other non-native speakers who are not fluent in Dutch, potentially leaving them at a permanent disadvantage with respect to the language. This may be one reason that ethnic minority citizens are more often unemployed than other members of Dutch society, and partly why minority children drop out of school more often than other students or become juvenile delinquents at a higher rate (a problem especially among Moroccan youth).

Other factors also play a role in politicians' insecurity, including the highly divergent views of the immigrant Muslim and Dutch-majority communities on moral issues, such as homosexuality and the status of women.[c] So does criticism by activist former Muslims – for example, Ayaan Hirsi Ali, who now resides in the United States – that (immigrant) Muslim children are being raised to be anti-Western and anti-Dutch. Anxiety only increased after the November 2004 murder of writer, master provocateur, and movie director Theo van Gogh by a Muslim fundamentalist. Van Gogh had made a short film based on a scenario by Hirsi Ali about the subjection of Muslim women.

Dutch politicians are permanently insecure about the right policy toward the country's Muslim citizens. Will kindness and understanding help minority citizens come to feel welcome and "at home" in their new country? Or is such a policy a misguided relic of the 1970s? Is it acceptable to be kind out of fear of terrorist attacks or riots like the ones that took place in the Parisian suburbs? (In October 2005 two North African juvenile delinquents were electrocuted when they tried to hide from the French police in an electricity plant. Thereupon riots broke out in the Parisian *banlieus*. Cars were set on fire and police officers were molested. French President Nicolas Sarkozy announced that he would clear the streets from scum). Or is it cowardice, which will only breed more resentment and contempt among the Muslim minority? Choosing a complicated compromise in the old Dutch way may lead to fierce criticism from the populist Party for Freedom.

What effect might this social and political turmoil have on the current euthanasia regime? Will the euthanasia regime become more conservative or more liberal in response to the Muslim minority or the uncertain Dutch policy toward that minority? To us, this does not seem likely. To be sure, the Muslim community is much more conservative on many morally charged issues than is the secular Dutch majority[17,d] and might be expected to support (political) action geared toward changing the Dutch "moral regime" and law. But

[c] More orthodox groups, especially among the (native) Christian population, are averse to the public manifestation and public recognition of homosexuality, too. Their aversion to homosexuality and homosexuals is a political issue as well, in that it has an effect, among other things, on hiring policies (orthodox Christians often do not want to hire employees with a homosexual lifestyle). But they do not vilify homosexuals in the public sphere, they do not shout abuse at them, and they do not behave violently toward homosexuals. And although the attribution of sex-specific roles to men and women by these orthodox Christian groups may lead others to denigrate their position as discriminatory toward women, their young males treat their own and other women with respect in the public sphere.

[d] Research among young people in Rotterdam has shown that Moroccan and Turkish youngsters are much more conservative with regard to abortion and euthanasia than native Dutch people. Among native Dutch respondents, about 75% thought that people should be able to get an abortion or euthanasia if they wanted to. Among Turkish youngsters, about one in three shared this opinion, among Moroccans less than one in five. The poll was taken in 1999. The results were published in 17. Phalet, van Lotringen, and Lotringen 2000.

euthanasia does not seem a viable starting point for promoting broad change in a conservative direction for either aspiring Muslim politicians (of whom there are now many at various levels of government) or for majority politicians who want to meet them halfway. A strategy with more promise would include efforts to seek special accommodation of Muslim religious beliefs in health-care institutions – perhaps, for example, *halal* hospitals that respect dietary rules, prohibit care by members of the opposite sex, and are also "euthanasia free." While such action wouldn't be popular among the Dutch majority, there is precedent in the country's tradition of consensus democracy[18] or, alternatively, in contemporary calls for "patient-centered" and "demand-oriented" health care.

It is imaginable too, however, that if the issue of euthanasia were to be taken up as a vehicle for changing the moral, and legal, climate of the Netherlands, the majority of secular Dutch might feel compelled to make a point of the native majority's positive, liberal, progressive stance toward euthanasia and strive for an even more liberal regime. But we do not think this is is a promising result either. There is a profound public debate going on about Dutch identity, provoked by the very question of what "we" should make immigrants and their descendents understand about the country in which they live. We make a point of enlightening immigrants about what are supposedly Dutch *traditions*:[19,20] male and female equality; tolerance toward homosexuals (albeit not a very ancient tradition); tolerance of recreational drugs, free euthanasia, and mercy killing by physicians. It does not make sense to argue that immigrants should embrace these traditions, or at least respect them, when one is planning to change them soon.

Dutch (political) culture is presented to "recent arrivals" as if it is more (or less) fixed; it is simplified, standardized, perhaps even canonized. It is not presented as something in flux. Today's positions on moral topics, whether euthanasia, homosexuality, or the substantive (as opposed to merely juridical) equality of men and women, are taken to be and are presented to others as "essentials" of Dutch culture and hallmarks of "Dutchness."

In our view, then, although major changes have indeed taken place in the Dutch culture of consensus, no changes are to be expected in the practice or legal framework of euthanasia – not because this cultural aspect appears to be unimportant after all but because of the specifics, the politics of this breakup of the culture of consensus: There is no majority to be found, no coalition of forces foreseeable, strong enough to tilt the regime in either a more conservative or a more liberal direction. Equally important, this has occurred, perhaps not accidentally, when the Dutch identity itself has become a focus of discussion and debate in which the present regime of euthanasia is being made to serve almost as an icon of Dutch culture and society.[21]

We now turn to the second aspect of the Dutch euthanasia regime: the Dutch GPs. What – if any – have been the consequences of changes in the role of GPs and their relationship with patients?

FAMILY PRACTICE IN MODERN TIMES

The classical image of the Dutch GP dates from the 1960s and 1970s: the dedicated male professional who takes an interest in his patients as human beings rather than as mere patients, who discusses and addresses their problems and needs, even if their complaints are, at heart, nonmedical – (e.g., because what they actually need is a steady job, a loving wife, or some appreciation from their boss); who makes house calls in order to treat and observe his patients in their natural habitat; and who works around the clock because he wants to be available for his patients whenever they need him. This is – was – the GP's rather rosy image. An image, of course, is different from an actual fact, but many GPs at least tried to live up to this ideal.[e,22,23]

This "modern classical" GP has become an endangered species. In the 1970s and 1980s, the practice began to change, although the GP's (self-)image was changing gradually even before that. In her 2008 review of all issues of the GPs' scientific journal in the Netherlands to trace changes in their professional ethics, Jolanda Dwarswaard observed that the image of total dedication had suffered its first blows as early as 1960, when a GP wrote:

> The group practice system allows every doctor a free afternoon in which he can practice a personal hobby.

In 1963, another GP expressed his opinion that

> [the family physician] will be less and less prepared to sacrifice his family life to his practice. For him too, the psychological well-being of his family has become more important. Hence he will strive to organize his practice in such a way as to give family life its due. One expression of this is the growing desire to have a vacation.

Another GP confessed in 1968:

> We are not that happy anymore with the role of the counselor available at all hours, even though some patients still expect us to fulfill that role.

About house calls, the GP journal wrote as early as 1968:

> One should investigate whether we could not save an enormous amount of time by reducing the number of house calls. No doubt this will entail lesser service, but this is what we see happening in all sorts of service activities, because of their labor-intensive character. We cannot ignore these economic considerations with regard to health care.

Moreover (again in 1968):

> We feel that the number of house calls should be strongly reduced in order to get a nicer life with rational working hours.[24]

[e] On the classical GP during the fifties, see F. J. A. Huygen, *Family Medicine: The Medical History of Families* (reprinted version of a book originally published in 1978), typically dedicated to "the families I had the privilege to serve so long as their personal doctor and whom I came to love" (22. Huygen 2006).

During the seventies and eighties, house calls were in fact reduced. In that same period, so-called group practices were introduced in which three, four, or more GPs together started to take care of a common clientele.[f,25] The group practice has become ever more popular in recent times. In 1993, 52% of the general practitioners worked in a solo practice and 17% in a group practice. Ten years later, in 2003, 39% of family doctors operated solo and 29% in a group practice. Of all GPs who graduated in 2002, 45% started work in a group practice and only 20% in a solo practice. The remaining 36% of GPs went to work in a two-physician practice.[26]

Ever more medical students (more than half) are female, and women in the Netherlands usually work only part time. Female medical doctors are no exception to this rule. In November 2002, 64% of all GPs in training were women.[26] Female doctors have an even stronger preference for group practices than do their male colleagues. In these group practices, doctors share their patients, and patients have to share their (increasingly frequently female) doctor's attention with the doctor's spouse, children, and children's after-school program, such as soccer and scouting activities.

Obviously, there is no need to assume that female doctors are not up to the professional task or that they tend to lack professional skills. One can be very good at what one does only three days a week. However, the continuous care and the intimate knowledge of the patient as a person, which has underpinned the euthanasia regime in the Netherlands, may suffer as a result of group practices and the more frequent occurrence of part-time GPs.

It was the more enduring, intimate relationship between patient and family doctor – the doctor's willingness to provide help and care to his or her (dying) patient on what at life's (approaching) end might be an almost daily basis for weeks at a stretch – that gave the GP, as the personal doctor, a very good reason to be granted a say in the joint decision of possible mercy killing, of euthanasia. Less frequent and more intermittent contact between doctor and patient may come to undermine the acceptance of euthanasia, which in fact was only recently established.

To put it differently, could this development of "collective care" by a group of part-time GPs for a "panel" of patients change the actual practice of euthanasia? Is it perhaps already changing this practice? It is possible that physicians who do not know their patients as well as the family doctors "of old" did will be more hesitant to perform euthanasia. Frances Norwood and other researchers, such as Robert Pool, Bert Keizer and Anne-Mei The, remind us that a euthanasia request must be made repeatedly and in a specific manner before it is acted upon.[27,28,29,30] The doctor has to be convinced that euthanasia is what the patient really wants. If the patient does not get as many chances to convince a GP as before, or if the patient has to convince two or three part-time GPs,

[f] The first GP group practice was registered in 1969.

he or she may not succeed in making a request that is up to this standard. If this logic prevails, patients, who under previously established standards would have been aided by their (personal) physician to shorten the span of their last days, would now be trying in vain to get "their" physician's ear.

Alternatively, one might hypothesize the following consequence: Taking a terminally ill patient's claim to a medically aided "soft death" to be essentially the patient's right, part-time GPs might be less meticulous about the standards for request and more inclined to go along with their patient's wish to die, without the proper reticence and without taking adequate precautions. They might be (dutifully) inclined to alleviate the patient's suffering by mercy killing without properly knowing him or her, because they have not been in a position to truly understand what the patient really wishes.

We may – indeed, we must – theorize about the possible consequences of major changes in the general practice of medicine and how GPs actually work. But theorizing cannot replace research into the effects of these changes on the actual practice of euthanasia. What does the research show so far?

At this point, the evidence we have does not yet point in the direction of any of these potential changes. So far the research shows that when patients get seriously or terminally ill, individual GPs often return to a practice that more closely resembles the personal, intimate doctor–patient relationship of old.[31] GPs find the provision of care for terminally ill patients a very important, rewarding part of their job.[32] They want to make house calls to their dying patients, and they feel a responsibility to be available outside office hours for these patients (an opinion that is shared by patients).[33] Seventy-five percent of GPs make themselves personally available to terminally ill patients at all times.[34] So when the situation arises that the patient might be willing to express his or her wishes as to a medically aided death, the GP in this respect can and does function again as the family doctor.

Researchers also point out that this may not last, however. Thus, for example, Sander Borgsteede and others studied the ideas of patients and GPs about what counts as "good care" with regard to terminally ill patients. Four values were identified: 1) the GP's availability for house calls and after-hours care, 2) medical competence and cooperation with other professionals, 3) personal attention to the individual patient, and 4) continuity of care.[33] The researchers observe that these values will be challenged by the ever-growing percentage of part-time doctors and the fact that after-hours care is increasingly transferred to large GP collectives that may or may not be able to call the dying patient's own GP, depending on how effectively the after-hours service is set up to coordinate care.

To conclude, it is feasible that the changing GP practice system will prompt change in the euthanasia regime, either in a more strict direction, because part-time doctors who do not know their patients as well as traditional family doctors do not dare to end their patients' lives, or in a more "consumerist" direction whereby doctors would go along with their patients' requests without further ado. However, to date, researchers have not found any evidence of change in either direction. In the next section we continue to explore the move toward consumerism because this tendency is fostered by government policy, as well as well as popular culture.

INCONSISTENT CIVICS

The third element of the social fabric underpinning the euthanasia regime in the Netherlands has been patients' willingness to submit to medical rationales for decision making and for doctors' authority. What has changed in this respect in the recent past and what might change in the years to come? For a better understanding of how attitudes toward doctors and the medical profession may have changed recently or are likely to in the future, we focus first on reforms in the formal, institutional set-up of health care, especially the financing of care.

In 2006, the government changed the health insurance system. Before 2006, the Dutch health-care system was extremely complicated. It consisted of three tiers. Long-term institutional care (in a psychiatric hospital, a geriatric ward, or an institute for the mentally disabled) was financed by means of a social insurance system, which covered the whole population. Less expensive home care for chronically ill, elderly, or handicapped patients also belonged to this first tier.

Acute care, including "ordinary" hospital care, visits to general practitioners, and midwives, as well as several other provisions broadly classified as curative, were financed differently for different segments of the population. In this second tier of the Dutch health-care system, roughly two-thirds of the population was legally obliged to pay income-dependent premiums into the state sickness fund. These patients never saw a medical bill because their sickness fund paid hospitals and other care providers directly. The remaining one-third of the population (the majority of whom were citizens with a high income) could choose a private health insurer.

There were some elements of solidarity built into this private insurance part of the second tier as well. Private insurers had to offer a so-called standard package to less healthy, higher-risk clients whom they might have preferred to refuse. Although these high-risk clients had to pay high premiums for the standard package, those premiums did not cover their health-care costs entirely. The healthier, privately insured clients had to pay a "solidarity bonus" on top of their premiums to make up for the losses that private insurers suffered as a result of being obliged to take in chronically ill or otherwise extremely expensive clients.

The third tier in Dutch health care was quite small and covered mostly elective medical services (such as cosmetic surgery) that people could do without or might choose to pay for out of pocket.

This health insurance system had always been considered a messy compromise that no political party really liked or considered its own. Most left-wing political parties would have liked to do away with the private insurance part of the system. They would have preferred a tax-funded national health insurance scheme for all citizens. On the other side of the political spectrum, the right wing never liked the income-dependent insurance premiums of the sickness fund(s). The Christian Democrats in the middle of the political spectrum sided with the Left on the issue of general health insurance but were much more concerned about cost containment and thus were favorably inclined to out-of-pocket payments, copayments, and other private ways to cofinance the general scheme. Thus, there was general discontent with the old system among politicians, some parties unhappy with the social components of the system and others objecting to the free market components. During the 1980s and 1990s and into the first years of the twenty-first century, Dutch politicians discussed the health-care system numerous times. Several minor changes were introduced, but for a long time, a real overhaul of the system seemed impossible – until 2006, that is, when a new system was finally introduced by the then-ruling center-right coalition.

Under the new regime, health-care insurance is offered by private insurers. However, insurers cannot offer whatever provision they want, to anyone who is willing to pay the premium. In the new system, they are compelled by law to offer the so-called standard health-care package (roughly comparable to the old sickness fund package) to their clientele and to charge the same price to everybody. Health insurers are not allowed to show preferences or attract younger, healthier clients by offering them cheap insurance. If they want to offer cheap insurance, they have to give it to old and young, sick and healthy alike. Insurers may try to achieve lower prices than their competitors by striking bargains with hospitals and other care providers. Clients are entitled to change insurers once a year, and so insurers have to compete for their favors constantly. Low-income clients get a tax rebate or tax bonus that enables them to pay for their health insurance premiums.

Although this present system mixes social insurance with a market orientation, it was introduced by a liberal minister in a center-right coalition government, who emphasized the importance of the elements of both regulated competition and market incentives in the new scheme. Patients were addressed as "consumers of care," who had to "shop around to find the best insurance package for themselves," "tailor made to their individual situation." Clients were invited not to restrict themselves to finding merely a good insurer; they were advised, almost admonished, to look for the very best hospital and the ultimate GP. A fancy government Web site (http://www.kiesbeter.nl) features patients shopping around in the health-care system. The Web site offers a short video about a recently widowed woman who did not take the trouble to look for a good GP; she just happened to pick one near her home from the yellow pages. The man turned out to be an inadequate doctor who did not diagnose her husband's skin cancer in time, and here she was now: a poor widow. Other patients are pictured as much more sensible. The video shows them interviewing one GP after another before finally choosing the one that fits their personal preferences. The government's rhetoric stresses individual choice and preferences and assertive consumer behavior, rather than the collective package, the tax refund, and the built-in elements of solidarity among individuals of all ages and health status.

This newly advocated consumerism sits uneasily with the traditional reticence toward ethically sensitive treatments. Remember: Dutch women could not get an epidural on request, nor could Dutch citizens simply ask for a genetic test or an MRI scan without medical approval. A similar regime held and still holds for euthanasia: Patients cannot obtain euthanasia unless their doctor and an independent colleague classify their suffering as unbearable. In practice, this means that many patients will not receive a euthanasia death if their suffering is mostly psychological or psychiatric or if they are tired of life because they have grown too old and lonely, because doctors do not classify these conditions as medical conditions or as unbearable.

One can see a potential tension here. If citizens are explicitly encouraged to be assertive consumers in health care, they may no longer be willing to practice restraint and accept the boundaries drawn by medical professionals. If in the future the patient as client is paramount, one can indeed imagine that patients will be inclined to behave less deferentially toward medical professionals. Is such a change of attitude, and a concomitant change in patients' behavior, likely to occur?

Successive governments have shown an ambivalent attitude toward (the importance and desirability of) individual choice in the health-care system. This ambivalence dates from even before 1987, when the government-commissioned Dekker Report laid out the contours of a new health-care system, a system that was basically very much like the one actually introduced in 2006. The Dekker Report introduced the concept of the health-care consumer who would bid on the market for health and happiness.[35] In 1991, however, another government-sponsored report advocated a "community-oriented" vision of health care, inspired by the works of the American communitarian philosopher Daniel Callahan. In the Dunning Report, people's health-care needs were to be determined by asking whether their illnesses prevented them from participating in the community, and if so, what treatment or provision would help restore their capacity to participate. Those treatments or provisions should then be financed collectively. Needs that did not undermine one's capacity to participate were classified as less important, as were treatments or provisions that would not restore one's capacities to participate in society. The Dunning committee recommended a government education program to teach citizens that they must not behave like spoiled consumers trying to get everything they want in the health-care mall. Citizens would have to be taught that "trees do not grow into heaven," as the Dutch saying goes – that is, that all good things (must) come to an end. They would have to learn to be frugal with health care.

Ever since the beginning of the 1990s, these two streams of government education have existed alongside each other, without much challenge and even without causing much wonder. On the one hand, the market rhetoric emphasizes individual choice and tailor-made care, and stresses the benefits of a demand-driven health-care system and consumer sovereignty. On the other hand, the community rhetoric stresses budget restraints, solidarity, equality before the doctor, equal treatment, and boundaries. "You can't always get what you want" indeed captures the essence of the community rhetoric. The acceptance of medical authority and the honoring of medical indications as limits to care clearly belong to the community rhetoric.[36]

Public opinion polls have consistently shown strong popular support for the community approach.[g,37] The Dutch have found it very desirable that doctors treat people according to medical need and not according to income or social class. They did not like the system of copayment. They did not favor the idea of changing the system in order to allow individuals to buy preferential treatment. They did not favor the liberalization and "marketization" of the public sector.[h,38] Whereas the community approach echoed shared understandings that exist in the Netherlands, the market rhetoric actually has been a form of government education, even of government propaganda, foisted on an unwilling populace.

At long last, however, the market propaganda (or "civic education," depending on one's political preferences) seems to be having an effect. Half of the respondents in a large-scale poll in 2007 indicated that they would find it acceptable if people could buy more luxurious forms of care in hospitals.[i] Almost half of the male respondents found it acceptable for people to be able to buy higher-quality care, a marked increase in percentage from a few years earlier; in female respondents no change was reported.[39] Another survey indicated that 50% of respondents agree with the idea that people should be allowed to buy extra care, for example, in order to get private facilities rather than a bed in a hospital ward. Yet the same recent poll still shows continuing support for the community value system: 92% of respondents find it unacceptable to allow people to buy a higher place on a waiting list, and 85% of all respondents agreed that social solidarity is "important" or "very important."[j]

[g] The opinion poll figures can be found at http://www.scp.nl.

[h] This goes for citizens in other Western countries as well. C. Pollitt and G. Bouckaert studied New Public Management measures in several European countries, Australia, and New Zealand. They concluded: "Certainly, there is no firm ground for the assertion that the public would like the welfare state to be 'rolled back' and replaced by private modes of provision" (see 38. Pollitt and Bouckaert 2004).

[i] The results of the poll were published in *NRC Handelsblad*, October 5, 2007, http://www.21minuten.nl.

[j] The results of the poll were published in *NRC Handelsblad*, October 5, 2007, http://www.21minuten.nl.

Perhaps the actual introduction of a new system (rather than endless debates about it, as in the 1990s) has changed people's attitudes after all. Citizens have constantly been addressed as *consumers* in health care by government education/government propaganda, and they are now actually being treated as consumers of health care in the "marketized" system. The growing emphasis in government policy on consumer sovereignty, individual choice, and tailor-made care could affect the traditional willingness to submit to medical authority. The Dutch association for midwives and gynecologists is currently considering a new guideline that would allow women to indicate their preference for an epidural without a clear medical indication. Hospitals in the Netherlands now give young, single, and/or career-oriented women the opportunity to freeze their eggs for later fertilization, a procedure that was riddled with ethical objections just a few years ago. In tune with the general development toward consumerism, the Dutch Association for Voluntary Euthanasia (NVVE) produced a new strategic statement in 2008, in which it is argued that patients should have a menu of choices regarding their death.[40] According to the NVVE, it should be possible to ask for physician-administered euthanasia as one option. One should also be able to choose palliative sedation, assisted suicide, or a do-it-yourself death by starvation, with a little help and information from your doctor.

In February 2010, a group of prominent citizens (former politicians, media personalities, and retired professors, among others) started a so-called citizens' initiative. They found that elderly people who are tired of life (though not terminally ill) should be able to end their lives without having to resort to gruesome means like hanging or jumping in front of a train. Their petition to Parliament was supported by more than 100,000 people. Parliament has to take a citizen's initiative into consideration although it is not obliged to go along with it.[41] In August 2010, the NVVE announced that it would like to investigate the feasibility of an end-of-life clinic, for people who are not eligible for physician-assisted euthanasia or suicide.[42]

CONCLUSION

We set out to study recent changes pertaining to three strands in the fabric of Dutch (political) culture that have (had) direct relevance for explaining how the legal framework and actual practice of euthanasia came about and have been maintained. To reiterate, these strands are the culture of consensus, the close relationship of Dutch GPs with their patients, and most people's willing submission to the medical elite. How much has changed in the social fabric, and what are the actual or likely effects of change on the euthanasia regime in the Netherlands? Let us try to summarize the competing pressures with which this regime is being confronted.

The corporatist, pragmatic, consensual political culture has changed to a considerable extent, mainly due to the settlement of a Muslim minority in the

Netherlands and the wave of populist politics in reaction to it. However, we have concluded that it is unlikely that these changes will lead to a change in the euthanasia regime. Although the legal framework of euthanasia evolved in a specific party-political setting, we have argued that law and actual practice nevertheless can be expected to endure in even quite different circumstances.

The emerging system of group practice and part-time GPs is gradually changing the doctor–patient relationship. It is plausible for one to think that part-time GPs have less contact with their patients and are more reluctant to grant their wishes with respect to euthanasia. Research indicates that, so far, this has not been the case.

Lastly, we pointed out that the change in the health insurance system toward a more market-oriented system may diminish people's willingness to submit to medical authority and professional decision making. If the government rhetoric continues to emphasize the importance of individual choice, demand-driven and tailor-made care, and consumer sovereignty while neglecting the competing discourse of solidarity, community, and frugality, citizens may decide to take up the consumer role laid out for them and demand tailor-made, end-of-life care according to their own preferences and principles. This could provoke a change of the current regime in a more liberal direction.

References

1. Cohen-Almagor, Raphael. 2001. Culture of death in the Netherlands: Dutch perspectives. *Issues in Law & Medicine* 17: 167.
2. Norwood, Frances. 2006. A hero and a criminal: Dutch huisartsen and the making of good death through euthanasia talk in the Netherlands. *Medische Antropologie* 18: 329–346.
3. Hendin, Herbert. 2002. The Dutch Experience. *Issues in Law & Medicine* 17: 3.
4. Andeweg, Rudy B., and Galen A. Irwin. 1993. *Dutch Government and Politics*. Houndmills: Macmillan.
5. Andeweg, Rudy B. 2000. From Dutch disease to Dutch model? Consensus government in practice. *Parliamentary Affairs* 53: 697–709.
6. Weyers, Heleen. 2004. *Euthanasie. Het proces van rechtsverandering*. Amsterdam: Amsterdam University Press.
7. Onwuteaka-Philipsen, Bregje D., Agnes van der Heide, Dirk Koper, Ingeborg Keij-Deerenberg, Judith A.C. Rietjens, Mette Rurup, Astrid M. Vrakking, Jean Jacques Georges, Martien T. Muller, Gerrit van der Wal, and Paul van der Maas. 2003. Euthanasia and other end-of-life decisions in the Netherlands in 1990, 1995 and 2001. *The Lancet* 362: 396–399.
8. Borgsteede, Sander D., Luc Deliens, Corrie Graafland-Riedstra, Anneke L. Francke, Gerrit van der Wal, and Dick L. Willems. 2007. Communication about euthanasia in general practice: Opinions and experiences of patients and their general practitioners. *Patient Education and Counseling* 66: 156–161.
9. Heide, Agnes van der, Bregje D. Onwuteaka-Philipsen, Mette Rurup, Hilde M. Buiting, Johannes J. M. van Delden, Johanna E. Hanssen-de Wolf, Anke G. J. M. Janssen, J. Roeline W. Pasman, Judith A. C. Rietjens, Cornelis J. M. Prins, Ingeborg

M. Deerenborg, Joseph K. M. Gevers, Paul J. van der Maas, and Gerrit van der Wal. 2007. End-of-life practices in the Netherlands under the Euthanasia Act. *New England Journal of Medicine* 356: 1957–1965.

10. Trappenburg, Margo. 2001. Paarse ethiek, In *Zeven jaar paars*, ed. F. Becker et al., 53–74. Amsterdam: De Arbeiderspers.
11. Oversloot, Hans. 2002. Van politiek naar economie, van staat naar markt en management. In *Democratie in verval?* ed. J. van Holsteyn and C.Mudde, 123–137. Amsterdam: Boom.
12. Andeweg, Rudy. 2001. Lijphart versus Lijphart: The cons of consensus democracy in homogeneous societies. *Acta Politica* 36: 117–128.
13. Katz, Richard, and Peter Mair. 1995. Changing models of party organization and party democracy: The emergence of the kartel party. *Party Politics* 1: 5–28.
14. Hakhverdian, Armen, and Christel Koop. 2007. Consensus democracy and support for populist parties in Western Europe. *Acta Politica* 42: 401–420.
15. Andeweg, Rudy, and Jacques Thomassen. 2007. *Binnenhof van binnenuit. Tweede Kamerleden over het functioneren van de Nederlandse democratie*, p. 16. http://www.rob.rfv.nl.
16. Dagevos, Jaco, and Merove Gijsberts. 2007. *Jaarrapport integratie 2007*. Den Haag: SCP. http://www.scp.nl.
17. Phalet, K., C. van Lotringen, and H. Entzinger. 2000. *Islam in de multiculturele samenleving. Opvattingen van jongeren in Rotterdam.* http://www.manavzw.be/_files/Islam%20in%20de%20multiculturele%20samenleving_%20Opvattingen%20van%20jongeren%20-%202000.pdf (accessed October 30, 2011).
18. Lijphart, Arend. 1968. *The Politics of Accommodation: Pluralism and Democracy in the Netherlands.* Berkeley: University of California Press.
19. Scheffer, Paul. 2000. Het multiculturele drama. *NRC Handelsblad*, January 29.
20. Scheffer, Paul. 2007. *Het land van aankomst.* Amsterdam: De Bezige Bij.
21. Mak, Geert. 2004. *In Europa: Reizen door de Twintigste Eeuw* Amsterdam: Atlas.
22. Huygen, F. J. A. 2006. *Family Medicine: The Medical History of Families*. Assen: Royal Van Gorcum.
23. Mol, A., and P. van Lieshout. 1989. *Ziek is het woord niet. Medicalisering, normalisering en de veranderende taal van huisartsgeneeskunde en geestelijke gezondheidszorg 1945–1985*. Nijmegen: Sun.
24. Dwarswaard, J. 2011. *De dokter en de tijdgeest. Een halve eeuw veranderingen in de beroepsethiek van huisartsen en chirurgen.* Amsterdam: Boom/Lemma.
25. Ree, J. W. van. 2005. *Eenmaal huisarts*. Farewell lecture, Maastricht University. http://www.google.nl/search?hl=en&source=hp&q=van+ree+eenmaal+huisarts&aq=f&aqi=&aql=&oq=&gs_rfai= (accessed August 23, 2010).
26. Kenens, R. J., and L. Hingstman. 2003. *Cijfers uit de registratie van huisartsen, Peiling*. Utrecht: NIVEL.
27. Pool, Robert. 1996. *Vragen om te sterven. Euthanasie in een Nederlands ziekenhuis*. Rotterdam: WYT.
28. Keizer, Bert. 1995. *Het refrein is Hein: dagen uit een verpleeghuis*. Nijmegen: Sun.
29. The, Anne-Mei. 1997. *Vanavond om 8 uur ... Verpleegkundige dilemma's bij euthanasie en andere beslissingen rond het levenseinde*. Houten: Bohn Stafleu Van Loghum.

30. Tol, D. G. van, S. van de Vathorst, and Bert Keizer. 2008. Euthanasie voor beginners. *Medisch Contact* 4, January 25.
31. Schers, Henk, Hans Bor, Wil van den Bosch, and Richard Gol. 2006. GPs' attitudes to personal continuity: Findings from everyday practice differ from postal surveys. *British Journal for General Practice* 156: 536–538.
32. Groot, Marieke, Myrra Vernooij-Dassen, Ben J. P. Crul, and Richard Grol. 2005. General practitioners (GPs) and palliative care: Perceived tasks and barriers in daily practice. *Palliative Medicine* 19: 111–118.
33. Borgsteede, Sander, et al. 2008. Goede zorg in de laatste levensfase volgens patiënten en hun huisarts. *Huisarts en Wetenschap* 51: 120–124.
34. Giesen, P. H. J, E. Terpstra, and B. P. M. Schweitzer. 2008. Terminale zorg buiten kantoortijd. *Medisch Contact* 63, 6: 240–243.
35. Achterhuis, Hans. [1979] 1983. *De markt van welzijn en geluk: een kritiek van de andragogie*. Ambo: Baarn.
36. Trappenburg, Margo. 2008. *Genoeg is genoeg. Over gezondheidszorg en democratie*. Amsterdam: Amsterdam University Press.
37. Trappenburg, Margo. 2005. *Gezondheidszorg en democratie*, rede EUR. Inaugural lecture, Erasmus Medical Center, Rotterdam.
38. Pollitt, C., and G. Bouckaert. 2004. *Public Management Reform: A Comparative Analysis*. Oxford: Oxford University Press.
39. SCP/Netherlands Institute for Social Research. 2007. *De sociale staat van Nederland 2007*, p. 179. http://www.scp.nl/dsresource?objectid=19574&type=org (accessed August 23, 2010).
40. NVVE (Nederlandse Vereniging voor Vrijwillige Euthanasie). 2008. *Perspectieven op waardig sterven*. http://www.nvve.nl/assets/nvve/nieuws/Perspectievennota.pdf (accessed August 23, 2010).
41. Uit vrije wil, burgerinitiatief Voltooid leven. 2010. http://www.uitvrijewil.nu/index.php?id=10 (accessed August 23 and 27, 2010).
42. NVVE (Nederlandse Vereniging voor Vrijwillige Euthanasie). 2010. NVVE onderzoekt mogelijkheid levenseinde kliniek. http://www.nvve.nl/nvve2/pagina.asp?pagkey=143915&metkey=375 (accessed August 23, 2010).

PART II

REGULATION AND PRACTICE DEFICIENCIES

7

The Unreported Cases

Bregje D. Onwuteaka-Philipsen

Effective regulation of euthanasia and physician-assisted suicide[a] in the Netherlands depends heavily on physicians, who are supposed to report all cases to the proper authorities. These practices have been subject to public oversight since 1991, with changes in review procedures over time as public debate and law evolved (summarized in Box 7.1).

Box 7.1. Evolution of Reporting Procedures 1991–2008

1991–1998

Beginning in 1991, physicians were required to report cases of euthanasia or physician-assisted suicide to the public prosecutor (through the medical examiner). Cases were reviewed first by the public prosecutor and then by the Committee of Prosecutors General and the minister of justice, which had final authority to decide whether to prosecute. Although euthanasia and physician-assisted suicide were punishable, physicians could expect not to be prosecuted if they met criteria of due care. This procedure was enacted into law in 1994 and evaluated in 1996 in a study of the notification rate, compliance with the criteria of due care, and characteristics of review by the public prosecution.[1]

(*continued*)

[a] Under Dutch law, the medical practice *euthanasia* is defined as a physician's purposefully ending a patient's life at that individual's explicit request. *Physician-assisted suicide* is defined as prescribing or supplying drugs with the explicit intention of enabling the patient to end his or her own life.

1998–April 2002

In 1998, a new procedure went into effect. Physicians were required to report to one of five Regional Review Committees for Euthanasia and Physician-Assisted Suicide (RRCs) (again through the medical examiner). These committees, consisting of a lawyer, an ethicist, and a physician, reviewed reported cases and advised the Committee of Prosecutors General. The latter still made the ultimate decision on whether or not to prosecute, and the legal status of euthanasia and physician-assisted suicide was similar to the previous procedure. This revised procedure was evaluated in 2001 in a study similar to the one in 1996.[2,3]

April 2002–Present

On April 1, 2002, a new law on euthanasia was enacted and the reporting and review procedure was changed again. All cases are still reviewed by the Regional Review Committees, but only those cases in which a committee concludes that criteria of due care were not met are subsequently reviewed by the Committee of Prosecutors General. Under the new law, euthanasia and physician-assisted suicide are allowed provided that the criteria of due care are met. This procedure was evaluated in 2005.[4,5]

Despite the changes since 1991, the central question for review under all procedures has always been whether established criteria of due care have been met. These requirements have remained unaltered: a voluntary and well-considered request of the patient, unbearable and hopeless suffering, no acceptable alternatives for treatment, a medico-technical appropriate performance (substantive requirements), consultation of another physician, and reporting the case as an unnatural death (procedural requirements).[6]

To ensure the quality of the practice of euthanasia and physician-assisted suicide, it is important that cases that are not reported not differ materially from the majority of cases, which are reported.

This chapter focuses on the empirical evidence available from research carried out in 1990, 1995, 2001, and 2005, which sought to determine the number of cases reported, the reporting rate, the reasons physicians do or do not report cases, and possible differences between reported and unreported cases. Box 7.2 shows the characteristics of the empirical studies. I conclude by discussing the implications of these data for the often-mentioned possibility that there may be a slippery slope in Dutch practices with respect to euthanasia and physician-assisted suicide.

Box 7.2. Characteristics of Empirical Studies

Around 1990, 1995, 2001, and 2005, nationwide studies on end-of-life practices took place; after 1995 they included evaluation of the euthanasia review procedure. The following substudies can be distinguished for all or some of the study years:[1,2,3,4,5,7,8]

Death Certificate Studies in 1990, 1995, 2001 and 2005

These studies were based on a stratified random sample of about 6,000 death certificates. The attending physicians of the deceased people were asked to fill in a four-page written questionnaire with predominantly prestructured questions (response between 74% and 78%). These studies were used to estimate the total number of cases of euthanasia and physician-assisted suicide in those years.

Interview Studies in 1990, 1995 and 2001

These studies, in which a stratified random sample of about 400 Dutch physicians was interviewed, were used to assess the opinions of Dutch physicians (response between 85% and 91%). The interviews were performed by trained physicians and consisted of predominantly prestructured questions. In 2005, a physician survey (stratified random sample of 2,100 Dutch physicians; response: 56%) took the place of the interview studies. The written questionnaire consisted of predominantly prestructured questions and was based on the earlier interview studies.

Reported Cases Study in 1995 and 2001

We interviewed approximately 200 physicians who had reported a case of euthanasia or physician-assisted suicide. This random sample of reported cases, stratified according to region and type of practice (general practice, hospital practice, nursing home practice), was taken from all reported cases in 1995 and 2001 (response 90% and 92%). In the structured interviews, which were conducted by trained and experienced physicians, questions were asked about the reported case and about the physician's opinions.

RRC and Public Prosecution Study

The per-year numbers of reported cases of euthanasia and physician-assisted suicide were derived from the *files* of the Public

(*continued*)

Prosecution (1990–1998) and the *annual reports* of the RRCs (1998–2001). Permission was granted to disclose the *minutes* of the Committee of the Prosecutors General (1995, 2001, 2005) in order to study the reasons for discussion of reported cases in the committee. The files of cases reported to the RRCs were used in order to obtain reasons for discussing cases.

REPORTED AND UNREPORTED CASES

Since 1990, it has been possible to derive the number of reported cases from records of the public prosecutor (until 1998) or the Regional Review Committees for Euthanasia and Physician-Assisted Suicide (since 1998), respectively. Estimating the total number of cases of euthanasia and assisted suicide (EAS), and thus the number of unreported cases and the reporting rate, is more complex. It requires large-scale, nationwide empirical studies. Such studies were carried out in 1990, 1995, 2001, and 2005 through a review of large stratified samples of death certificates representative of all deaths in each year studied.[1,2,4,7,8] (Box 7.2) Figure 7.1 shows the number of reported cases per year between 1990 and 2005 and, for the four years studied, the estimated total number of cases of euthanasia and physician-assisted suicide.

Data indicate that the number of reported cases increased from 480 in 1990 to 1,460 in 1995 and 2,216 in 1999. After that, the numbers decreased somewhat, to 1,815 in 2003, but rose again to 1,933 in 2005. The estimated total number of cases of euthanasia and assisted suicide was about 2,700 in 1990 and increased to about 3,600 in 1995 and about 3,800 in 2001. In 2005, the total number of cases decreased substantially, to about 2,400 cases. For the reporting rate, this meant an increase through the years from 18% in 1990 to 80% in 2005, as shown in Figure 7.2.

PHYSICIANS' RATIONALE FOR REPORTING OR NOT REPORTING

It's also important to understand *why* physicians do or do not report cases of euthanasia or assisted suicide. The interview studies, physician survey, and reported cases studies (Box 7.2) were carried out so that the reasons cited by physicians for reporting or not reporting could be understood.

What Reasons Do Physicians Give for Reporting Cases of Euthanasia and Assisted Suicide?

The data show that an increase in the reporting rate coincided with the evolution of review procedures for euthanasia and assisted suicide, with a sharp rise from 18% to 41% after the enactment of the first procedure, when it was made

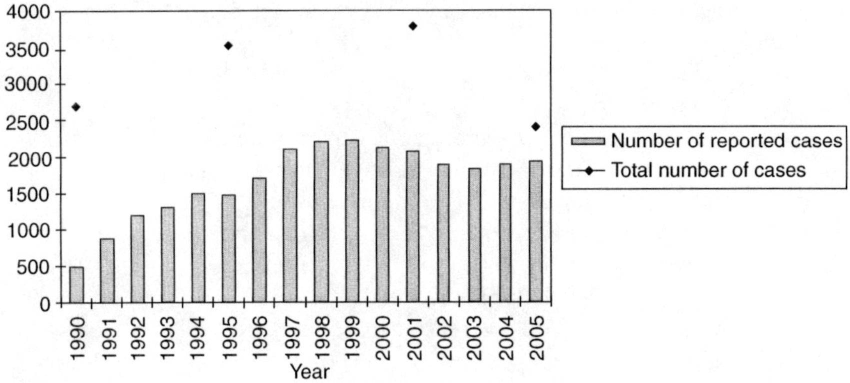

FIGURE 7.1. Numbers of reported cases of EAS and total number of cases of EAS.
Source: 5. Onwuteaka-Philipsen, et al., 2007.

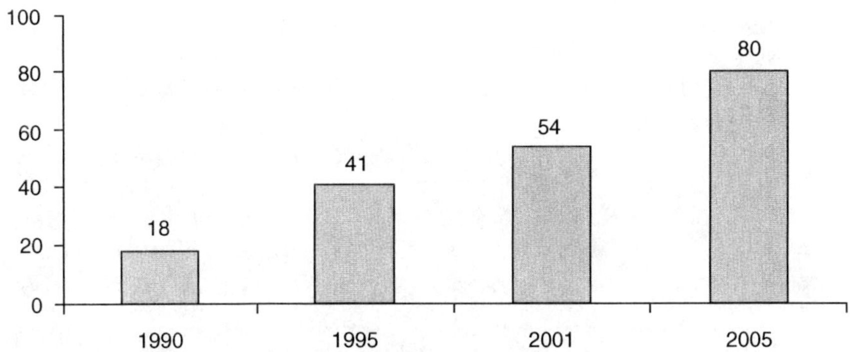

FIGURE 7.2. Reporting rate in 1990, 1995, 2001, and 2005.
Source: 5. Onwuteaka-Philipsen, et al., 2007.

clear that these practices should be reported. Subsequently, there was a modest rise after the start of the Regional Review Committees, and another, larger, rise again after the enactment of the euthanasia law.

The idea behind the changes in reporting procedures was to put the public prosecution at a greater distance, which may have encouraged physicians to report more frequently.

In 2001, the interview study (Box 7.2) was carried out among a representative sample of Dutch physicians to explore this question. The majority of respondents considered reporting through the Regional Review Committees to be an improvement over the original procedure. When asked whether reporting through the RRCs would help achieve the goals of reporting – that is, to promote disclosure, verifiability, and adherence to criteria of due care – the majority indicated that to various degrees they believed it would. When asked whether the new euthanasia law would further help in reaching the goals of the reporting procedure, most respondents, also to a greater or lesser extent, said that they thought the law would do so.[3]

Another, more direct, way of finding out why physicians report cases is to ask them what reasons they had to report a specific case. This was done in the interview studies carried out in 1995 and 2001 (Box 7.2). In 1995, "I always report" was mentioned most frequently (75% of respondents), followed at a distance by "reporting is obligatory" (17%), "accountability to society" (13%), and "it is the official policy of our institution" (13%).[3] (Percentages total more than 100% because more than one reason could be given.)

In 2001, all reasons were mentioned more often than in 1995. The most frequently mentioned reason for reporting a case of euthanasia or physician-assisted suicide was again "I always report" (91%). Compared to 1995, higher percentages of respondents also cited "accountability to society" (33%) and "it is the official policy of our institution" (11%) as reasons for reporting. More importantly, in 2001, significant numbers of respondents indicated additional reasons for reporting: "legal obligation" (64%), "moral obligation" (53%), "disclosure is important for achieving acceptance of the practice of euthanasia or physician-assisted suicide" (44%), and "contributing to the development of the review procedure" (22%).

In 2005, focus groups of physicians were used in order to get more insight into the practice of euthanasia.[5] They revealed several motivations for reporting. Thus, several physicians indicated that they report because not reporting really isn't an option. According to one, it is not possible to hide the fact that euthanasia was performed:

> I do not know how to perform euthanasia without reporting, since there is a whole team involved, including the nurses. I have no clue how I could avoid it (a medical specialist).

Another reason given for reporting is that doing so is a way of taking public responsibility:

> I like to report because it helps me in emotionally processing it, in a way by taking responsibility for it (a general practitioner).

A third reason physicians report is because the law requires them to do so:

> The rules are quite clear. In all institutions I worked in, the euthanasia guideline mentioned that reporting is necessary by law. I am actually very surprised that there are physicians who say, "We do not report" (a nursing home physician).

Finally, some physicians indicated that they didn't really have to think about it; it was simply clear that one should report:

> I just report. It is self-evident to report (a general practitioner).

What Reasons Do Physicians Give for Not Reporting Cases of EAS?

Looking at why physicians do report makes it clear that most physicians have positive opinions toward the euthanasia regulations, the extent to which the regulations would achieve their goals, and the influence they would have on physicians' willingness to report.

There is also a minority that is less positive, however. Here, the most direct way of understanding why some physicians do not is also to ask them what reasons they had for not reporting a specific case. In 1995, 27 respondents (out of 410) indicated that they had not reported one or more cases of euthanasia or assisted suicide. The reasons these physicians most frequently mentioned were practical ones: to avoid the fuss and bother that comes with judicial inquiry for themselves and their family (56%) or for the patients' relatives (30%), as well as relatives' wish to avoid a judicial inquiry (33%); physicians' doubt about having met all criteria for due care (30%); and fear of prosecution (11%). The more philosophical reason mentioned by three physicians (11%) was the belief that euthanasia is something between a physician and patient in which others should not be involved.

In the 2001 study, the number of physicians who described an unreported case was even lower. However, in this study, physicians who had reported a case (n = 158) were asked whether they would also have reported it if certain conditions had been different. Physicians most frequently stated that they would (probably) not report "if the chance of being prosecuted was greater" (25%), "if notification was via the Public Prosecution instead of the Regional Review Committee" (17%), "if no consultation had taken place" (14%), "if it would not have been possible to clarify the case to the Regional Review Committee if necessary" (13%), "if the patient's request had not been adequately documented" (10%), or "if there had not been a physician in the Regional Review Committee" (10%).

An important methodological change was made for the 2005 study. Instead of interviewing physicians about their reasons for not reporting, data were gathered from a review of death certificates, which require physicians to indicate whether death was the effect of the use (by patient or physician) of a drug that was prescribed, provided, or administered by a physician with the explicit intention of hastening the patient's life on the explicit request of the patient. In the 1995 and 2001 interview studies, physicians were asked to describe a case of euthanasia or assisted suicide that they had not reported. In the death certificate study, researchers classified a case as euthanasia or assisted suicide on the basis of the physician's answer to specific questions on the death certificate – that is, if the physician answered affirmatively that his or her action had played a role in the patient's death. This means that the terms *euthanasia* and *physician-assisted suicide* were not mentioned, making it possible that physicians themselves would not label their act as either practice. In interviews with the 30 physicians who had answered affirmatively on the death certificate but had not reported the death as euthanasia or assisted suicide, most (87%) indicated that they did not report because they thought it was not required in this case. Only two of the nonreporting physicians labeled their act as euthanasia and knew that they should have reported. In addition, two who labeled their act as "sedation" appeared to realize that it should have been reported but had not done so, one because the criteria for due care had not been met and the physician feared judicial consequences, and the other because the physician considered it a confidential matter between physician and patient.[9]

Finally, in the 2005 focus groups physicians revealed several motivations for not reporting,[5] including the fuss and bother that goes with reporting a case, negative experiences with reporting, lack of fulfillment of all criteria for due care, and ignorance of the requirement to report.

DIFFERENCES BETWEEN REPORTED AND UNREPORTED CASES

Another important concern for effective regulation of euthanasia and assisted suicide is whether cases that are not reported differ from those that are, and if so, in what ways they differ. As the aforementioned data indicate, one reason physicians give for not reporting is that they doubt whether all criteria for due care have been met. Another is that not all physicians understand which clinical practices fall within the category of euthanasia/assisted suicide.

Do Reported and Unreported Cases Differ in the Extent to Which the Criteria for Due Care Are Met?

Whether or not there actually were differences between reported and unreported cases in the extent to which the criteria for due care were met was studied in 1995 as part of the physician study (Box 7.2). All physicians who were in a sample of reported cases were asked to describe not only the reported case that was sampled but also a case that they did not report, if any. It turned out that with regard to the substantive criteria for due care (the patient's request being explicit, the suffering being unbearable and hopeless, and the absence of realistic alternatives for treatment), there were no differences between the reported and unreported cases.

With regard to the procedural criteria for due care, however, several differences emerged. In addition to the obvious difference with respect to reporting itself, it was found that the physicians more frequently had consulted another physician in reported than in unreported cases (94% versus 11%). Further, it was found that patients more often had a written will in reported cases as compared to unreported cases (74% versus 44%) and that the physician more frequently documented the decision making in the medical record or in a separate document (97% versus 57%). Although the latter two practices are not

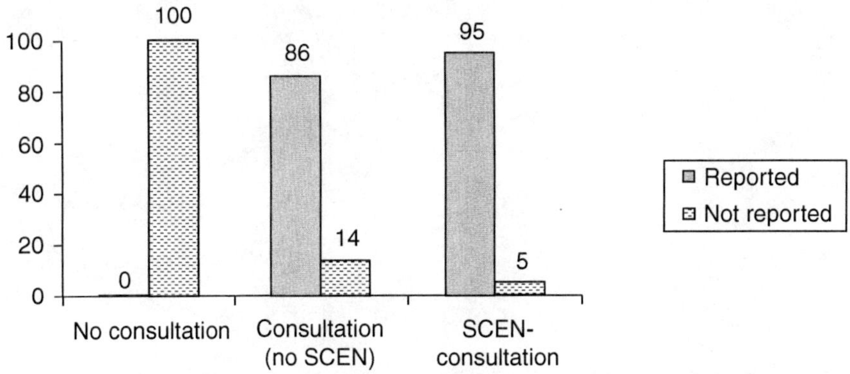

FIGURE 7.3. Reporting of EAS by physicians who did or did not organize a (SCEN) consultation.
Source: Death certificate study in 2005; 5. Onwuteaka-Philipsen, et al., 2007.

required under official criteria for due care, they give an indication about procedural aspects of the decision making.[1] A limitation of this comparison, of course, is that it does not give information on unreported cases by physicians who never report.

The relation between consultation with another physician and case reporting has been found consistently since 1995. Essential in consultation is that the consultant be independent from the physician, the patient, and the situation and be knowledgeable and experienced in acting as a consultant with respect to euthanasia and assisted suicide.

Important in professionalizing consultation is the SCEN project (Support and Consultation Euthanasia Netherlands), which started in 1997 with a pilot project in Amsterdam and reached full coverage of the Netherlands in 2002. This project provides specially trained, independent consultants for euthanasia and assisted suicide. Until 2003, the program focused on providing consultation for general practitioners. Since then, it is being gradually extended to medical specialists and nursing home physicians.

Evaluation of the pilot program revealed that consultation through SCEN is positively associated with reporting. In four general practitioner districts in which both a pretest (in 2000) and a post-test (in 2001/2002) took place, the reporting rate increased from 52% before the implementation of SCEN to 66% 18 months after implementation.[3] Data from the 2005 study based on a review of death certificates bring this relationship out clearly, as Figure 7.3 shows.[5] Among the group of actual euthanasia/assisted suicide cases identified on the basis of the death certificate, when no consultation took place, no cases were reported; however, when the physician had consulted another physician, a large majority of cases *were* reported. This was even the case when the consultant was a SCEN physician.

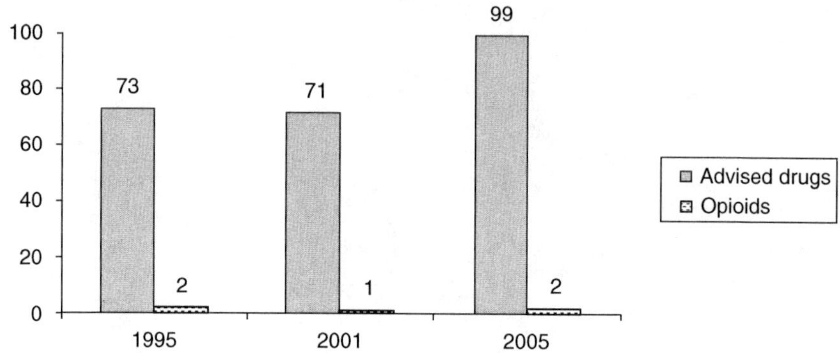

FIGURE 7.4. Reporting rates for euthanasia by drugs used.
Source: 5. Onwuteaka-Philipsen, et al., 2007.

Reporting and Physician Knowledge of Which Clinical Practices Fall Within the Category of Euthanasia/Assisted Suicide

The data from the death certificate study also indicate that the primary reason physicians gave for not reporting cases of euthanasia or assisted suicide was their belief that the case did not need to be reported, not unwillingness to report. This was related to the way the physicians themselves labeled their act. They almost always labeled the cases of euthanasia that they did not report as something else, such as palliative sedation or increase in pain and symptom control.

This was also found to be related to the drugs that were used by the physician in cases of euthanasia (see death certificate studies, Box 7.2).[b] The Royal Dutch Society for the Advancement of Pharmacy (KNMP) recommends the use of certain drugs for euthanasia and physician-assisted suicide: the administration of a barbiturate to induce a coma, followed by a muscle relaxant, which causes the death of the patient.[10] If the patient is in very poor condition, the barbiturate may bring about death before the muscle relaxant is administered.

In 2005, the recommended drugs were used in about three-quarters of the euthanasia cases. In addition to these recommended drugs, opioids (whether or not in combination with benzodiazepines) are sometimes used in performing euthanasia (see death certificate study, Box 7.2) though not according to the recommendation of the KNMP. Figure 7.4 shows the reporting rates for cases of euthanasia in which the recommended drugs were used and cases in which opioids were used for the years 1995, 2001, and 2005. It shows clearly that the reporting rate for cases of euthanasia in which opioids were used is

[b] This does not concern physician-assisted suicide, since a mix-up between cases of physician-assisted suicide (where the patients take the drugs themselves) and palliative sedation or increase in symptom control is not likely.

consistently very low for all of these years. For cases of euthanasia in which the recommended drugs were used, the reporting rate was a little over 70% in 1995 and 2001 and rose to 99% in 2005.

The increase in total reporting rate between 1995 and 2001 can be explained mainly by an increase in the use of the recommended drugs, from 59% to 76%. The increase in total reporting between 2001 and 2005 can be explained mainly by physicians' increased willingness to report cases that they consider euthanasia: By 2005, practically all cases that the physician clearly understood to be euthanasia, as indicated by both the drugs used and how the cases were labeled, were being reported to one of the Regional Review Committees. The same holds true for cases of physician-assisted suicide, which are obviously always labeled as such by physicians. For physician-assisted suicide, the reporting rate, which was 23% in 1995, increased to 54% in 2001 and then to 100% in 2005.

CONCLUSIONS

The Unreported Case

From the empirical evidence presented here, it becomes clear that over the years the nature of "the unreported case" has changed. Up until at least 2001, unreported cases could be divided roughly into two groups: those that physicians knew they had to report but were reluctant to do so and those they did not consider to be euthanasia and therefore did not report. In 2005, almost all of the unreported cases fell into the latter group.

Two points with respect to these findings call for discussion: first, the weight given in the death certificate studies to the effect of drugs used at the end of life, and second, the possible relation between euthanasia and palliative sedation.

The Relative Importance of Drugs Used

In reaction to the 2001 study, it was argued that the nationwide studies put too much emphasis on the physician's intention and too little on the effect of the drugs he or she had used, allowing for acts in which the physician intended to end a patient's life on the explicit request of the patient but did not do so because of the medication used (e.g., opioids titrated against pain).[11] Critics have maintained that as it is debatable whether opioids really have a life-ending effect,[12, 13,14] cases involving opioids should not be classified as euthanasia. If they were. the reporting rate would go up dramatically, as Figure 7.4 suggests.

In the 2005 study, however, the researchers rejected this suggestion for several reasons. For one thing, in the death certificate study, the physicians were asked in the interviews about the effect of the drugs used. The category of euthanasia included cases in which the attending physician indicated that the drugs used had hastened death.

More importantly, the intention to end life is an essential element in the definition of euthanasia. That physicians sometimes use drugs that do not seem very appropriate is a question about the quality of clinical practice, not about how to classify the action. Finally, although it's debatable whether opioids are appropriate drugs for ending life, it cannot be ruled out that in some cases, depending on the patient's condition and the dosage used, administering opioids *does* end the patient's life. For these reasons, the total reporting rate of 80% includes euthanasia performed with opioids.

Nevertheless, by calculating separate reporting rates for euthanasia with recommended drugs and those with opioids, and by asking physicians to label their act themselves, it has been possible to distinguish two groups of euthanasia cases. One is the large group of "clear" cases (i.e., cases that meet the definition of euthanasia, are labeled as such by the physician, and involve use of the recommended drugs). These cases are almost always reported. The other is the smaller group of less clear cases that meet the definition of euthanasia but are labeled as another act by the physician and involve the use of opioids, with a debatable life-ending effect. These cases are almost never reported.

Palliative Sedation and Euthanasia

In 2005, the total number of cases of euthanasia and assisted suicide decreased, compared to the earlier years. At the same time, the number of cases of palliative sedation increased. Especially in the media, it has been argued that this change must have occurred because physicians wanted to avoid reporting euthanasia/assisted suicide and therefore turned to palliative sedation instead.

If this were the case, it would not be a positive development for the continued public control of EAS. However, it is debatable whether the desire to avoid reporting euthanasia is the main cause for an increase in palliative sedation. The results of the 2005 study cannot answer the question definitively since the study was not designed to examine this relation. Nonetheless, the 2005 data offer some indications that the increase in palliative sedation mostly reflects positive choices in favor of palliative sedation, rather than negative choices against EAS. First, together with the decrease in cases of euthanasia/assisted suicide, there was a decrease in the number of requests from patients for assistance in dying. Second, in only 9% of cases of palliative sedation had there been a request for EAS earlier in the disease process. More research is needed to fully understand the relation between euthanasia/assisted suicide and palliative sedation.

Safe Ground or Slippery Slope?

Slippery slope arguments have often been raised about euthanasia and assisted suicide practices in the Netherlands, but they can be looked at from many different angles. From the angle of reporting, one could argue that the Netherlands was on a slippery slope if there was evidence that a large and increasing number of cases were not being reported and if the unreported cases differed from the reported ones in the extent to which the criteria for due care were met. In fact, however, the data make clear that the reporting rate has gone up significantly throughout the years. They also give us no reason to think that the cases that aren't reported systematically fail to meet criteria for due care. Therefore, with regard to reporting there is no evidence for a slippery slope.

Nevertheless, there has always been discussion about the extent to which the fact that there are unreported cases is cause to doubt the feasibility of regulating euthanasia and assisted suicide. Especially in 1995 and 2001, the news of an increase in the reporting rate was accompanied by discussion about whether the glass was half full or half empty. Now that the reporting rate is 80%, it is clear that the glass is more than half full. Moreover, by far the largest difference between reported and unreported cases lies in the drugs used, in combination with the designation given by the physician. This is not necessarily a sign of going down a slippery slope since it does not seem to involve differences in the substantive requirements for due care.

It remains important, of course, that the procedural requirements of consultation and reporting continue to be met. Thus, it's also important to strive for a higher reporting rate among the less clear cases of euthanasia and assisted suicide in order to ensure optimal public control.

Ensuring Effective Oversight

The data show a positive evolution since 1995: The frequency of euthanasia and assisted suicide has decreased while the percentage of cases reported has increased.

It is important to note that unwillingness to report seems no longer to be a significant reason for not doing so. When a case of euthanasia is not reported today, it is mainly because the physician did not classify the case as euthanasia and therefore did not believe it needed to be reported, a misperception related largely to the nature of the drugs used. Although this lack of clarity seems to have decreased in recent years, it is still desirable to decrease it further. To achieve this, physicians should receive additional education on the effects of opioids and benzodiazepines so that they can select the correct drugs if the intent is to bring about the patient's death. In this way, intention and effect can be brought into alignment.

References

1. Wal, Gerrit van der, Paul J. van der Maas, Jacqueline M. Bosma, Ilinka Haverkate, Carmen L. M. de Graaff, John G. C. Kester, Bregje Onwuteaka-Philipsen, Agnes van der Heide, Dick L. Willems, and Piet Kostense. 1996. Evaluation of the notification procedure for physician-assisted death in the Netherlands. *New England Journal of Medicine* 335: 1706–1711.

2. Onwuteaka-Philipsen, Bregje D., Agnes van der Heide, Dirk Koper, Ingeborg Keij-Deerenberg, Judith A. C. Rietjens, Mette Rurup, Astrid M. Vrakking, Jean Jacques Georges, Martien T. Muller, Gerrit van der Wal, and Paul J. van der Maas. 2003. Euthanasia and other end-of-life decisions in The Netherlands in 1990, 1995 and 2001. *The Lancet* 362: 395–399.
3. Onwuteaka-Philipsen, Bregje D., Agnes van der Heide, Martien T. Muller, Mette Rurup, Judith A. Rietjens, Jean-Jacques Georges, Astrid M. Vrakking, Jacqueline M. Cuperus-Bosma, Gerrit van der Wal, and Paul J. van der Maas. 2005. Dutch experience in monitoring euthanasia. *British Medical Journal* 331: 691–693.
4. Heide, Agnes van der, Bregje D. Onwuteaka-Philipsen, Mette L. Rurup, Hilde M. Buiting, Johannes J. M. van Delden, Johanna E. Hanssen-de Wolf, Anke G. J. M. Janssen, H. Roeline Pasman, Judith Rietjens, Cornelis J. M. Prins, Ingeborg Deerenberg, Joseph K. M. Gevers, Paul van der Maas, and Gerrit van der Wal. 2007. End-of-life practices in the Netherlands under the Euthanasia act. *New England Journal of Medicine* 356: 1957–1965.
5. Onwuteaka-Philipsen, Bregje D., Joseph K. M. Gevers, Agnes van der Heide, et al. 2007. *Evaluatie Wet Toetsing Levensbeëindiging op verzoek en hulp bij zelfdoding* [Evaluation of the Termination of Life on Request and Assisted Suicide (Review Procedures) Act]. The Hague: ZonMw.
6. de Haan, J. 2002. The new Dutch law on euthanasia. *Medical Law Review* 10: 57–75.
7. Maas, Paul J. van der, Johannes J. M. van Delden, L. Pijnenborg, and C. W. N. Looman. 1991. Euthanasia and other medical decisions concerning the end of life. *The Lancet* 338: 669–674.
8. Maas, Paul J. van der, Gerrit van der Wal, Ilinka Haverkate, Carmen L. M. de Graaff, John G. C. Kester, Bregje Onwuteaka-Philipsen, Agnes van der Heide, Jacqueline M. Bosma, and Dick L. Willems. 1996. Euthanasia, physician-assisted suicide, and other medical practices involving the end of life in the Netherlands, 1990–1995. *New England Journal of Medicine* 335: 1699–1705.
9. Rurup, Mette L., Hilde Buiting, Roeline W. Pasman, Paul J. van der Maas, Agnes van der Heide, and Bregje D. Onwuteaka-Philipsen. 2008. Differences between reported and unreported cases of euthanasia. *Medical Care* 46: 1198–1202.
10. Koninklijke Nederlandse Maatschappij ter bevordering der Pharmacie (KNMP). 1998. *Toepassing en bereiding van euthanatica* [Application and preparation of drugs for euthanasia]. The Hague: KNMP.
11. Den Hartogh, Govert. 2003. Mysterieuze cijfers: meldingspercentage kan niet meer stijgen [Mysterious numbers: Notification percentage cannot increase further]. *Med Contact* 58: 1063–1066.
12. Morita, Tatsuya, Junichi Tsunoda, Satoshi Inoue, and Satoshi Chihara. 2001. Effects of high dose opioids and sedatives on survival in terminally ill cancer patients. *Journal of Pain and Symptom Management* 21: 282–289.
13. Thorns, Andrew, and Nigel Sykes. 2000. Opioid use in last week of life and implications for end-of-life decision-making. *The Lancet* 356: 398–399.
14. Sykes, Nigel, and Andrew Thorns. 2003. The use of opioids and sedatives at the end of life. *The Lancet Oncology* 4: 312–318.

8

Physician Assistance in Dying Without an Explicit Request by the Patient

Agnes van der Heide

INTRODUCTION

Dutch euthanasia policy is often thought to be ultimately grounded in physicians' obligations of beneficence. A key element in the six criteria for due care relates to the suffering of the patient: Euthanasia and physician-assisted suicide are allowed only if the physician is convinced that the patient is suffering unbearably without any hope of relief and that there are no alternatives to address the suffering. However, a second key element in the criteria for due care relates to patient autonomy: Unbearable suffering without hope of relief can only be a ground for assistance in dying if the patient makes a voluntary and well-considered request to his or her physician to do so.

A generally appreciated essential safeguard for the practice of euthanasia under Dutch law is that the request is voluntary, that is, free from pressure by others, and well considered, that is, based on complete information and adequate insights. Nevertheless, in the periods both prior to and after the enforcement of the law, it has been proven that physicians have sometimes provided assistance in dying to patients who have not made an explicit voluntary and well-considered request.[1,2,3,4] These cases may have involved patients who were not able to express their wishes, such as neonates or comatose patients; patients whose competency to express well-considered preferences was doubtful, such as patients with dementia or psychiatric disorders; or competent patients for whom physician assistance in dying was the result of an implicit request or agreement to hasten death. Physician assistance in dying without an explicit patient request is illegal in the Netherlands, as well as in other countries.

The existence of a practice of physician assistance in dying without the patient's explicit request was first acknowledged in 1991, as a result of the studies that were done for the Dutch Commission Appointed to Carry Out Research Concerning Medical Practice in Connection with Euthanasia (the Remmelink Commission).[4,5] The commission's findings provoked much debate.[6,7,8,9,10,11] In particular, the finding of "nonvoluntary euthanasia," as the practice is also called, was cited as proof that a liberal policy toward euthanasia was leading inevitably to a slippery slope. However, findings from subsequent studies showed that the occurrence of physician assistance in dying without an explicit patient request did not increase in the Netherlands after 1991.[1,2,3] In fact, the enactment of the euthanasia law in 2002 was followed by a notable (though not statistically significant) decrease. Further, the rate of involuntary euthanasia has been found to be as high or higher in other countries, such as Belgium and Australia, where it cannot be seen as resulting from years of public tolerance of euthanasia.[12,13]

Even if they do not prove the existence of a slippery slope, however, cases of physician assistance in dying without an explicit patient request should be regarded cautiously because they are in principle very problematic, as is widely recognized within and outside of the Netherlands. Cases of physician assistance in dying without an explicit patient request are obviously not justified by the principle of respect for patient autonomy. It is, therefore, extremely important to understand why this practice occurs, even where euthanasia is not permitted, and why some see it as an ethically justifiable option of last resort in end-of-life care.

This chapter summarizes empirical data on the key characteristics of physician assistance in dying without an explicit request from the patient that are available from the Netherlands and other countries.

THE NETHERLANDS

The Studies

The nationwide study carried out in 1990 for the Remmelink Commission was the first to yield data on the practice of physician assistance in dying without an explicit patient request.[4,5] Written questionnaires were sent to a sampling of physicians who had filled out a death certificate for a deceased patient from a total of more than 5,000 cases between August and November 1990, to be answered anonymously. This death certificate study, which was repeated in 1995, 2001, and 2005, was aimed at assessing the main characteristics of decision-making practice at the end of life in the Netherlands.[1,2,3] About three-quarters of the physicians sampled responded to each survey: 76% in 1990, 77% in 1995, 74% in 2001, and 78% in 2005.

In addition to the questionnaires, in 1990, 1995, and 2001 more than 400 physicians were interviewed personally in order to gain a deeper understanding of their end-of-life practices. In 2005, interviews were replaced by a written survey among 1,135 physicians.

Frequencies and Patient Characteristics

The 1990 death certificate study found that physician assistance in dying without an explicit patient request had been the cause of death in about 0.8% of all

TABLE 8.1. *Characteristics of Patients Whom the Physician Assisted in Dying Without an Explicit Patient Request, in 1990, 1995, 2001, and 2005 (Death Certificate Study)*

	1990 N = 47 %[a]	1995 N = 64 %	2001 N = 60 %	2005 N = 24 %	All Deaths in 2005
Total[b]	0.8	0.7	0.7	0.4	
Age					
0–64 years	43	34	31	47	19
65–79 years	23	31	22	28	32
80 years or more	34	36	47	25	48
Gender					
Male	69	49	47	49	49
Female	31	51	53	51	51
Diagnosis					
Cancer	61	40	44	23	29
Cardiovascular disease	10	5	22	16	32
Other	29	55	34	61	39
Type of physician					
General practitioner	26	31	33	22	41
Clinical specialist	69	55	55	59	32
Nursing home physician	5	13	13	19	25
Estimated shortening of life					
Less than one week	86	95	77	86	
One week or more	14	6	18	12	
Unknown	0	0	5	3	

Notes: [a] All percentages weighted and rounded percentages.
[b] Percentage of all deaths in the Netherlands in the year concerned.

deaths in the Netherlands, or about 1,000 cases in one year (see Table 8.1).[4] In 1995 and again in 2001, 0.7% of all deaths were the result of physician assistance in dying without an explicit patient request; in 2005, the figure was 0.4%.

In the personal interviews in 1990, 27% of all physicians reported having been engaged in this practice at least once in their career (see Table 8.2). After 1990, physician involvement in this practice declined, and physicians increasingly expressed their unwillingness to intentionally hasten a patient's death without his or her explicit request; by 2005, only 6% of physicians responding to the survey reported having done so at least once in their careers.[14]

The main characteristics of the patients who died as a result of physician assistance in dying without having made an explicit request largely remained similar over the years; however, we should note that the small numbers of

TABLE 8.2. *Physicians' Experiences with Assistance in Dying Without an Explicit Patient Request, in 1990, 1995, 2001, and 2005 (Interview Study)*

	1990	1995	2001	2005
	N = 405	N = 405	N = 410	N = 1,032
	%[a]	%	%	%
Ever assisted in dying without an explicit patient request	27	23	13	6
Never assisted in dying without an explicit patient request but can imagine doing so	32	32	16	7
Never assisted and cannot imagine doing so	41	45	71	86

Note: [a] All percentages weighted and rounded.

patients per year only allow for imprecise estimates here. These cases involved male and female patients in all age categories, although patients under the age of 65 were somewhat overrepresented (Table 8.1). The practice was most common among patients with cancer. This overrepresentation of patients dying under the age of 65 and of those with cancer also characterizes the practice of (voluntary) euthanasia and physician-assisted suicide. However, whereas euthanasia and physician-assisted suicide are predominantly performed by general practitioners in the patient's home, assistance in dying without an explicit patient request was found to be more commonly carried out by clinical specialists, who mainly provided inpatient care in hospitals.

For all five study years, in the large majority of cases, physician assistance in dying without an explicit patient request shortened life by less than one week. It's important to remember that these data represent physicians' estimations of the degree to which life was shortened, estimations that are notoriously difficult to make. However, since physicians most frequently overestimate the survival time of their patients, the finding that, in general, life was shortened by less than one week suggests that this practice is typically performed very late in the disease process.

The Decision-Making Process

The majority of patients whose deaths resulted from physician assistance that had not been explicitly requested at the time it was carried out did not have decision-making capacity. With a quarter to nearly half of these patients, the possibility of euthanasia had been discussed at an earlier time. Some of the patients with whom physicians didn't discuss the particular treatment decision that led to the patient's death had expressed a wish for assistance in dying at an earlier point in their disease process.

In all study years, the reason most commonly reported by physicians for not discussing the decision at the time it was made (31%–48%) was that the patient had been comatose or unconscious. Less common reasons were that the patient had been a neonate (5%–22%), that the patient was incompetent due to dementia (1%–16%), that assistance in dying had clearly been in the best interest of the patient (0%–15%), that the patient lacked decision-making capacity because of a psychiatric disorder (0%–15%), that the patient was mentally handicapped (0%–5%), or that discussion would have been harmful to the patient (0%–4%) (see Table 8.3).

The extent to which physicians had discussed assistance in dying for a particular patient with their colleagues seems to have increased over the years, from 31% of all cases in 1990 to 65% in 2005. The involvement of nursing staff also rose, from 30% to 65%. Family members were involved in 39% of all cases in 1990, but this percentage seems to be substantially higher in the subsequent years (67%–98%).

Looking at the type of drug administered can be helpful for understanding the practice of physician-assistance in dying without an explicit patient request. The use of a neuromuscular relaxant, for example, suggests that ending life was the exclusive goal, whereas providing opioids with the aim of ending life may involve the concurrent goal of alleviating symptoms. Thus, physician-assistance in dying by administering highly dosed opioids, more than by administering neuromuscular relaxants, seems a practice that approaches alleviation of symptoms while merely taking into account the hastening of death as a possible concurrent effect. Beginning with the 1995 study, the questionnaires also asked about the types of drugs that had been used to end the patient's life. The majority of cases in which physicians hastened death involved the use of opioids: 80% in 1995 and 59% in 2005. Muscle relaxants were used in 18% of all cases in 1995 and in 23% in 2005, whereas sedatives were used in 2% of all cases in 1995 and in 8% in 2005.

Consider the following examples drawn from the physician interviews:

A 60-year-old man was admitted to a nursing home with a brain tumor that had increased in size after initial surgery. The patient was hemiplegious, had cognitive problems, and had increasingly serious epileptic insults despite treatment with carbamazepine, as well as general deterioration in his health status. One evening, the patient developed seizures that did not respond to highly dosed diazepam and diphantoin. A neurologist was consulted and clonazepam was given upon his advice, but this did not have any effect. It was then decided to further increase the dosages of diazepam and diphantoin with the aim of hastening the patient's death.

A 68-year-old man was admitted to the hospital because of increasing problems due to a malignant lung tumor. He had severe dyspnea, was very tired, and lacked any appetite. Treatment focused on palliation and consisted of morphine patches,

TABLE 8.3. *Decision Making about Assistance in Dying Without an Explicit Patient Request, in 1990, 1995, 2001, and 2005 (Death Certificate Study)*

	1990	1995	2001	2005
	N = 47	N = 64	N = 58	N = 24
	%[a]	%	%	%
Competency				
Patient was competent	37	21	16	15
Patient was (partly) incompetent	63	79	84	85
Discussion with patient				
Yes	46	37	26	35
No, but patient had previously expressed a wish	40	16	10	25
No, and patient had never expressed a wish	14	47	64	40
Reasons for not discussing assistance in dying with patient				
Patient was comatose/unconscious	42	31	48	35
Patient was neonate	5	11	12	22
Assistance in dying was clearly in the best interest of the patient	15	15	0	15
Patient had a psychiatric disorder	2	6	0	15
Discussion would harm the patient	0	2	0	4
Patient had dementia	3	14	16	1
Patient was mentally handicapped	0	0	5	1
Other	3	5	0	0
Discussion with others				
Other physician(s)	31	59	60	65
Nurses	30	65	62	42
Relatives	39	70	98	67
Drugs used	N.A.			
Muscle relaxants[b]		18	2	23
Barbiturates[c]		1	0	5
Opioids[d]		80	75	59
Benzodiazepines[e]		1	4	3
Other		0	0	5
Unknown		0	19	6

Notes: [a] All percentages weighted and rounded.
[b] In any combination.
[c] In any combination, except neuromuscular relaxants.
[d] In any combination except neuromuscular relaxants and barbiturates.
[e] In any combination except neuromuscular relaxants, barbiturates and opioids.
N.A. Data not available.

metoclopramide, and corticosteroids. On several occasions, he had requested assistance in dying should his situation deteriorate. Morphine dosages were gradually increased because of severe pain; as a result, the patient became drowsy and was no longer able to participate in decision making. The patient seemed to suffer severely, without any hope of improvement, and his family asked the physician to grant his earlier request for assistance in dying. The physician discussed the case with several colleagues and decided to hasten death, starting with the administration of high doses of morphine. The patient died several days later.

An 80-year-old man was admitted to the hospital with a colon carcinoma and widespread peritoneal metastases. The attending surgeon stated that no curative options were left. The patient was in extremely poor condition, with severe pain, intractable constipation, nausea, and frequent vomiting. He was not able to discuss treatment options. The main treatment consisted of morphine. After several days, the attending physicians, together with the family, assessed the patient's suffering as being unbearable without any hope of improvement. The decision was jointly made to end life by administering 1 gram of morphine intravenously. The patient died shortly afterward as a result of respiratory depression.

OTHER COUNTRIES

The practice of physician assistance in dying for patients without their request was found to occur in other countries as well as in the Netherlands.[13,15] For example, a 1996 survey similar to the Dutch death certificate study found that 3.5% of all deaths in Australia resulted from physician assistance in dying without an explicit patient request.[13] A similar study in 1998 in Flanders, Belgium, found that 3.2% of all deaths in the region involved assistance in dying without the patient's request.[12] In 2004, a somewhat differently designed study carried out in the United Kingdom found a percentage of 0.33% of deaths.[16]

A comparative study carried out in 2001 showed that 0.60% of all deaths in the Netherlands resulted from physician assistance in dying without the patient's request; in Belgium that number was 1.5%, in Denmark 0.67%, in Switzerland 0.42%, in Sweden 0.23%, and in Italy 0.06%.[15] The numbers found in Sweden and Italy were too small to allow for comparison of their characteristics, but in the other countries, cancer was the diagnosis reported most often. In the Netherlands and Belgium, physician assistance in dying without an explicit patient request occurred relatively often in hospitals (47% and 51%, respectively), whereas it was more often performed outside the hospital in Denmark (percentage in hospital 27%) and in Switzerland (22%). In all countries, assistance in dying was estimated to shorten life by less than one week in about 80% of cases.

Decision-making factors were largely comparable across countries: In about one-third of the cases, physicians had discussed the possibility of hastening death with the patient at some point before the actual decision was made. In two-thirds of the cases, physicians had no opportunity to talk with the patient about hastening death, nor were patients able to request it, because they had lost decision-making capacity earlier in the course of their disease. Physicians in Denmark (26%) and Switzerland (36%) – more frequently than physicians in other countries – stated that they had not discussed their decision with the patient because the act had so clearly served the best interest of the patient. In this 2001 study, this particular reason was not mentioned by any of the Dutch and Belgian physicians, which probably reflects a different attitude toward involving patients in, or burdening them with, making such difficult decisions. It cannot be ruled out that the attitudes of Dutch and Belgian physicians are influenced by the fact that in both countries, euthanasia and physician-assisted suicide are regulated by law. However, the similarities and differences between countries in the characteristics of the practice of physician assistance in dying without an explicit patient request must be interpreted cautiously. Due to the small number of cases, at least part of the variation is likely to be random. Further, physicians may be inclined to justify their acts when answering questions about so sensitive a topic, especially in countries where any type of euthanasia is illegal.

CONCLUDING REMARKS

Understandably, and rightly, the practice of physician assistance in dying without an explicit patient request often provokes heated debate. Both advocates and opponents of particular end-of-life practices use empirical data to support their views. However, the debate is sometimes flawed by misinterpretations of the meaning and role of empirical research.[17] Observational studies on the characteristics of practice cannot be used to prove that physicians who engage in practices that hasten death were right or wrong. Nor are such studies aimed at suggesting conditions in which assistance in dying is indicated; they merely provide insight into the reasons that physicians act the way they do. Observational studies on decision-making practices at the end of life are thus descriptive, not prescriptive. They are aimed at informing the medical community and supporting well-considered debate.

Arguments maintaining that the available data demonstrate that permitting physicians to perform euthanasia at a patient's request leads inevitably to a slippery slope seem seriously flawed. Often, such arguments rest selectively on data from the 1990 study by the Remmelink Commission and neglect trends found by subsequent studies.[18,19,20] Further, the fact that physician assistance in dying without an explicit patient request is also practiced in countries where euthanasia is not legal suggests that other factors may be as, or more, important. Despite improvements in medical care for the dying and increasing awareness that careful patient–physician communication is an important aspect of end-of-life care, physician assistance in dying without an explicit patient request seems to be a part of medical end-of-life care in the Netherlands, as well as in other countries.

On the one hand, this practice may reflect ineffective or delayed communication between patients and physicians about the dying process.[5] Obviously, a patient's situation sometimes deteriorates rapidly, so that he or she loses decision-making capacity before having an opportunity to discuss further medical treatment options. But patients and physicians may also avoid such discussions because of reluctance on the part of the patient, the physician, or both to confront the expected unfavorable course of the disease, the suffering that may be the result, and the imminence of dying.

On the other hand, the existence of this practice demonstrates that physicians feel that their obligation to relieve suffering sometimes takes precedence over their obligation to preserve life, even if the patient cannot make a request to support such decision making.

References

1. Heide, Agnes van der, Bregje D. Onwuteaka-Philipsen, Mette Rurup, Hilde Buiting, Johannes J. M. van Delden, Johanna E. Hanssen-de Wolff, Anke Janssen, H. Roeline Pasman, Judith A. Rietjens, Cornelis Prins, Ingeborg Deerenberg, Joseph C. Gevers, and Gerrit van der Wal. 2007. End-of-life practices in the Netherlands under the euthanasia act. *New England Journal of Medicine* 356: 1957–1965.
2. Onwuteaka-Philipsen, Bregje, Agnes van der Heide, Dirk Koper, Ingeborg Keij-Deerenberg, Judith Rietjens, Mette Rurup, Astrid M. Vrakking, Jean Jacques Georges, Martien T. Muller, Gerrit van der Wal, and Paul J. van der Maas. 2003. Euthanasia and other end-of-life decisions in the Netherlands in 1990, 1995, and 2001. *The Lancet* 362: 395–399.
3. Maas, Paul J. van der, Gerrit van der Wal, Ilinka Haverkate, Carmen L.de Graaff, John G. Kester, Bregje D. Onwuteaka-Philipsen, Agnes van der Heide, Jacqueline M. Bosma, and Dick L. Willems. 1996. Euthanasia, physician-assisted suicide, and other medical practices involving the end of life in the Netherlands, 1990–1995. *New England Journal of Medicine* 335: 1699–1705.
4. Maas, Paul J. van der, Johannes J. M. van Delden, L. Pijnenborg, and C. W. N. Looman. 1991. Euthanasia and other medical decisions concerning the end of life. *The Lancet* 338: 669–674.
5. Pijnenborg, L, Paul J. van der Maas, Johannes J. M. van Delden, and C. W. N. Looman. 1993. Life-terminating acts without explicit request of patient. *The Lancet* 341: 1196–1199.
6. Crisci, C. 1993. Life-terminating acts without explicit request of patient. *The Lancet.* 341: 1598.
7. Forde, R., and K. W. Ruyter. 1993. Life-terminating acts without explicit request of patient. *The Lancet* 341: 1598–1599.
8. Hug, G. 1993. Life-terminating acts without explicit request of patient. *The Lancet* 341: 1598.
9. Lindtjorn, B. 1993. Life-terminating acts without explicit request of patient. *The Lancet* 341: 1599.
10. McCallum, R. 1993. Life-terminating acts without explicit request of patient. *The Lancet* 341: 1599.
11. Pollard, B. 1993. Life-terminating acts without explicit request of patient. *The Lancet* 341: 1598.

12. Deliens, L., F. Mortier, J. Bilsen, M. Cosyns, R. Vander Stichele, J. Vanoverloop, and K. Ingels. 2000. End-of-life decisions in medical practice in Flanders, Belgium: A nationwide survey. *The Lancet* 356: 1806–1811.
13. Kuhse, Helga, Peter Singer, Peter Baume, Malcolm Clark, and Maurice Rickard. 1997. End-of-life decisions in Australian medical practice. *Medical Journal of Australia* 166: 191–196.
14. Onwuteaka-Philipsen, Bregje D., J. K. M. Gevers, Agnes van der Heide, et al. 2007. *Evaluatie Wet Toetsing Levensbeëindiging op verzoek en hulp bij zelfdoding.* Den Haag: ZonMw.
15. Heide, Agnes van der, Luc Deliens, Karin Faisst, Tore Nilstun, Michael Norup, Eugenio Paci, Gerrit van der Wal, Paul J. van der Maas. 2003. End-of-life decision-making in six European countries: Descriptive study. *The Lancet* 362: 345–350.
16. Seale, Clive. 2006. National survey of end-of-life decisions made by UK medical practitioners. *Palliative Medicine*. 20: 3–10.
17. Delden, J. J. M. van, L. Pijnenborg, and Paul J. van der Maas. 1993. Dances with data: Reports from the Netherlands. *Bioethics* 7: 323–329.
18. Hendin, Herbert. 1997. Euthanasia and physician-assisted suicide in the Netherlands. *New England Journal of Medicine* 336: 1385.
19. Hendin, Herbert. 2002. The Dutch experience. *Issues in Law & Medicine* 17: 223–246.
20. Keown, John. 2002. *Euthanasia, ethics and public policy: An argument against legalisation.* Cambridge: Cambridge University Press.

9

When Requests Do Not Result in Euthanasia or Assisted Suicide

H. Roeline W. Pasman

When a patient requests euthanasia or assisted suicide (EAS), there is no guarantee that his or her physician will fulfill that request. Patients have a right to ask a physician for aid in dying, but neither euthanasia nor assisted suicide is a right in the Netherlands. Beyond the patient's request, Dutch law requires the patient's situation to meet specific criteria for due care.[a] Moreover, the physician must be willing to fulfill the request: Physicians are not obliged to perform euthanasia or assist in suicide and can refuse on grounds of personal conscience, even when the criteria for due care have been met. In that case, however, the physician must refer the patient to another physician. When a physician rejects a request for EAS, it is important that he makes this decision carefully and that he explains his decision to the patient.

To understand euthanasia in the Netherlands, it's important to examine not only the situations in which requests are fulfilled but also those in which they are not. In particular, it's important to understand the differences between the two patient populations: Apart from legal considerations, do all patients or patient groups have equal chances of receiving euthanasia or assisted suicide when legal criteria are otherwise met, or do some have less chance of receiving aid in dying? This chapter examines available empirical data in the Netherlands about the incidence of requests for euthanasia or assisted suicide that are not fulfilled, the reasons euthanasia/assisted suicide is not performed, and the characteristics of patients whose requests are not fulfilled (see Box 9.1). The chapter also examines evidence concerning the reasons for rejecting a request, from the perspectives of both physicians and patients.

[a] See Chapter 3 in this volume.

Box 9.1.

Data about requests for euthanasia and assisted suicide that are not fulfilled come from several different empirical studies carried out in the Netherlands: reviews of death certificates, physician interviews, a general practitioner survey, and (qualitative) interviews with patients (or family members) whose requests were not fulfilled and with their physicians.

Death Certificate Studies

In 1990, 1995, 2001, and 2005, a stratified sample of deaths was drawn from the central death registry of Statistics Netherlands, which receives death certificates for all deaths that occur in the Netherlands. For all sampled cases in which the cause of death did not preclude physician assistance in dying, attending physicians were mailed a four-page questionnaire. One of the questions concerned whether the patient had asked for euthanasia or assisted suicide and if the request was not fulfilled, why it was not. Response rates were as follows: 1990 – 76% (of a total of 8,500 questionnaires mailed); 1995 – 77% (6,632 total questionnaires mailed); 2001 – 74% (5,617 total questionnaires mailed); and 2005 – 78% (6,860 total questionnaires mailed).[1,2,3,4]

Physician Interviews

In 1995 and 1996, Dutch physicians, randomly sampled nationwide and stratified by specialty and region, were interviewed by more than 30 specifically trained and experienced physicians who used a structured questionnaire. A total of 405 physicians were interviewed (89% of those initially contacted). All interviewees were asked to describe the most recent case in which they had fulfilled a request for euthanasia or assisted suicide (134 physicians had had such a case) and the most recent case in which they had not fulfilled such a request (148 physicians).[5]

General Practitioner Survey

From April 2000 to December 2002, written questionnaires were sent to 6,596 general practitioners (GPs) in the Netherlands, 3,614 (60%) of whom responded.[6,b] Among other topics, the

(*continued*)

[b] Of those originally approached, 556 were no longer in practice and not eligible to participate.

questionnaire asked about the number of requests received in the previous 12 months and how the GP had dealt with them. In addition, questions were asked about the characteristics of the most recent explicit request (if any) received within the last 18 months. Respondents also answered questions regarding the patient's reasons for requesting euthanasia or assisted suicide, his or her symptoms, the extent to which the patient's situation met criteria for due care, and the decision-making process.

Patient/Family–Physician Interviews

From December 2005 to September 2007, in-depth interviews were conducted with patients who had explicitly requested euthanasia or assisted suicide but whose requests had not been fulfilled. Family members were interviewed for patients who had died in the interval. If the patient/relative gave consent, the physician who received the request was also interviewed. Patients were first asked about their current situation and their request for euthanasia or assisted suicide. Subsequent questions were based on what the respondent said, drawing on a list of general topics that included reasons for requesting aid in dying and reasons why the request was not fulfilled. The interviews with physicians started with a general question about the patient's request. At the end of each interview, the researcher checked that all topics had been covered. In total, 10 patients and 8 relatives were interviewed, 15 of whom allowed us to approach their physician. We interviewed 16 physicians (in two cases, two physicians were interviewed; in one case, the physician refused because of lack of time). The result: 14 cases in which both the patient/relative and the physician was interviewed and 4 cases in which only the patient/relative was interviewed. Patients were interviewed in their homes for 60–120 minutes and the physicians in their offices for 30–60 minutes.[7]

INCIDENCE OF REQUESTS FOR EUTHANASIA/ASSISTED SUICIDE THAT ARE NOT FULFILLED

From the different death certificate studies we know that in the Netherlands, about 3 to 4 per 10 explicit requests for euthanasia or assisted suicide will be granted and performed (Figure 9,1).[1,2,3,4] Most requests (about three-quarters) are made to GPs, who tend to fulfill them more often than do other physicians.[3,4,5] Respondents in the GP survey indicated that they had not fulfilled requests for euthanasia/assisted suicide in about half of the cases.[6]

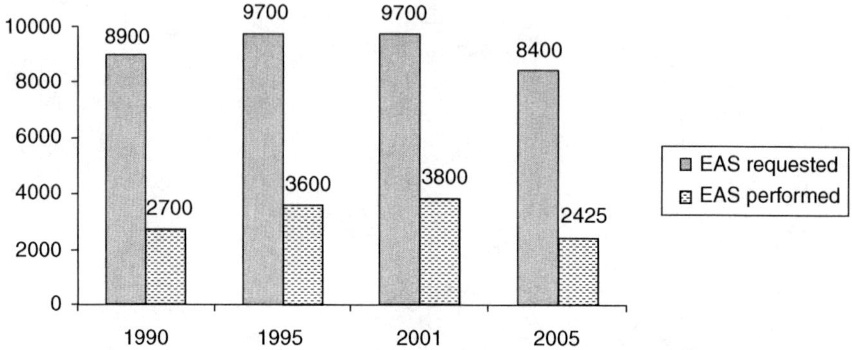

FIGURE 9.1. Total requests for euthanasia and assisted suicide versus requests granted in 1990, 1995, 2001, and 2005.
Source: 3. Onwuteaka-Philipsen, et al., 2007.

Reasons for Not Fulfilling Requests for Euthanasia or Assisted Suicide

The available data suggest several situations in which requests for euthanasia or assisted suicide are not fulfilled: those in which physicians refuse to fulfill the request for either legal reasons or on grounds of personal conscience; those in which the patient dies before a decision is reached or the procedure can be carried out; and those in which the patient withdraws the request.

In the death certificate studies, the reason for not *performing* euthanasia or assisted suicide that physicians mentioned most often was the death of the patient before the request could have been fulfilled (8% in 2001; 39% in 2005).[1,3]

In the general practitioner survey, respondents cited variants of these situations about equally: In 13% of cases, the patient died after the GP accepted the request but before he or she could perform euthanasia. In another 13%, the patient died before the physician had made the final decision to grant or refuse the request. In a further 13%, the patient no longer wanted euthanasia or assisted suicide, and in 12%, the physician refused to fulfill the request.[6]

The patient–physician interviews suggest the same underlying reasons for not fulfilling a patient's request for euthanasia or assisted suicide. In each of the cases in which the patient died before a final decision was made (2) or before euthanasia could be performed (2), the patient's condition deteriorated very rapidly. Both the family members and the attending physicians were of the opinion that this situation probably could not have been foreseen and could not have been prevented.

In any given case, however, the reasons for not fulfilling a request can be difficult to ascertain. The patient–physician interviews indicated that patients (or family members) and physicians can sometimes have different perspectives on a situation and on the reason that euthanasia/assisted suicide was not performed (see Table 9.1.). For example, in one case, the relative said that the physician had rejected the patient's request for euthanasia, but the physician indicated that the patient had not made an explicit request. The physician had interpreted what the patient said as a possible future situation. In another case, the partner of the deceased patient thought the patient had withdrawn the request because he had not continued to mention euthanasia when he was close to death. The physician said that the patient never asked for euthanasia explicitly, however, although they had talked about it intensively.

Characteristics of Patients Whose Request for EAS Was Not Fulfilled

In both the 1995 and 1996 physician interviews and the GP survey, patients whose request for euthanasia or assisted suicide were rejected tended to be older than 80, to have a diagnosis other than cancer, and not to have had a clear diagnosis but, rather, to have suffered from "old age or general deterioration."[5,6] In both studies, physicians reported that pain was not the most frequent reason for the patient's request; they also indicated that these patients often had symptoms of depression.[6]

In the GP survey, both patients who received euthanasia/assisted suicide and those whose requests were granted but who died before euthanasia could be performed seemed to be highly similar in age (the minority in both groups was older than 80), diagnosis (cancer in 90% of the patients in both groups), and reasons for requesting euthanasia or assisted suicide ("pointless suffering": more than 70% of the patients in both groups; "loss of dignity": just under 67%).

In the patient–physician interviews, patients whose requests were rejected differed from patients whose requests were not fulfilled for other reasons, especially with respect to diagnosis. Of the 12 cases in which the patient (or surviving family member) indicated that the request was rejected, only one patient had cancer. Of the remaining 5 cases in which the patient died before a final decision was made or before euthanasia was performed or withdrew his or her request, the patient did have cancer.

Rationale for Rejecting a Request for Euthanasia or Assisted Suicide: Physicians' Perspectives

In the 1995 and 1996 physician interviews, for about half of the cases in which the physician had rejected the request, the physician stated that he or she had done so because there were still alternatives for (palliative) treatment available. In 70% of these cases, the physician assessed that the patient's situation did not truly meet the criterion of unbearable suffering.[5]

The GP survey revealed similar reasons for rejecting a request for euthanasia/assisted suicide.[6] Asked why they had been reluctant to fulfill a request,

TABLE 9.1. *Characteristics of Patients and Interviewees and Reasons for Not Granting/Performing EAS (Patient and Physician Perspective)*

Case No.	Patient Characteristics	Interviewees	Reason EAS Not Performed: Patient/Relative Perspective Physician's Perspective
1	Man, age 47, cancer (glandular cell)	Patient's mother General practitioner (woman, age: 40–50)	Died before performance Died before performance
2	Woman, age 88, cancer (pancreas)	Patient's daughter General practitioner (man, age: > 50)	Died before performance Died before performance
3	Man, age 72, cancer (Kahler)	Patient's wife/partner (No consent to interview physician)	Died before final decision Unknown
4	Man, age 78, cancer (lung)	Patient's daughter General practitioner (man, age: > 50)	Died before final decision Died before final decision
5	Man, age 41, Crohn's disease	Patient himself Clinical specialist (man, age: 40–50)	Request refused Request refused
6	Woman, age 85, paralyzed after stroke	Patient herself Current nursing home physician (woman, age: < 40) Former nursing home physician (woman, age: > 50)	Request refused Request refused
7	Woman, age 68, Alzheimer's disease	Patient's husband Nursing home physician (man, age: 40–50) Geriatrician (woman, age < 40)	Request refused Request refused
8	Woman, age 82, Alzheimer's disease	Patient's husband Nursing home physician (woman, age: < 40)	Request refused Request refused
9	Woman, age 89, rheumatism	Patient herself General practitioner (woman, age: < 40)	Request refused Request refused/ request withdrawn

(*continued*)

Case No.	Patient Characteristics	Interviewees	Reason EAS Not Performed: Patient/Relative Perspective Physician's Perspective
10	Man, age 69, several strokes, Parkinson's disease, depressive symptoms	Patient himself General practitioner (man, age: 40–50)	Request refused Request refused
11	Man, age 91, Parkinson's disease, severe constipation	Patient's wife/partner General practitioner (man, age: > 50)	Request refused No explicit request
12	Woman, age 81, colon cancer, rheumatism, asthma, heart failure, Ménière's	Patient herself (No consent to interview physician)	Request refused Unknown
13	Woman, age 84, stroke, neurological problems	Patient herself (Physician refused because of lack of time)	Request refused Unknown
14	Man, age 88, stroke, depressive symptoms	Patient himself General practitioner (man, age: 40–50)	Request refused Request refused
15	Man, age 85, Parkinson's disease	Patient himself General practitioner (man, age: > 50)	Request refused Request refused
16	Woman, age 87, heart failure	Patient herself (No consent to interview physician)	Request refused Unknown
17	Man, age 63, cancer (prostate)	Patient's wife/partner General practitioner (man, age: > 50)	Request withdrawn No explicit request
18	Woman, age 86, weak sighted	Patient herself General practitioner (man, age: 40–50)	No explicit request No explicit request/ request withdrawn

GPs cited doubts about whether the criteria for due care had been met. For instance, half of the GPs who rejected a request doubted whether the patient's suffering was hopeless and unbearable, and about 1 in 3 GPs believed that there still were alternatives for treatment available. About 1 in 3 GPs also were concerned that the patient was depressed. In 24% to 30% of cases in which patients died before a decision was made about their request or before euthanasia could be performed, or in which the patient withdrew his or her request, the GP had doubts about the hopelessness and unbearableness of the patient's suffering. In 23% to 37% of these cases, the GP believed that alternatives were still available. Overall, the GP survey concluded that physicians' rationale for rejecting a request of euthanasia or assisted suicide was associated with concerns that the patient was not fully competent; that he or she did not truly meet the criterion of unbearable, hopeless suffering; or that alternatives were available to address the patient's situation.[6]

In the patient–physician interview study, for the 6 cases of refusal in which we interviewed both the patient and the physician, the physician doubted whether the criteria for due care had been met at the time of the request.[7] In all 6 cases, the physicians had doubts about at least two criteria: In 5 cases, the physician felt that there were still alternatives available that would probably address the patient's reasons for requesting euthanasia or assisted suicide. These alternatives included treatment for malnutrition, more attention provided to the patient to resolve loneliness, psychiatric consultation and treatment of depressive symptoms, and watchful waiting to see whether aphasia associated with a cerebro-vascular accident improved over time. Five physicians also doubted whether patients'suffering was unbearable – in the view of these physicians, the patients were not very ill and continued their daily life. In 3 of the 6 cases, the physician doubted whether patients' requests were well considered – the patients had not convinced them that their wish to die was sincere and serious and had not mentioned the subject again after the initial request. Only one physician mentioned that he would never perform euthanasia or assist a patient in suicide himself on personal grounds. If his patient had met the criteria for due care, he would have referred the individual to another physician.

Rationale for Rejecting a Request for EAS: Patients' Perspectives

All patients in the patient–physician interview study whose request for EAS had been refused said that their physician had indicated that their situation did not meet the criteria for due care and that, therefore, euthanasia or assisted suicide was not possible. Three patients agreed with the physician; however, their wish to die had remained after the request was refused. Two patients explicitly stated that they did not want their physician to perform euthanasia or assist their suicide because of the legal consequences for him.

In the cases in which the physician doubted whether the patient's suffering was unbearable, two patients themselves questioned whether their suffering in fact met the criterion. One patient said about his suffering:

RESPONDENT: No, my pain isn't unbearable. I sometimes have pain in my back, and then at other times it's somewhere else. And all sorts of problems with my body – awful trouble with my bowels, for instance, and pain in my neck – I do have that so I go to a physiotherapist who massages my neck. That does help a bit.

INTERVIEWER: But it's not unbearable?
R: No, I wouldn't even call that unbearable, no.
I: But your whole situation?
R: I find it really horrible. But not unbearable, because I go on living every day, and each day comes and goes. Tomorrow is another day.

Another patient had similar considerations:

R: I don't know, myself, whether it's unbearable. I sit here all day doing nothing – yes, I got the sports channel because my daughters suggested it.... I can't really say it's unbearable suffering. I've got this awful trouble with my hips so I don't sleep at all well at night. I wake up at about 1 o'clock and I get painkillers. But I take painkillers and I take four paracetamols; they help me in the daytime, because now I haven't got any pain at all when I sit like this all day. And then at night the pain comes, and then I lie on my back. I've got one of those hospital beds that you can raise the top end of, and then I sleep again for about an hour. Usually, at 4 o'clock I'm sitting in this chair – I can almost lie flat in the chair and the catheter bag hangs on my chair, that just reaches. And there's a blanket there that I pull over me, I put on my dressing gown, and then I often sleep for three hours until 7 o'clock when the sisters come. So, is that unbearable suffering, that I can't lie in bed?

A third patient was of the opinion that she suffered unbearably, but not all the time:

I: And do you yourself think that you suffer unbearably?
R: Yes, sometimes, but not every day.

Unlike the previous two cases, in this third case, the patient disagreed with the physician in rejecting her request for euthanasia.

Two other patients disagreed with their physician's assessment that their suffering was not unbearable, however. One patient described

R: that every day is the same, waking up every day, pain, sleeping ... and pain and waking up and eating and sleeping, not being able to do anything. [Silence; she drinks something.]

About her physician's reason for rejecting her request:

I: Because you also asked for it six months ago [euthanasia]?
R: Yes.
I: And the doctor said the same thing again [that euthanasia was not possible]?
R: Yes.
I: Because you can still read?
R: Because I'm still interested in things. But it's only that I try to fill in the time, by what I call "eating up letters."
I: She [the nursing home doctor] uses that as an argument against euthanasia?
R: Well, they don't say it quite like that. [Silence.]

Her physician said about the patient's suffering:

R: I also have to observe on the unit, and then I see her sitting at the table with a book, she's just sitting there reading ... and when I see her like that, well, then I think that she's reasonably well. [Silence, thinking.] Yes, in any case she doesn't seem to be suffering unbearably.
I: Because she ...
R: Because of what she doesn't say, yes, just from what you see.

The fifth patient also deemed his own suffering to be unbearable:

I: The second, and that is usually much more difficult, is that the patient must suffer unbearably, and that is often the problem.
R: Yes, well, no, because you could say that mentally it's unbearable for me. it's mentally unbearable that I bloody well have to get worse than I am already and worse than I used to be.

Among three cases in which the physician refused the patient's request, we could not interview the physician, either because the patient gave no consent or the physician did not have time for an interview. In two of these cases, the patients said that the physician had rejected their request because he or she feared legal consequences. In the third case, the patient reported that the physician had said he would only perform euthanasia at the moment when he was certain that the patient was dying.

DISCUSSION

Depending on the physician's specialty, between half and two-thirds of explicit requests for euthanasia and assisted suicide are not fulfilled. These rates have been fairly stable over the last 15 years. The complexity of decision making around euthanasia and assisted suicide is reflected in the fact that beyond the clear categories of requests granted and requests refused, three other situations can be distinguished: The patient dies before the physician has made a final decision about the request, the patient dies after the physician agrees to the request but before he or she can perform euthanasia, and the patient no longer wants euthanasia or assisted suicide.

It is interesting to consider in particular why patients come to die before their request is either rejected or fulfilled. Did the patients request euthanasia or assisted suicide too late in their illnesses (were they already close to death)? Did the physician take too much time in deciding whether to grant the request? Or did the physician overestimate survival? From the GP survey, we know that the situation of patients in this category met the official criteria for due care somewhat less often than did patients who received euthanasia/assisted suicide. Thus, it is possible that in general, the patients died before the performance of euthanasia and assisted suicide not because they were more ill but because the decision-making process took longer.[6] (As noted previously, there seems to have been concern among the physicians involved that these patients had mental health problems, in comparison to patients who received euthanasia or assisted suicide.)

The reasons given by physicians for rejecting requests for euthanasia and assisted suicide do seem to be in line with the criteria for due care. In the studies described here, physicians had doubts whether the criteria for due care had been met in those cases in which they refused patients' requests. This doubt most often concerned either of two requirements: that there be alternatives for treatment or that the patients' suffering be unbearable.

Unbearable suffering is, in fact, the most debated criterion and the one physicians experience as the most difficult to determine.[1,c] Even some patients themselves were uncertain whether their suffering was truly unbearable. On the one hand, it might be that the patients' suffering indeed was not that severe. On the other hand, it might also be that physicians – and even patients – may set a very (even unreasonably) high threshold for what is "unbearable." Some patients doubted whether their suffering was unbearable, although they stated that it was serious and that they still had a strong desire to die. In several cases, their physicians could also understand this desire, despite the fact that they did not consider the patients' suffering to have met the criterion of being unbearable.

The data suggest that there are differences between patients whose requests for euthanasia or assisted suicide are or are not fulfilled. Even among the latter, patients whose requests are refused seem to form a distinct subgroup.

In all studies described here, cancer was positively associated with requests that resulted in euthanasia or assisted suicide. (This was also found in studies done in the United States in Oregon.)[8,9] Some of these distinctions are likely due to differences in how closely physicians adhere to the criteria. However, differences in diagnosis may also be taken into account, at least partly, in the following way: Physicians may be more inclined to grant a request from a patient who has a diagnosis, like cancer, for which adherence to the criteria is generally good, than from a patient with a less clear-cut diagnosis or one who is a member of a vulnerable group, such as elderly people and people with chronic, nonterminal illnesses. Although these patients do not fall outside the scope of the Euthanasia Act per se, data suggest that physicians are less inclined to fulfill their requests. Thus, there is inequality with respect to the kinds of patients who are likely to receive euthanasia or assisted suicide among those for whom it would be permitted.

It is possible that physicians are not aware of what is permissible under the act. For instance, in the patient–physician interview study, it appeared that some physicians defined unbearable suffering more stringently than do the authorities in the Netherlands – for example, by defining it as "physical

[c] See Chapter 21 by Wijsbek.

suffering" or even more narrowly as "extreme pain." Similarly, one physician said that the patient had to be in the terminal phase before euthanasia is permissible, although this is not a legal prerequisite.

The data strongly indicate that physicians use the criteria for due care in their decision-making process, which is positive. However, it could be argued that since it seems that if anything, physicians are likely to apply the criteria for due care more rather than less strictly, some patients or groups of patients have less chance of receiving euthanasia or assisted suicide when they request it.

References

1. Onwuteaka-Philipsen, Bregje D., Joseph K. M.Gevers, Agnes van der Heide, et al. 2007. *Evaluatie Wet Toetsing Levensbeëindiging op verzoek en hulp bij zelfdoding* [Evaluation of The Termination of Life on Request and Assisted Suicide (Review Procedures) Act]. The Hague: ZonMw
2. Heide, Agnes van der, Bregje D. Onwuteaka-Philipsen, Mette L. Rurup, Hilde M. Buiting, Johannes J. M. van Delden, Johanna E. Hanssen-de Wolf, Anke Janssen, H. Roeline W. Pasman, Judith A. C. Rietjens, Cornelis Prins, Ingeborg M. Deerenberg, Joseph K. M. Gevers, Paul van der Maas, and Gerrit van der Wal. 2007. End-of-life practices in the Netherlands under the euthanasia act. *New England Journal of Medicine* 356: 1957–1965.
3. Wal, Gerrit van der, Agnes van der Heide, Bregje D. Onwuteaka-Philipsen, and Paul J. van der Maas. 2003. *Medische besluitvorming aan het einde van het leven* [Medical decision-making at the end of life]. Utrecht: Uitgeverij De Tijdstroom.
4. Onwuteaka-Philipsen, Bregje D., Agnes van der Heide, Dirk Koper, Ingeborg Keij-Deerenberg, Judith A. C. Rietjens, Mette Rurup, Astrid Vrakking, Jean Jacques Georges, Martien T. Muller, Gerrit van der Wal, and Paul J. van der Maas. 2003. Euthanasia and other end-of-life decisions in The Netherlands in 1990, 1995 and 2001. *The Lancet* 362: 395–399.
5. Haverkate, Ilinka, Bregje D. Onwuteaka-Philipsen, Agnes van der Heide, Piet J. Kostense, Gerrit van der Wal, and Paul J. van der Maas. 2000. Refused and granted requests for euthanasia and assisted suicide in the Netherlands: Interview study with structured questionnaire. *British Medical Journal* 321: 865–866.
6. Jansen-van der Weide, Marijke C., Bregje D. Onwuteaka-Philipsen, and Gerrit van der Wal. 2005. Granted, undecided, withdrawn, and refused requests for euthanasia and physician-assisted suicide. *Archives of Internal Medicine* 165: 1698–1704.
7. Pasman, H. Roeline W., Mette L. Rurup, Dick L. Willems, and Bregje D. Onwuteaka-Philipsen. 2009. Concept of unbearable suffering in context of ungranted requests for euthanasia: Qualitative interviews with patients and physicians. *British Medical Journal* 339: b43–b62.
8. Hedberg, Katrina, David Hopkins, and Melvin Kohn. 2003. Five years of legal physician-assisted suicide in Oregon. *New England Journal of Medicine* 348: 961–964.
9. Chin, Arthur E., Katrina Hedberg, Grant K. Higginson, David W. Fleming. 1999. Legalized physician-assisted suicide in Oregon – the first year's experience. *New England Journal of Medicine* 340: 577–583.

10

Dutch Euthanasia in Retrospect

John Griffiths

INTRODUCTION

For some, the euthanasia discussion begins with the Greeks, for some in the late nineteenth century, and for yet others somewhere just before or just after World War II. For me, it began in 1987 when more or less out of the blue I was asked by the editors of the *Nederlands Juristenblad* (a weekly journal for Dutch lawyers) to write an article looking at the euthanasia discussion in the Netherlands from an "outsider's" point of view.[1] At the time, I was an outsider in three senses: I was an American; I had never paid any attention to euthanasia other than as a casual reader of the newspaper; and as a sociologist of law, I was professionally committed to an observer's rather than a participant's perspective on matters legal.

As it happened, the article was very well received, and among other things it gave rise to possibilities for research funding. A decade – and a variety of research projects and a number of articles – later, our research group in Groningen published *Euthanasia and Law in the Netherlands*[2] in which we gave a full account of Dutch euthanasia law, the history of legal change, the public debate, what was known about medical practice, and in particular the successes and limitations of legal regulation.

This first book led to further possibilities of research and, as a result of increasing contacts with scholars in other countries, to an ever more international and comparative approach to the problems of effective regulation. Another 10 years, many articles, and several dissertations later, we have recently published a new book, *Euthanasia and Law in Europe*,[3] not only covering the Netherlands and Belgium but also including chapters by local experts on eight other Western European countries.

In the course of two decades of continuous and concentrated research into the regulatory aspects of euthanasia, I gradually shed two of the three outsider qualities just mentioned. I have now lived and worked in the Netherlands for over 30 years and, in the course of time, have become pretty thoroughly acculturated, including acquiring Dutch nationality. And I have been actively, if only intermittently, involved in the public discussion. But while I cannot any longer claim the first two, I have done my best to preserve the third of my outsider characteristics. Like everyone else I have personal views concerning euthanasia, but as a sociologist of law my professional interest in it has from the beginning concerned a general theoretical question: How and under what circumstances can the regulation of a socially problematic sort of behavior be effective? In my public utterances I have tried to stick closely to data and analysis concerning the effectiveness – or, as I would prefer to call it, the "social working"[4] – of euthanasia law.

I burden the reader with this bit of autobiography because it provides the latent structure to what follows. I shall return to my 1987 article about the public euthanasia discussion, and consider what developments there have been in the intervening decades with regard to the ideas discussed there and in what respects the situation now is different. The predominant perspective remains the same throughout: What can we say about the effectiveness of legal control?[a]

THE EUTHANASIA DISCUSSION IN 1987

The public discussion of euthanasia and the possibility of making it legal seemed to me remarkably civilized. Apart from a handful of fringe characters, no one was using the "Nazi" argument, insinuating hidden motives or dishonesty, or disqualifying opponents in other ways. On the other hand, the argumentative quality of the public debate was rather low. With a few exceptions,[b,5] public discussion did not consist of much more than arguments from authority (the Bible); *ipse dixit*-isms, such as "euthanasia *is* murder"; and the ritual invocation of slogans, such as "self-determination" and "sacredness of life."

While rife with supposition and speculation and rich in uncontrollable anecdotes, public discussion was almost entirely free from grounding in serious empirical information. This is probably because it was not really a public policy discussion at all but a debate about the ideal norm. Such a debate assumes that a norm that perfectly reflects the values on which it rests will be implemented in behavior and produce results that optimally realize those values. The participants do not worry whether in regulatory practice the best may well be the

[a] With a couple of unavoidable exceptions, I will make reference only to literature in English. The basic sources for most of this chapter are two books: 2. Griffiths, Bood, and Weyers 1998 and 3. Griffiths, Weyers, and Adams 2008. All literature and data referred to are current as of 2010.

[b] A report of the Health Council of 1982 (5. Gezondheidsraad 1982), meant to prepare the way for the State Commission on Euthanasia, which reported in 1985 (6. Staatscommissie Euthanasie 1985), is an important exception. However, it had little effect on the public discussion.

enemy of the good. In such a debate, empirical information is essentially irrelevant, and the State Commission on Euthanasia considered the relevance of empirical information for its work too limited to justify having it carried out.[c]

In particular, public debate paid essentially no attention to the problem of effective control. As we will see, the "medical exception" was generally thought not to cover euthanasia, and this entailed that control would take the form of criminal investigations and prosecutions. Nothing but the criminal law was "good enough" for so serious a matter of control.[d,7] But no one seemed much interested in how such a system would work in practice. Whether the duty of doctors to report a "non-natural" death could support an adequate system of control was not discussed. Other possible forms of control – in particular, guidelines of professional associations and protocols of hospitals and nursing homes – played no role in the discussion at all.

One of the most important contributions of the State Commission to a fruitful public discussion of euthanasia was to give it a clear, narrow, official definition: ending the life of another person at that person's request. This made it possible to argue about the desirability of legalizing euthanasia, free from the Babylonian confusion that had heretofore plagued the debate. But however important for the sake of debate, definitional clarity is a different matter from effective control. No attention was addressed to the question whether excluding other forms of medical behavior that potentially shorten the life of a patient from the control system being worked out for euthanasia might in practice undermine the regulation of euthanasia.

In short, as I wrote in 1987, the public discussion seemed to be "floating in an ideological ether," essentially unconnected with the social practices that it ostensibly was about. The lack of attention in the public and political discussion to the ways in which the legal rules – whatever they became – could effectively regulate medical practice was echoed in the process of legal change taking place concurrently in the courts. Dutch judges legalized euthanasia by means of the justification of necessity. But finding sensible practical solutions in individual cases is not a way of creating an effective general system of control.

I identified two other weaknesses in the public discussion as of 1987, matters that were already giving rise to problems that are still with us. In the first place, euthanasia was conceived as a problem of doctors, and the solutions being discussed involved allowing doctors, and only doctors, to do something that had theretofore been forbidden to everyone. No one seemed aware of the fact that offering a new mode of dying to patients who want it, by giving a new behavioral possibility to doctors willing to perform it, was going to lead to problems. I predicted that the monopoly of the medical profession over legal euthanasia would inevitably lead to the imposition of some sort of obligation

[c] 6. Staatscommissie Euthanasie 1985, vol. 1, p. 21. The minority, in a dissenting report, appeared to agree (id. at p. 326).

[d] See 7. Griffiths 2007 on this assumption and how it was falsified in practice.

on doctors – or, at least, on the profession as a whole – to make sure that it is, in fact, available to individual patients.

In the second place, no attention was being paid to the differences between euthanasia and physician-assisted suicide.

THE SITUATION MORE THAN 20 YEARS LATER

Almost a quarter of a century later, the most dramatic change in the public discussion is that the legality of euthanasia has vanished as an issue from the political agenda. A decade and a half after the courts had effectively made it legal, the euthanasia law of 2002 essentially codified what the courts had already accomplished. For the first time since the early 1980s, euthanasia legislation was no longer pending in Parliament. There is now no significant public voice calling for a return to the legal past, and occasional criticisms from abroad tend to be shrugged off. Of course there remain people – and politicians – who regret what happened and who might want to turn back the clock if there were suddenly a majority to be found for such a proposal. But forbidding euthanasia is not high on anyone's list of priorities. Most of the continuing discussion has become professionalized and technical and has to do either with refinements of the system of control or with one or another unforeseen consequence of the key role of the doctor, in particular in the case of people who request euthanasia although they are not suffering from a "medical" condition. The legitimacy and effective control of other kinds of medical behavior that potentially shorten the life of a patient (most recently, so-called terminal sedation, about which more later) has also gradually begun to attract attention.

A Wealth of Reliable and Not-So-Reliable Information

Serious discussion of euthanasia policy nowadays is based not on ideological oppositions but on the vast amount of empirical information that has become available over the last two decades (some of which is presented in this book).[e] The quantitative data (I will say a few words on qualitative data further on) concern such matters as the frequency of euthanasia and related behavior, the diseases and other characteristics of those who request it and those who receive it, the decision-making process involved, the extent to which the applicable rules are being followed, and the operation of the legal control system. It seems useful to say a few words about the strengths and weaknesses of this information.

Quantitative Studies

The strengths of the available quantitative data lie in the careful, responsible methodologies used to collect them, in particular in the so-called death

[e] For an extensive presentation of the available data, see 3. Griffiths, Weyers, and Adams 2008.

certificate studies; in the large national samples on which these studies are based, the high response rates achieved (partly due to the watertight guarantees given by the Ministry of Justice that facts revealed would not be used for purposes of criminal prosecution), and the resulting high levels of statistical significance; and in the fact that not only "euthanasia" in the narrow sense, but also all medical behavior that potentially shortens the life of the patient is studied at the same time and in the same way – that is, in the fact that euthanasia is studied in the context of its behavioral alternatives. A final strength lies in the fact that the national studies have been repeated four times since 1990, roughly every five years. These are formidable strengths, to the credit largely of those who first designed the death certificate studies in 1990. Their approach has become the international standard for this sort of research, used in recent years in similar surveys in a number of other countries so that comparable data are now available (albeit nowhere of equal quality).[f]

What is not generally appreciated is that the death certificate approach has some important shortcomings. The data collected in such studies derive from doctors. About the "medical" facts of individual cases (the patient's medical situation, the drugs and other treatments used or withheld, and so forth) there is probably little reason to question the accuracy of the data.[g] But data on the number of requests (and of refused requests), on patients' reasons for their requests, on whether the request was discussed with those close to the patient and with nurses, on why a request was or was not carried out, and so forth are known to be the subject of substantial differences of view between the various participants (for example, a doctor may think a patient withdrew his or her request, whereas the patient thinks the doctor refused it). It is thus essential to keep the source of the data in mind when interpreting the results of death certificate studies.

Another problem with existing quantitative data concerns the way in which different sorts of medical behavior have been classified by the investigators. I have already noted how important it is that "euthanasia" was not studied in isolation from other medical behavior that causes a patient to die at another time or in a different way from what otherwise would have been the case. But the value of this approach has been undermined by insufficient critical attention to the definitions used and to the way they are operationalized in research. Nor have the investigators responsible for the four national studies proven receptive (until recently) to external criticisms on this point.

[f] For a more detailed presentation of the methodology of the "death certificate" approach in Dutch research and in studies elsewhere using the same or slightly different methodologies, see 3. Griffiths, Weyers, and Adams 2008, specifically pp. 149–152 and Chapter 17.

[g] Such complacency is, however, out of place as far as the cause of death and the effects of drugs are concerned, and even more so regarding doctors' estimates of a patient's life expectancy and the amount of life shortening due to a particular treatment. Doctors' assessments of voluntariness and competence, and even more so of suffering, are also probably subject to a great deal of interpersonal – and intercultural – variability.

The classification of medical behavior in the Dutch studies (and in a major international, comparative study)[8] depends on essentially subjective (and uncontrollable) statements by doctors about what their intention was in administering pain relief in a potentially life-shortening dose: to shorten the patient's life or to relieve his or her pain.[h] In effect, for research purposes, the investigators adopted the basic idea (but not the crucial restrictions) of the doctrine of double effect, which treats the intention of the actor as determinative of the morality of his or her act. Thus, the criticism that some foreign observers[9] have made of the Dutch data – to the effect that much of what is classified as "pain relief" (because of what doctors report about their intentions) may "really" be euthanasia or termination of life without a request – is correct as far as it goes. But the convenient supposition of such critics, that the problem only arises when "euthanasia" is legal, overlooks the fact that the very same classification problem may to a significant extent account for the apparently low level of "euthanasia" in countries where it is illegal but where the level of death due to "pain relief" is often higher than it is in the Netherlands.[i] Dutch doctors may well simply be blunter about their "real" intentions.

A second objection to the way the investigators approach the classification of medical behavior that potentially shortens life is that it does not correspond to the applicable legal classifications. In particular, the subjective conception of intention that they use to distinguish between pain relief and euthanasia (or termination of life without a request) has no foundation in the criminal law.[j] To make a long story short, the relevant distinguishing criterion is not the doctor's intention but the existence of a medical indication.[3] Pain relief, when indicated and given in indicated doses, does not amount to termination of life even if it causes the patient's death. On the other hand, giving pain relief that is

[h] How the questions were posed will be discussed. A similar but probably less critical problem concerns the classification of behavior as withholding/withdrawing treatment or as termination of life.

[i] For comparative data, see 3. Griffiths, Weyers, and Adams 2008, p. 489. Ironically, some vociferous opponents of legal euthanasia (e.g., 9. Keown 2002), convinced that it is impossible to keep euthanasia under control, contribute to that very situation by emphasizing what they take to be a fundamental difference between euthanasia and pain relief, namely, the doctor's subjective intention. In every country where the difference is so defined, we can be quite sure that "euthanasia" – while illegal and barely visible in available data – is in fact taking place under the guise of "pain relief," with doctors adjusting their (stated) "intention" to the exigencies of local law and morality. Under such circumstances, it is unlikely that euthanasia practice will be surrounded by significant safeguards.

[j] The "doctrine of double effect," important in Catholic moral teaching (which has the benefit of an omniscient judge who can know precisely with which of various externally unobservable "intentions" an act was done), has never been recognized for legal purposes, for the excellent reason that mere mortals have no way of making the required judgments. The criminal law works with an objectified intention (knowledge of the probable consequences of behavior), which means that medical behavior known to the particular doctor to be likely to cause death is always "intentional."

expected to cause death does amount to termination of life if it is not medically indicated. It is quite clear from recent research[k,10] that if looked at by a prosecuting attorney, a considerable amount of what the investigators in the Dutch studies have classified as pain relief would be regarded as termination of life.

Ethnographic Studies

The strengths of the information produced by the sort of quantitative surveys I have been discussing lie in their representativeness and their supposed "hardness" and "objectivity." These are more or less counterbalanced by the classificatory problem just noted and by the fact that such survey data give little insight into the question why, and as a result of what processes, the data are distributed as they are (for example, why the ratio of physician-assisted suicide to euthanasia is so small and steadily declining). Further, as we have seen, the available quantitative data derive almost exclusively from doctors. Ideally, for every quantitative survey, one would like to have a companion ethnographic study – interviews and observations – of the same matter, and for every study from the doctor's perspective, one from that of the other participants (patient, family, nurses, etc.). Unfortunately, such studies are expensive and time consuming, generally carry less prestige, and require expertise not widely available. They are therefore rare.

Nevertheless, in recent years there have been a handful of good ethnographic studies of the problematic communication between doctors and dying patients;[l,11] of the "euthanasia talk" among doctor, patient, and family made possible by legalization;[m,12,13] and of the participation by parents in the decision making concerning end-of-life treatment of extremely premature newborns in a Dutch and a Belgian neonatal intensive care unit (NICU).[n,14,15]

Despite these and a few other studies,[o,16,17,18,19,20] more than a quarter century into the euthanasia discussion in the Netherlands, we still know far too little

[k] See 10. van Tol 2005 (which unfortunately is not yet available in English; see 3. Griffiths, Weyers, and Adams 2008 for a brief summary).

[l] See 11. The 1999. This study of communication between doctors and patients in a cancer ward where an experimental therapy was being offered to patients with incurable lung cancer shows how the structure of communication systematically undermines the autonomy of patients.

[m] See 12. Norwood 2005 and 13. Norwood 2007. Norwood's findings show that the legality of euthanasia has made possible a cultural practice in which "euthanasia is more often a discussion than it is a life-ending act." And this discussion includes far more than "the immediate, the obvious (planning for death) [but also serves] to affirm social bonds and social life at the end of Dutch life" (see 12. Norwood 2005, pp.8–9).

[n] See 14. Vermeulen 2001 and 15. Vermeulen 2004. Vermeulen's research shows that involvement of the parents was expected and generally achieved in both NICUs. He further confirms the impression from quantitative data that medical practice in relation to very ill newborns is similar in the two countries. Termination of life is not an acknowledged practice, although medical behavior that fits the definition of termination of life does occur in connection with the withdrawal of treatment.

[o] See 16. Chabot 1996, 17. Chabot 2001, and 18. Chabot 2007 (Chabot's research concerned suicide without the help of a doctor as a reaction to various forms of avoidance by doctors).; 19.

about the perspective of the patient (and his or her family and intimate social surroundings). What patients want and why, whether they succeed in getting it and when and how they do, what their experiences are of the process of dying in various ways, how all this resounds in their immediate social surroundings – all this is still largely uncharted territory. Politicians, publicists, and others invoke shopworn slogans with no known empirical foundation (e.g., that a request for euthanasia is a "cry for help," or, on the other hand, that it is an exercise of "self-determination"), but apart from a handful of determined individual researchers, very few people give evidence of being seriously interested in knowing what euthanasia means in practice for those who do or do not receive it.

The Question of Adequate Control

If euthanasia is to be legalized, one of the most important points of concern is whether as a practice it can be kept under adequate societal control. Often, adequate control is (wrongly) identified with adequate *legal* control or even with control by means of *criminal law*.[7] Unfounded "doubts" that adequate legal control is possible, and tendentious interpretations of the Dutch experience as "proof" that it is not, are the most widespread form of foreign criticism of legalization of euthanasia. It is interesting to note that the Dutch themselves are not overly troubled by the issue, although the transparency of euthanasia practice – which, in practice, usually means accurate reporting by doctors who perform it – has been a key objective of Dutch policy from the very beginning.[p]

The "Reporting Rate"

How frequently doctors are reporting euthanasia can be calculated by comparing the numbers of reports received with the total amount of euthanasia estimated in the national death certificate studies. In these studies, the classification of a doctor's behavior as amounting to one or another of the different medical behaviors that potentially shorten life is not done by the doctor who provides the basic data but by the researcher according to a standard scheme. There is an obvious advantage to this approach: It enables varying interpretations of terms like *euthanasia* to be excluded. Unfortunately, there are also powerful objections.

van Dam 2005 (Van Dam's interviews with family and intimates revealed a considerable level of ignorance, avoidance, and procedural errors on the part of doctors); 20. Thomasma, et al., 1998 (Thomasma and his colleagues report largely positive accounts of euthanasia by family members).

[p] For the current system of reporting and review, see 3. Griffiths, Weyers, and Adams 2008, pp. 126–127, and Chapter 4.2.4.3. For the history of the reporting procedure through 1997, see 2. Griffiths, Bood, and Weyers 1998, Chapters 2.3.3 and 3.2; for the origins of the idea of reporting outside the sphere of the criminal law, see id., pp. 278–282.

To appreciate the problem, it is essential to revisit the question of how the investigators classify the behavior of doctors. Roughly speaking, the procedure is as follows:[q] For every death certificate included in their sample, the responsible doctor is asked whether the patient's death was due to withholding or withdrawing treatment or to administration of a drug, whether the patient asked for this, and what the doctor's intention was. If the doctor reports that the patient died from administration of a drug, that the patient had asked for this, and that the doctor's "explicit intention" was to cause death, the investigators classify the case as one of "euthanasia." If there was no request from the patient, it is one of termination of life without a request. If the doctor says that his or her intention was not principally to cause death but to relieve pain, the case is classified as one of "pain relief with life-shortening effect."

Such classifications made by researchers do not always correspond to doctors' own ideas about what sort of behavior they were engaged in, ideas that determine whether they report a case as euthanasia. There are a number of pieces of internal evidence in the Dutch quantitative data that doctors do not necessarily regard a case as one of euthanasia just because they "intended" to cause the death of the patient; they may nevertheless consider it to be a case of pain relief. There are also external qualitative indications (observations of the way doctors describe their own behavior) to the same effect. Research by Donald van Tol, specifically directed at the way that doctors and others classify medical behavior, demonstrates beyond a shadow of a doubt that this is the case:

> Doctors classify as "euthanasia" prototypical cases in which a doctor administers by injection an immediately lethal substance (not morphine) to a patient on his request at a moment agreed upon beforehand.[r]

In the most recent national survey, the investigators themselves have finally responded to criticism based on all these indications. They conclude that when morphine is the drug used, doctors almost never consider the case to be one of euthanasia, regardless of how they describe their intention.

This finding is of critical importance in connection with the so-called reporting rate. Doctors are required to report cases of euthanasia as such, and reporting is the basis of the whole system of legal control.[s] The supposed fact that they do not always do so has for years been regarded, understandably, as the Achilles' heel of Dutch euthanasia policy. The reporting rate calculated on the basis of the national surveys was 18% in 1990, 41% in 1995, 54% in 2001, and

[q] For a detailed account, see 3. Griffiths, Weyers, and Adams 2008, pp. 150–152.

[r] See 3.Griffiths, Weyers, and Adams 2008, p. 203.

[s] Technically, a doctor may not report a death due to "intentional termination of life" as a "natural death" on a patient's death certificate – to do so is a criminal offense (in effect, a form of perjury). Cases described as "not reported" are, in fact, cases that are *falsely* reported as natural deaths. Hence, the expression "lying doctor" in the text.

most recently almost 80% (in itself a progression that is no mean accomplishment). The "missing cases" were taken to be cases, in effect, of "lying": Doctors know that what they have done is euthanasia but willfully fail to report it as such.[t] International and domestic criticism of Dutch euthanasia policy focused on the weaknesses of a control system where so much lying seemed to be going on, and for more than a decade the Dutch policy discussion was addressed to the question of how to reduce the rate of lying by making honest reporting more attractive to doctors. The Regional Review Committees, which since 1998 have taken over from the prosecutorial service the task of assessing reported cases for conformity to the "requirements of due care," were supposed to contribute to honest reporting by forming a "buffer" between doctors and the criminal law system (in which doctors were thought to have little confidence).[u]

How then is a reporting rate calculated? It is a fraction whose numerator is precisely known: the number of reports. The denominator is the number of actual cases of euthanasia revealed in the national surveys, using the methodology already described. In other words, the numerator is determined by *doctors'* interpretations of the concept "euthanasia" when deciding whether to report a case, but the denominator is determined by the *researchers'* interpretation. Doctors obviously only report a case as one of euthanasia if that is what they think it was. So a disappointing reporting rate may not reflect dishonesty by doctors but simply the fact that they interpret "euthanasia" in a way different from that of the researchers. And that is in effect precisely what the investigators in the national studies ultimately concluded, although they have not exactly trumpeted the fact that their earlier, disappointing reporting rates are based on classificatory quicksand.

The results of the 2005 research, adjusted to take account of the problem of classification, led to the conclusion that the rate of honest reporting nowadays is close to 100%. And whether it is 80% (measured in the old way) or almost 100% (measured in the new way), it has ceased to be seen as a major policy problem. An issue that dominated the public debate for about 15 years has largely vanished from the scene. This is a pity, since while it is true that "lying doctors" are (and probably for quite some time have been) a rare phenomenon, this does not mean that nothing troublesome is going on.

The fact that "lying" is not (any longer) the crux of the matter does not mean that the problem of nonreporting has been solved. But it does turn the problem into something rather different from what it has been thought to be. Since doctors are now reporting virtually all cases that they themselves consider to be euthanasia, trying to make them honest will not increase transparency. The need is to *educate* them about the legal differences between euthanasia

[t] See 3. Griffiths, Weyers, and Adams 2008 on the "lying doctor hypothesis."

[u] There is in fact little or no evidence that the committees had such an effect (3. Griffiths, Weyers, and Adams 2008, p. 201), although in other important respects there is much to be said in their favor (id., p. 137).

and pain relief. Doctors need to learn that the euthanasia they are required to report concerns cases in which the patient dies due to the intentional administration of a *nonindicated dose* of a potentially lethal drug.[v] And the national researchers need to be persuaded to redesign the death certificate studies in the same way. Only then will we have legally accurate data on the frequency of euthanasia, and a reporting rate whose numerator and denominator are based on the same classification of behavior.[w]

The Flight into "Pain Relief" and "Terminal Sedation"

Euthanasia has permeable borders with other behavior that potentially shortens the life of the patient: pain relief (which I have already addressed), as well as withholding/withdrawing treatment and "terminal sedation."[x] When one of these (euthanasia) is subject to strict and, for a doctor, burdensome control while the others are not, one can expect doctors to prefer the path of least resistance when it is available, and to choose to shorten life in a way not subject to such control. Instead of performing euthanasia, they can accomplish the same result in a slightly different and more convenient way. In our 1998 book, we referred to this possibility as the "constructibility" of medical behavior that shortens life. At the time, there was plenty of indirect evidence in the Dutch data that it was going on.[y] The consequences for the effectiveness of legal control of euthanasia are obvious: If we think that allowing doctors to shorten the lives of their patients is dangerous – as it plainly is – we should not be satisfied to control only those ways of doing so that bear a given name. The seeming success of the Dutch system of legal control of euthanasia is made somewhat illusory by the phenomenon of constructibility. The same applies a fortiori to legal systems in which euthanasia (but not its alternatives) is entirely illegal.

[v] Similar problems exist in the case of withholding or withdrawing treatment (3. Griffiths, Weyers, and Adams 2008, pp. 73–75).

[w] Another problem in the classification of causes of death (and hence with regard to the duty to report "non-natural" deaths) is the role of *post hoc ergo propter hoc* reasoning in such cases, especially when a drug with notoriously unpredictable and generally exaggerated lethal effect (morphine) is used with the expectation that death will result. Since in a significant number of cases the patient's death will actually not be due to the morphine but to the patient's underlying condition, attributing the expected result (death) to the behavior concerned will, to a greater or lesser extent, overestimate the amount of termination of life actually going on. The same problem of causation underlies the classification of cases of death as due to pain relief or to withholding and withdrawing treatment. In short, the sum total of all deaths due to something a doctor intentionally does or does not do, as measured in death certificate research, is probably inflated.

[x] The terms "terminal" and "palliative" sedation have yet to acquire settled meanings. Both involve deep, continuous sedation of a dying patient. I reserve the term *terminal sedation* for the situation in which, because artificial feeding and hydration is withheld for a period long enough that this is expected to be the cause of the patient's death, the behavior must be considered potentially life shortening.

[y] See 2. Griffiths, Bood, and Weyers 1998, pp. 254–257.

The early years of this century saw an apparent decline in the frequency of euthanasia, and there may have been a concurrent increase in the frequency of death due to "terminal sedation."[z] Anecdotal evidence suggests that such a shift may have been largely a matter of constructibility, doctors preferring not to perform euthanasia where there was a less onerous alternative.[aa] But in the absence of research directly addressed to the question, it seems wise to reserve judgment on whether palliative sedation was or is being used "instead of" euthanasia. There are those, of course, who would welcome such a shift, because it would seem to confirm their view that euthanasia is not really necessary at all if adequate pain relief (including terminal sedation) is given. But there are others who would be troubled by it, since they argue that "slow euthanasia," as terminal sedation is sometimes referred to, is – from the point of view of public policy, if perhaps not of morality – quite as dangerous as euthanasia.[21] It follows from that view that it ought to be subjected to a similar control regime.[bb]

Review and Sanctions

Beginning informally in 1997 and continuing formally under the 2002 statutory legalization of euthanasia, legal review of reported cases of euthanasia is the responsibility of the five Regional Review Committees, each consisting of a lawyer, a doctor, and an ethicist. The committees have been a stunning success. They address careful and expert attention to more than 2,000 cases per year, something the prosecutorial authorities had proven neither capable of nor competent in doing themselves. In the period before the establishment of the Regional Review Committees in 1998, about 9,000 cases had been reported to the prosecutorial authorities, of which (in the later years) only 1% to 2% had actually been discussed each year by the College of Procurators General, the body responsible for decisions whether to prosecute. From 1991 through 1995, the College gave full consideration to only 120 of more than 6,000 cases. There seems to have been a total of about 20 prosecutions to date.[cc]

[z] 3. See 3. Griffiths, Weyers, and Adams 2008, p. 201 (euthanasia reporting data through 2006); p. 165 (data on palliative and terminal sedation together). The downward trend in the number of reports of euthanasia since 1998 has recently come to an end, and since 2007 the numbers are increasing again. According to the annual reports of the Regional Review Committees, 2,120 cases were reported in 2007, 2,331 in 2008, 2,636 in 2009, and 3,136 in 2010.

[aa] In theory, a patient does not have to accept his or her doctor's preference. The Regional Review Committees have held that euthanasia in the case of a patient who refuses terminal sedation does not violate the due care requirement that there be no available alternative treatment (see 3. Griffiths, Weyers, and Adams 2008, p. 92 n. 179).

[bb] See the argument to this effect in 7. Griffiths 2007.

[cc] See 2. Griffiths, Bood, and Weyers, p. 244, and 3.Griffiths, Weyers, and Adams 2008, pp. 207, 505.

The committees rarely find a doctor to have violated the "requirements of due care," a finding that under the Law of 2002 is a prerequisite to criminal prosecution. In the few cases in which the committees have found a doctor in violation of the requirements, the prosecutorial authorities have so far never decided to bring criminal charges.[dd] There are, however, several more informal sanctions that the committees make use of frequently. And in most of the really troublesome cases, either a prosecutor or a medical inspector discusses the case with the doctor(s) concerned. In particularly serious cases, medical disciplinary proceedings are brought.

RESURRECTION OF THE "MEDICAL EXCEPTION"?

Early on in the legal developments concerning euthanasia, the idea that it should be regulated in the context of the so-called medical exception was roundly rejected. The medical exception is an implicit exception for normal medical practice (e.g., injections and surgery) from the literal coverage of the criminal law provisions that protect bodily integrity. Legal regulation of normal medical practice is largely left to the law of contracts and torts and to medical disciplinary law. In 1998, I argued that treating euthanasia in the same way would ultimately be more effective than regulating it in the context of the criminal law.[ee] The Law of 2002, however, continued on the path already chosen: Euthanasia is regulated in the form of a qualified exception to the relevant sections of the Criminal Code. A doctor whose behavior does not fall within the exception is guilty of a very serious criminal offense (a form of homicide).

While the medical exception has thus been formally rejected, it seems to have entered informally through the back door. As we have seen, initial review of all reported cases is in the hands of the Regional Review Committees and a case can only be prosecuted if a committee decides that the doctor has violated the requirements of due care. The committees almost never do this, and even if they do, prosecutions are – so far, at least – not brought. Instead, a number of less drastic forms of control are used.

At the same time, the burden of control seems to be shifting from after the fact to before the fact. Since 1997, a system of professionalized consultation has been in place, providing expert, independent consultants to doctors considering euthanasia.[ff] The 2005 national study shows that these so-called SCEN[gg] consultants are now used in about 90% of cases of euthanasia. Both the Royal Dutch Medical Association (KNMG) and the Regional Review Committees have repeatedly stressed the importance they attach to SCEN consultation.

[dd] See 3.Griffiths, Weyers, and Adams 2008, 214–215.

[ee] See 2. Griffiths, Bood, and Weyers, pp. 285 ff.

[ff] See 3.Griffiths, Weyers, and Adams 2008, pp. 138–140.

[gg] Steun en Consultatie Euthanasie Nederland (Support and Consultation Euthanasia Netherlands).

And it is clear from research data that the SCEN consultants play an increasingly key role in the system of control of euthanasia practice.[hh]

In the meantime, there has been continuous production of professional guidelines covering both euthanasia and related end-of-life medical practice (in particular, withholding and withdrawing treatment and palliative/terminal sedation).[ii] Generally, these cover both the substantive criterion ("medical indication") that a doctor is expected to apply and the decision-making procedures he or she should follow. In this way, the medical profession has taken seriously the regulatory responsibility placed in its hands by the Supreme Court in the *Schoonheim* case, in which the defense of justification was held to be applicable to euthanasia performed by a doctor. The court, in referring to "responsible medical opinion" and "the applicable norms of medical ethics," plainly relied on the expressed willingness of the organized medical profession to play a regulatory role.[jj]

In short, as it actually functions, Dutch euthanasia practice seems a very nice example of how decriminalized regulation – in effect, the medical exception – can work in practice. Despite the concerns often expressed about such a development, there is every indication that regulation of this sort of precarious medical practice is far more effective in the Netherlands than in countries where euthanasia remains illegal.

SOME IMPORTANT UNFINISHED LEGAL BUSINESS

Lest the foregoing paragraphs paint all too rosy a picture, it is important to note some legal business that was already apparent in 1987 when I first addressed the subject and that remains unfinished.

From the beginning, the Dutch have been principally concerned with what doctors legally may do, not (directly) with the legal position of patients or others. As we have seen, such an exclusive focus on doctors has been reflected both in the Dutch national surveys and in all comparable international studies, and data from and about doctors have dominated the public discussion. The most important unfinished legal business has to do in one way or another with the limitations of such a narrow focus.[kk]

[hh] See 3.Griffiths, Weyers, and Adams 2008, pp. 194–196.

[ii] See, for examples, 2. Griffiths, Bood, and Weyers 1998, Chapters 3.3 and 3.4 (discussing reports of the Medical Association's Committee on the Acceptability of Life-Ending Treatment [CAL], the Dutch Association for Pediatrics [NVK], and the Dutch Association for Psychiatry [NVP]). See also 3. Griffiths, Weyers, and Adams 2008, Chapter 4.2.2.4 (Medical Association report on palliative/terminal sedation) and Chapter 6 (various reports on neonatology).

[jj] See 2. Griffiths, Bood, and Weyers 1998, p. 328, for the relevant passage of the Supreme Court's decision. See id. at p. 31 for the court's reliance on the Medical Association's willingness to assume responsibility.

[kk] In addition to the matters discussed in the text, the highly unsatisfactory situation concerning the legal position of nurses is also connected with the historic focus on doctors. See 3. Griffiths, Weyers, and Adams 2008, pp.108–111, for discussion of this.

The Responsibility of Doctors and the Rights of Patients

There has, of course, been a great deal of lip service paid to patient self-determination, but as a practical matter, the only role this principle has played in Dutch euthanasia law is as a limiting condition on the empowerment of doctors to perform euthanasia in order to relieve suffering due to a "medical" disorder. It is absolutely clear that no patient, whatever his or her suffering, has a "right" to euthanasia (with a corresponding "duty" on the part of a doctor to perform it). Nor is it permissible for a doctor to perform euthanasia only on the basis of a voluntary request, as in the case of patients who are not "suffering" or whose suffering is not "medical" in nature.[ll] In the long run, as I predicted in 1987, given the monopoly of the medical profession over legal euthanasia (the doctor, as the Dutch put it, has the "keys to the medicine cabinet"), such restrictions on the availability of euthanasia will not be sustainable.

The easiest problem to solve – at least legally speaking – will concern the right of a patient who is suffering due to a medical disorder and who meets all the other legal requirements for euthanasia, but whose doctor is unwilling for personal reasons to perform it. The medical profession as a whole will be regarded as being responsible for ensuring access, and a doctor not willing to perform euthanasia will be required to refer his or her patient to a doctor who is willing. This is arguably the legal position already, and if not, there are definite signs of movement in that direction.[mm] Enforcement will be difficult, of course, but organizations such as the Dutch Association for Voluntary Euthanasia (NVVE) and probably the Medical Association itself, will come to play a facilitating role.

Assistance in Dying by Laypersons, and "Auto-Euthanasia"

It seems pretty clear that the solution to the problem of those who want to die in a humane way[nn] but who are not "sick" or not "suffering" will have to be found outside the medical profession. There are basically two paths that such people could take in order to end their lives in a way that is, or could be made, legal: with the assistance of laypersons or by doing it themselves.

The first possibility involves – technically – not euthanasia but assisted suicide. In Western European countries, assistance with suicide has generally not been illegal since the Napoleonic codifications, except when specifically made illegal at some time thereafter. The Netherlands is an example of the latter case, assistance with suicide having been made an offense late in the nineteenth century in reaction to a notorious case in which the accused was charged with murder for his participation in a suicide pact that he survived, but was acquitted

[ll] See 3.Griffiths, Weyers, and Adams 2008, pp. 122–123.

[mm] See 3.Griffiths, Weyers, and Adams 2008, pp. 107–108.

[nn] Chabot defines "humane" suicide as suicide without violence or physical disfiguring, and not carried out in isolation from family and friends (see 18. Chabot 2007).

because assisting suicide was not a crime.[oo,22] In Dutch euthanasia law, assistance with suicide – when given by a doctor – is subject to essentially the same requirements and control as euthanasia in the strict sense (I have included both of them under the term *euthanasia* in this chapter).[pp,23]

By contrast, in countries like France, Belgium, and Germany, assistance with suicide is not in itself punishable, and a lay practice could in theory come into being.[qq] However, only Switzerland in fact has a regular, institutionalized practice of assisted suicide.[24] Doctors are involved only to the extent that they must check the physical and mental condition of a would-be suicide before prescribing the necessary lethal drugs. Actual assistance is given by an experienced volunteer from one of several Swiss right-do-die organizations. In general, the circumstances under which Swiss law permits a doctor to write a prescription, and the internal rules of the right-to-die organizations, limit assisted suicide to persons who, roughly speaking, meet the requirements of the Dutch euthanasia law (medical condition and suffering).

Limitations of the Dutch and the Swiss sort on the availability of euthanasia to the nonsick and the nonsuffering generally derive from a single ethical and legal problem: The right to self-determination of the person concerned can justify his or her suicide but is not sufficient to justify another person's assistance. This problem can be circumvented if the person carries out a humane suicide him- or herself. One way – not so easy in practice and easily afoul of the line separating suicide from assisted suicide – is to acquire the necessary drugs in some way (e.g., by saving up sleeping pills or some other potentially lethal drug acquired on prescription, or by traveling to a country where effective drugs are more readily available). One can then consume them either alone or in the presence of (but without any assistance from) those dear to one.

Another effective method, especially for the elderly, is to refrain from drinking and eating. From the point of view of self-determination, this has the advantage that it does not need to involve the active participation of anyone else, and by contrast with violent and disfiguring forms of suicide (hanging, shooting, drowning), it meets the requirement of being humane. It is also entirely legal, and there is nothing to prevent a doctor or anyone else from giving palliative assistance.

Recent research by Chabot using a very conservative methodology shows that what he calls "auto-euthanasia" (nonviolent suicide in continuous contact with others) accounts for about 3.2% of all deaths in the Netherlands (2.1% the stopping of eating and drinking, 1.1% sleeping pills). This is more

[oo] See 22. Weyers 2004, pp. 23–27, for the legislative history of the prohibition.

[pp] One piece of unfinished business, in my view, is to distinguish more clearly between the two and to give a "preferred" legal status to physician-assisted suicide (see 23. Griffiths 2007). As a matter of fact, Dutch doctors strongly prefer euthanasia (see 3. Griffiths, Weyers, and Adams 2008, pp. 178–180).

[qq] For Belgium and France, see 3. Griffiths, Weyers, and Adams 2008.

than the annual total of euthanasia and physician-assisted suicide (2.8% in the same period).[rr]

In short, if the current limitations on the involvement of a doctor in euthanasia remain in place – and there is no reason to think they will not – then it seems likely that those who fall outside the current arrangements will increasingly make use of the support of laypersons. Such support might take the form of institutionalized assistance by experienced volunteers (as in Switzerland), which can offer as much by way of safety and control as the current Dutch "medical" approach, but which in the Netherlands would require significant legal change. More likely – in countries like the Netherlands – nonmedical support will be in the context of "auto-euthanasia," in particular when it takes the form of stopping eating and drinking.

CONCLUDING REFLECTIONS

In 1987, the Dutch discussion of euthanasia was still very naive. This despite several reports of the Medical Association, a report of the State Commission on Euthanasia in 1985, several court decisions leading up to the recognition of a defense of necessity in 1984, legalization bills pending in Parliament since 1984, and extensive attention in the academic and professional literature and the popular press.[ss] But all of this had taken place in the absence of the sort of detailed knowledge that can only emerge once there exists an active, institutionalized practice. The modern world's first legalization of euthanasia was therefore a bit of a leap in the dark, accompanied by euphoric hopes and apocalyptic fears.

In the intervening years, euthanasia practice has become normalized, and naïveté has given way to considerable sophistication. A great deal is now known about how euthanasia looks when it goes well, and about all the things that can go wrong even when the practice is legal and out in the open.[tt,25] The rudimentary contours of a regulatory system that already existed in 1987 ("voluntary request," "unbearable suffering," "prospect of improvement," "independent consultation," "due care in performance," "duty to report") have all been fleshed out in great detail. There is now in place a system of review outside the context of the criminal law. It processes about 2,000 cases a year, is the main locus of legal interpretation and development, and, through its production of individual case reports and annual reports, and in more informal ways, is responsible for a highly transparent medical and regulatory practice.

Wild speculations concerning the extent and characteristics of euthanasia practice have given way to sober estimates based on careful – if, as we have seen, imperfect – research.

[rr] See 18. Chabot 2007; for a summary, see 3. Griffiths, Weyers, and Adams 2008, pp. 182–184.

[ss] See Chapter 2 in 2. Griffiths, Bood, and Weyers 1998 for a full discussion of all of this.

[tt] For a grim picture of euthanasia practice when it is entirely illegal, see 25. Magnusson 2002.

Fears of a slippery slope into abhorrent practices have proven unfounded. But at the same time, the assumption that legal euthanasia would be readily available to those "entitled" to it has faded as the great reluctance of doctors to perform it has become increasingly apparent and Dutch politics has proven unwilling to provide relief for those who fall outside the current "medical model."

The international discussion of euthanasia and its possible legalization has become more open, more honest, more respectful. On both sides, the ideological shouters have largely quieted down, making room for more dispassionate consideration of the pros and cons of the Dutch approach. The Dutch have become much less defensive, no longer feeling the need to misrepresent Dutch euthanasia law to make it palatable for external consumers.[uu] Policymakers no longer consider it important to minimize the voices of those who express criticisms of one or another aspect of Dutch euthanasia policy.[vv] Observers in many other countries now seem genuinely interested in the Dutch experiment in all of its cultural specificity and medico-legal complexity.

In 1987, euthanasia was radical, exciting, a little dangerous. It seemed a part of a general cultural revolution that was leading to a freer, opener, more uninhibited way of life, in which death followed sex, drugs, psychiatric disorders, and other things as subjects that could be discussed in public. With the benefit of hindsight, the shadow side it shares with other successful revolutions is now readily apparent. The emancipation of the dying has been partial, at best, and institutionalized euthanasia practice can perhaps better be seen in a nonromantic light: as part and parcel of the increasing juridification of the doctor–patient relationship.[ww] A service to their patients that doctors have (more or less secretly) performed in one form or another since time immemorial has been brought out into the open and subjected to legal rules and formal legal review.

References

1. Griffiths, John. 1987. Een toeschouwersperspectief op de euthanasiediscussie [An observer's perspective on the euthanasia discussion]. *Nederlands Juristenblad* 62: 681–693.

[uu] The most egregious example of such misrepresentation was, in the past, the Dutch inclination to deny, for external consumption, that euthanasia had become legal in the Netherlands after the Supreme Court's decision in 1985. Statements abounded to the effect that "euthanasia is still illegal, but in certain circumstances a judge can let the doctor off" – as if the judge had any choice in the matter, given the fact that the behavior was legally justifiable.

[vv] For example, many years ago the then–minister of health was personally responsible for sabotaging a proposal I had submitted for a qualitative/quantitative evaluation of the reporting procedure, on the grounds that the proposal came from someone "who was always criticizing" her policy (confidential communication). The main lines of such "criticism" are contained in the present contribution and are now widely shared.

[ww] See 3.Griffiths, Weyers, and Adams 2008, Chapter 18.

2. Griffiths, John, Alex Bood, and Heleen Weyers. 1998. *Euthanasia and Law in the Netherlands.* Amsterdam: Amsterdam University Press.
3. Griffiths, John, Heleen Weyers, and Maurice Adams. 2008. *Euthanasia and Law in Europe.* Oxford: Hart.
4. Griffiths, John. 2003. The social working of legal rules. *Journal of Legal Pluralism* 48: 1–84.
5. Gezondheidsraad. 1982. *Advies inzake euthanasia* [Advice concerning euthanasia]. The Hague: Ministry of Health.
6. Staatscommissie Euthanasie. 1985. *Rapport van de Staatscommissie Euthanasie* [Report of the State Commission on Euthanasia]. The Hague: Staatsuitgeverij.
7. Griffiths, John. 2007. Criminal law is the problem, not the solution. In *The Criminal Justice System and Health Care*, ed. C. Erin and S. Ost, 119–135. Oxford: Oxford University Press.
8. Heide, Agnes van der, Luc Deliens, Karin Faisst, Tore Nilstun, Michael Norup, Eugenio Paci, Gerrit van der Wal, and Paul J. van der Maas. 2003. End-of-life decision-making in six European countries: Descriptive study. *The Lancet* 362: 345–350.
9. Keown, John. 2002. *Euthanasia, Ethics and Public Policy: An Argument Against Legalization.* Cambridge: Cambridge University Press.
10. Tol, Donald van. 2005. Grensgeschillen: een rechtssociologisch onderzoek naar het classificeren van euthanasie en ander medisch handelen rond het levenseinde [Boundary disputes: A legal-sociological study of the classification of euthanasia and other medical behavior at the end of life]. Ph.D. diss., University of Groningen.
11. The, Anne-Mei. 1999. *Palliatieve behandeling en communicatie* [Palliative care and communication]. Houten: Bohn Stafleu Van Loghum.
12. Norwood, Frances. 2005. Euthanasia talk: Euthanasia discourse, general practice and end-of-life care in the Netherlands. Ph.D. diss., University of California, Berkeley and San Francisco. Later published as *The Maintenance of Life: Preventing Social Death through Euthanasia Talk and End-of-Life Care: Lessons from the Netherlands.* Durham: Carolina Academic Press, 2009.
13. Norwood, Frances. 2007. Nothing more to do: Euthanasia, general practice, and end-of-life discourse in the Netherlands. *Medical Anthropology* 26: 139–174.
14. Vermeulen, Eric. 2001. Een proeve van leven: praten en beslissen over extreem te vroeg geboren kinderen [A test of life: Talking and deciding about extreme premature children]. Ph.D. diss., University of Amsterdam.
15. Vermeulen, Eric. 2004. Dealing with doubt: Making decisions in a neonatal ward in the Netherlands. *Social Science and Medicine* 59: 2071–2085.
16. Chabot, Boudewijn. 1996. *Sterven op drift* [Dying adrift]. Nijmegen: SUN.
17. *Chabot, Boudewijn.* 2001. *Sterfwerk* [The work of dying]. Nijmegen: SUN.
18. Chabot, Boudewijn. 2007. *Auto-euthanasie. Verborgen stervenswegen in gesprek met naasten* [Auto-euthansia. Talking to those left behind about hidden ways to death]. Amsterdam: Bert Bakker.
19. Dam, Hans van. 2005. *Euthanasie. De praktijk anders bekeken* [Euthanasia: The practice from another perspective]. Amsterdam: NVVE.
20. Thomasma, David C., Thomasine K. Kushner, G. L. Kimsma, and C. Ciesielski-Carlucci. 1998. *Asking to Die: Inside the Dutch Debate about Euthanasia.* Dordrecht: Kluwer.

21. Orentlicher, D. 1997. The Supreme Court and physician-assisted suicide: Rejecting assisted suicide but embracing euthanasia. *New England Journal of Medicine* 337: 1236–1239.
22. Weyers, Heleen. 2004. *Euthanasie – het proces van rechtsverandering* [Euthanasia – the process of legal change]. Amsterdam: Amsterdam University Press.
23. Griffiths, John. 2007. Physician-assisted suicide in the Netherlands and Belgium. In *Giving Death a Helping Hand: Physician-Assisted Suicide and Public Policy: An International Perspective,* ed. D. Birnbacher and E. Dahl, 77–86. Dordrecht: Springer.
24. Bosshard, Georg. 2008. Switzerland. In John Griffiths, Heleen Weyers, and Maurice Adams, *Euthanasia and Law in Europe*, 463–81. Oxford: Hart.
25. Magnusson, Roger. 2002. *Angels of Death: Exploring the Euthanasia Underground.* New Haven, CT: Yale University Press.

PART III

QUALITY ASSURANCE

11

Euthanasia Consultants

Professional Assessment Before Euthanasia and Physician-Assisted Suicide in the Netherlands

Gerrit K. Kimsma

I. INTRODUCTION

One of the safeguards built into the Dutch system is the use of consultants to physicians who are seriously considering physician-assisted death. In a sense, this is a prospective check and balance that is required before any act of PAD. Formal review by a Euthanasia Review Committee (ERC), the subject of Chapter 10, is a form of retrospective review. In this chapter, I will explain why consultants were thought to be necessary in the Dutch regulatory system and the problems that were associated with their early use. Next I will describe the systematic effort to train and deploy trained consultants throughout the country, beginning in 1996. Finally, I will present the results of studies that demonstrate how this effort has had a positive influence on Dutch euthanasia practice.

Why Consultants Were Thought Necessary

The idea of involving medical consultants in complex medical problems is as ancient as the development of medical specialization. From the beginning, the Dutch acknowledged that euthanasia/PAD consultation is different from the usual intercollegial consultation. Given the gravity of the facts and the non-reversibility of the course of events, the consultation requires a connection between facts and conclusions, in addition to an assessment of the facts of a case.

Problems with the Initial Use of Consultants

This new aspect of consultation and its legal origin led to "spontaneous" practices that, in retrospect, were unacceptable – even though physicians seemed to be comfortable with them. Criticism was aimed more at procedural conditions than material outcomes. Some physicians tended to use those colleagues who had asked for their opinion in prior cases as consultants; this resulted in the appearance of "pairs of physicians" who were consulting each other. A more serious issue was posed by physicians who provided consultations based on the case description, without having seen the patient. In some cases, there would be no consultation at all because the physician believed that the facts of a case were so self-evident that outside consultation would be superfluous.

In the early 1990s, Gerrit van der Wal investigated compliance with the procedural conditions by comparing several sources: police records of reported cases of euthanasia in the province of North Holland and data from a survey of two groups of family physicians, one from the province of North Holland and one from the rest of the country. The police records, which covered only reported cases, mainly from family physicians, showed that the rate of consultations ranged from 75% in 1986 to 89% in 1989. The two surveys of family physicians showed that an average of 20% of physicians did not have a consultation before PAD; 12% did not have any type of deliberation with another caretaker. Van der Wal's research, based on data from 1986 through 1989, indicated that at that time there were no adequate rules or regulations to check the independence of a consultant. For example, 60% of the consultants "knew" the patients before the consultation. The fact that some consultants happened to work at the same institution as the physician who requested the consultation is another reason for concern with respect to the desired consultant independence. On the basis of these accumulated data from various sources, van der Wal concluded that a substantial number of family physicians did not act according to the "operative conditions of due care"[1] in cases of PAD over these years.

Creation of a Network of Consultants in the Netherlands

The Dutch network of consultants was facilitated in 1997 as part of a project by the Amsterdamse Huisartsen Vereniging (Amsterdam Society of General Practioners), a regional branch of the Royal Dutch Medical Society (RDMA). The project was christened with the acronym SCEA, Steun en Consultatie bij Euthanasie in Amsterdam, meaning Support and Consultation with Euthanasia in Amsterdam. It was later expanded to include the other regions of the RDMA under the acronym SCEN, meaning Support and Consultation Euthanasia Netherlands.[2]

This interest among family physicians reflected their high level of involvement in the practice of euthanasia. The Remmelink Report showed that 80% of PAD was done by family physicians. The network started in the Amsterdam area with about 20 family physicians, selected on the basis of interest, experience, and good standing in the profession. The SCEN project changed from a regional into a "national" project in 1999; by the year 2002, SCEN consultants were available for the whole country. At present, the project involves more than 600 physicians. Two training sessions are organized each year for about 20 new consultants in each regional group.

In the beginning, participants were exclusively from family medicine, which, in the Netherlands, is a totally outpatient practice. Since 2005, the number of participating clinical specialists and nursing home physicians has grown to 20%. The consultants have always been observed closely through a government-supported research project of the EMGO Institute at the Vrije Universiteit in Amsterdam.[3]

The official goals of SCEN[3] are

1. *to offer expert advice as meaningful support for physicians, in order to help them to answer questions and solve problems (of patients requesting euthanasia).* The activities are primarily targeted for consultation and support for physicians and only indirectly aimed at patients, especially where it concerns an assessment of available palliative options.
2. *to realize easy access to a consultant* by developing a low-threshold approach with the assurance of an independent consultant.
3. *to improve the quality of a formal consultation in the context of reporting* by providing special training to learn all the angles and pitfalls of a request and its assessment.
4. *to improve medical interventions of physicians faced with a request for euthanasia or physician-assisted suicide,* including the evaluation of options for palliative care and adequate knowledge of how to end life in a medically careful way.
5. *to improve palliative knowledge and expertise in order to access palliative care for physicians in general.* This is accomplished by cooperating with the five government-financed centers for palliative care.

II. PROTOCOL AND PROFESSIONAL SUPERVISION

The RDMA developed a protocol to streamline the functioning of euthanasia consultants and to maximize the quality of the practice. This protocol provides the core of a three-day course for candidate SCEN consultants. The work of consultants is differentiated into material and procedural aspects. Procedural aspects involve the implementation of: 1) consultant independence and 2) actions that are required for a well-constructed report that ends with an opinion about whether the legal requirements have been fulfilled.

Independence is guaranteed by implementing the general legal conditions for expert witnesses in courts of law. Thus, a consultant and consultee should not be direct colleagues in a medical practice, have a personal relationship, or be in a hierarchical professional relationship. The consultant should not have been involved in the past treatment of the patient, and should not have a personal relationship with the patient.

Before the establishment of SCEN, 24% of the consultation physicians acted as "couples," each taking turns being the attending physician or consultant. Even though coupling did not seem to affect outcome – 90% of coupled cases had positive outcomes versus 80% for noncoupled cases – this procedure was seen as undesirable because of its potential to diminish independence or the appearance of independence.[4]

A "call-in system" for accessing SCEN was developed to promote independence, as well as to make the system more user friendly and efficient. A physician in need of a consultation or support calls a regional SCEN phone number and receives a return call from the SCEN consultant on duty. Two consultants are available for direct consultation, and a third is available as a backup in case there is a request overload. SCEN is accessible seven days a week from 8 A.M. through 5 P.M., and in some areas until 10 P.M.

Consultants perform the following services:

1. answer the first phone call requesting consultation;
2. study the medical reports;
3. make an on-site visit to see the patient, either at home or the clinic;
4. write a consultation report and fax it to the consultee;
5. touch base with the requesting physician.

First Phone Call

SCEN physicians aim to answer a phone call as soon as possible, usually after office hours when there is adequate time for a lengthy exchange. PAD should never be a "rush job," and there must be sufficient time for a consultation. The nature of the request is established during the first contact. Is there a need for an actual euthanasia consultation or is a more general issue of support needed? A typical issue that arises in this first conversation concerns the correct timing of a consultation. Other important issues include whether the physician has already set a date and time for PAD, whether the legal conditions have been fulfilled, and whether there is a hidden agenda in the request.

Timing is essential. A request for a consultation may come either too early or too late. Early consultations are often instigated because patients want to be sure that help in dying will be a realistic option at some point. A request that comes too early often ends in the conclusion that the condition of a request being voluntary and well considered is met, but that the condition of suffering is not. This situation may lead to a repeat consultation later. A request comes too late when the consultant doesn't become involved until the patient is suffering but has now lost the ability to communicate. Such a problem complicates the assessment and could terminate the PAD procedure.

Sometimes the physician requesting a consultation has a hidden agenda. He or she may think that the conditions for intervention have not been fulfilled; because of pressure by the family (and an unwillingness to be the "bad guy"), this physician may wish to use the consultant as a messenger of refusal.

If consultants conclude that the conditions have not been fulfilled, they can provide support for the requesting physician but never intervene directly with the family or take responsibility for the decision. Moreover, consultants never perform the procedures leading to PAD.

After determining the nature of the request, the consultant asks the physician for details of the case history and whether he or she thinks the case fulfills the conditions of request and suffering. Past and present treatments are reviewed, including available options; if applicable, treatment refusals are analyzed. It is important to learn the history of the request in order to evaluate voluntariness and whether the request is well considered.

Studying Medical Reports

After the phone call, a consultant studies faxed information such as medical data, communications, and the medical status. Most of the time there will be correspondence from a specialist who was managing the patient's care before concluding that the end of curative treatment in the hospital had been reached and that the palliative phase had started.

Seeing the Patient

After the initial inventory, the consultant decides if there is sufficient justification to visit the patient. Since more than 80% of the PAD cases are performed by family physicians, the consultant will most likely go to the patient's home. Other venues include hospitals and, to a much smaller extent, nursing homes or hospices. These visits usually occur after office hours, in the late afternoon or the early evening.

Home visits are full of emotions and potential pitfalls. It is not uncommon for patients to view a consultant's visit as a kind of examination that, if passed, allows PAD to proceed. A consultant seeks to prevent those unnecessary and disturbing images by making sure that the physician correctly introduces the consultant as his or her advisor – no more, no less.

The RDMA has prepared an information letter for patients that explains the reasons for the visit and what can be expected from the consultation. It is not clear, however, how often the requesting physician provides this printed information.

Upon arrival, a consultant introduces him- or herself and begins by asking about the patient's expectations for the visit. Adult children and other family and friends are almost always present. Their presence is justified because they have been part of the care team and have witnessed the day-to-day developments, and they have a close personal relationship with the patient and family. Coffee is often served. The physician asks the patient to describe the history of the disease, treatments, effects, symptoms, loss of function, and how he or she has coped with the illness. Family or friends will often jump in with additional details.

The central issue is the reason the patient has decided that the suffering has become unbearable and wants his or her life ended. This self-description often provides insights into the personal views and biographical elements that play a role in patients' decisions. Patients are usually quite willing and able to answer these questions – but not always. Sometimes patients are weak and too tired to speak very much or to reflect at length on the course of events; their suffering is evident. In such cases, the assessment of their suffering is completed by reviewing all the information that has been received from the physician in charge and any reports by health professionals. Patients do, however, have to answer questions with regard to their request and why they feel that their suffering has become unbearable. The RDMA strongly recommends that the consultant speak to the patient alone at least part of the time.

Writing a Report

The consultant's report is usually based on a checklist of items. These include

1. names and qualifications of consultant, physician, and patient;
2. relationship to the physician in charge regarding independence;
3. actions:
   a. the first contact, the nature of the request, the medical data;
   b. the visit with the patient, observations, impressions;
   c. description of previous history;
   d. the present situation: the signs and symptoms of suffering, the loss of functions, reasonable alternatives, and reasons for acceptance or rejection of those alternatives;
   e. focus on suffering and the request: What makes this suffering unbearable for the patient and why is it hopeless? Is the request well considered or are there reasons to doubt the competency of the patient? How did the process of decision making proceed? In other words, is the patient fully aware of his or her situation and the consequences of the request?
   f. finally, the consultant's judgment: I come to the conclusion that ...

Touching Base after the Consultation

It is customary to touch base and discuss the results of a consultation with a requesting physician in order to resolve any uncertainties and to find out what the physician will do with the consultant's assessment. Some consultants routinely call a physician after the PAD to ask how the procedures went. The rationale behind this idea is that it is helpful to share the emotional burden of the intervention by having a physician talk about events and feelings.

Consultations typically involve three to five hours of work. Consultants are paid by the insurance companies, regardless of their conclusions.

III. TRAINING, EDUCATIONAL CONCEPTS, AND CONTINUED SHARING OF EXPERIENCES

The RDMA has developed a three-day course to train the SCEN consultants. The course is spread over eight weeks in order to allow time for digestion of the contents. The relatively small size of the Netherlands makes this plan feasible – that is, anyone can travel to the RDMA seat in Utrecht within roughly two hours. The first trainees in the Amsterdam area were selected on the basis of experience with PAD and their interest in becoming SCEN consultants. Trainees should have at least five years of experience in medical practice in order to develop the level of communication skills and ability required to deal with highly charged emotions in relatively short periods of time. The course stresses that a consultant is an advisor to the requesting physician, nothing more. Nowadays there is a special application procedure for aspiring consultants.

Two major tasks are emphasized during the consultation. First, the consultant must make certain that the legal requirements have been fulfilled. Part of that assignment is a medical judgment about whether all available palliative options have been addressed and whether the patient is depressed. In a sense, the consultant uses medical knowledge to fulfill a law-based task – that is, making sure that the legal conditions are fulfilled. Finally, the consultant writes a report that is used in the final assessment by the Euthanasia Evaluation Committees.

On the first day, the students begin by sharing experiences and emotions concerning PAD. These accumulated experiences are expanded and developed to establish links with the formal aspects of the SCEN consultation: independence, expertise, required procedures and pitfalls, impediments, and the final report. Representatives of a Euthanasia Review Committee present the function and workings of the committees as part of the training (see Chapter 12). They tell the consultants about the important facts and issues that committees need in order to make a fair judgment. The emphasis is on clear descriptions of suffering and a reflective assessment of the patient's competency.

On the second day, the focus is on communication with consultees, patients, and families in a variety of possible dilemmas. One example concerns dealing with consultees who are either ambivalent or confused. Another features manipulative families who try to pressure the patient or the physician to end a life.

Special attention is paid to the analysis of the nature of depressive feelings in terminal patients and the symptoms of clinical depression. A series of case scenarios are presented, with professional actors in the roles of physicians and patients. The participants are required to write a final report treating one of the simulated cases as if it were a real request. These reports are assessed by the course staff and used as the basis for Day 3.

Day 3 has three lessons: how to report, how to assess unbearable suffering, and the role of palliative care as a potential means to alleviate suffering. With the "checklist" of the course as a guide, the written reports are assessed in terms of completeness and the depth of their descriptions. Participants evaluate each other's reports and then receive an assessment by a staff member.

The heart of consulting is the assessment of unbearable suffering and the presence of a voluntary and well-considered request. The request has a primal position in the Dutch definition of PAD. There cannot be a PAD without a well-considered request. PAD is never simply the act of ending life. It is best understood as the final stage of a longer process between patient and physician. This process has several phases: the initial request, the discussion of treatment options, the actual request for the near or immediate future, the agreement to ask for a consultation, the actual consultation, and the intervention to end life. One prospective study found that patients, rather than physicians, initiate the shift from one phase to the next. This process involves continuous deliberation and discussion.[5]

It is important to realize that an assessment of suffering with the aim of helping to relieve it is very different from an assessment of suffering with the possible aim of ending life. The physician in charge and the consultant assess suffering by cataloging the signs and symptoms, seeing the developments over time, and recognizing which signs will get worse or stay static.

The following list is used in the course to assess suffering:[6,7]

1. Time and Suffering
   - 1.1. Actual suffering
     - 1.1.1. Synchronous aspects: What symptoms and loss of functions at present?
     - 1.1.2. Diachronous aspects: What is the expected/projected course of symptoms and loss of function?
   - 1.2. Future suffering/fear of future suffering: What type of suffering? Is this fear realistic? Are there treatment refusals? How do you anticipate a refusal?
2. Suffering and Personality: What does the patient find unbearable and how does it relate to the patient's personality?
3. Suffering and Personality over Time/Biography: What are the disease experiences of this patient? What type of work has the patient done? How autonomous has the patient been socially? Is the patient religious and what does religion contribute to the patient's understanding of his or her situation?
4. Suffering and Context: Where does the patient reside? Is the care sufficient? What does the length of the suffering/disease process mean with respect to the place where care is provided? In what way does the context add to the nature of suffering?

The normal professional distance of objective observation has an additional aspect in the course of a request to help a patient die. The objective perspective implies a clear eye for the signs and symptoms of suffering; the "close reading" of a patient's suffering implies the necessity in order to get close to a patient to find out what the suffering means for this particular person and why. The intention is to find out how a patient feels about these ailments in a more existential sense. The approach combines two academic traditions. The inventory is analytic, but the question of what the symptoms and loss of functions mean for a patient involves a hermeneutic moment of understanding – that is, discovering what the situation means for an individual patient.

IV. CONTINUED PROFESSIONAL EVALUATION AND TRAINING OF SCEN PHYSICIANS

Once they are trained, SCEN physicians meet four times a year as a form of continuing medical education. Each meeting lasts two and a half hours as SCEN physicians share experiences, discuss new developments, and agree on policies. The meetings, which also offer emotional support, are chaired by experts, and notes are kept and filed for review by the SCEN organization at the RDMA office in Utrecht.

V. THE EFFECT OF SCEN

During the tenth-year celebration of SCEN in 2007, there was general satisfaction that its goals had been fulfilled and that the quality of SCEN as an institution was good.

The effects of SCEN have been studied by Bregje Onwuteaka-Philipsen [8,9] and in a report for the RDMA in 2003.[6] SCEN is highly appreciated by Dutch physicians in general. Even those physicians who had not used the service said they felt supported and would use it if the need arises. In 2002, up to 85% of the physicians with a case of PAD had used the SCEN consultants; the other 15% of the consultations were carried out by physicians without SCEN qualification. In general, Dutch physicians feel supported by SCEN consultants and are more than satisfied with the quality of information, both in issues of procedures and assessment, to fulfill the legal conditions.[3] The reports submitted by physicians to the Euthanasia Review Committees are higher in quality than before SCEN was employed because they are more systematic and detailed, resulting in a better overall view of cases. Even though it is difficult to determine whether SCEN consultations improved the quality of medical care, it is clear that they are timed better – that is, before a date has been set or promises have been made.

The 2007 report on the evaluation of the Termination of Life on Request and Assisted Suicide (Review Procedures) Act indicated that reporting has increased to 80%. It is likely that SCEN has significantly added to this increase. That impression is confirmed in one of the subgroups of the national survey. Interviews were conducted on the basis of randomly selected death certificates. There were also interviews of 248 physicians who were identified as having been involved in euthanasia. The 248 interviews revealed that in 14 cases there was no consultation, in 13 cases the consultation was by a non-SCEN physician, and in 221 cases the consultation was by a SCEN physician. None of the 14 cases without a consultation was reported. Of the 13 cases in which the consultation was from a non-SCEN physician, 12 (85%) were reported while one was not. Of the consultations by a SCEN physician, 95% were reported and 5% were not.[10] Thus, SCEN consultation substantially promoted and increased reporting.[10]

VI. CURRENT AND FUTURE DEVELOPMENTS

Further steps have been taken to professionalize SCEN as an institution since early 2007. The RDMA established an Advisory Council to describe the terms of SCEN schooling, a system of registration, procedures for quality control of SCEN consultations, and professional sanctions after complaints or malpractice. Most of these items had received official recognition by 2008, or were being finalized within the RDMA and delegated as a responsibility of the RDMA Department of Policy and Advice. Quality control of the written SCEN consultation reports is an important item for future development, requiring the cooperation of the Euthanasia Review Committees.

VII. CONCLUSIONS

Since 1995, the official response to PAD has focused on evaluating whether the legal conditions have been met, before and after the act. This is consistent with an overall strategy of keeping a formal judicial and criminal approach at a distance. The evaluation *before* the act of euthanasia and PAD has become a physician procedure via SCEN; it is organized by the RDMA, which is supported by the government. Surveys reveal that the SCEN is highly appreciated, both by the medical profession and the political establishment. Its presence is likely a major factor in the increase of reporting. Ongoing professionalization makes it likely that SCEN consultation will become a permanent feature of the Dutch system for responsible PAD.

References

1. Wal, Gerrit van der. 1992. *Euthanasie en hulp bij zeldoding door huisartsen* [Euthanasia and assisted suicide by family physicians]. Rotterdam: Wyt Uitgeefgroep.
2. Wijlick, E. H. J. van. 2003. Consultatie en kwaliteitsbewaking: SCEN. In *Levensbeeindigend handelen door een arts op verzoek van de patient* [Life ending by a physician after a request from a patient], ed. Johan Legemaate and Robert Dillmann, 61–77. Houten: Bohn Stafleu Van Loghem.
3. Onwuteaka-Philipsen, Bregje D., M. C. Jansen-vander Weide, H. R. W. Pasman, and Gerrit Van der Wal. 2003. *Steun en Consultatie bij Euthanasie in Nederland* [Support and Consultation in Euthanasia in the Netherlands. Amsterdam: KNMG-LHV.
4. Onwuteaka-Philipsen, Bregje. 1999. Consultation of another physician in cases of euthanasia and physician-assisted suicide, 127. Ph.D. diss., Vrije Universiteit.

5. Norwood, F. 2005. Euthanasia talk: Euthanasia discourse, general practice and end-of-life care in the Netherlands: The role of family in euthanasia decision making. Ph.D. diss, University of California at San Francisco/Berkeley.
6. Kimsma, Gerrit K. 2000. Het lijden beoordeeld: een voorstel voor een conceptueel kader [The assessment of suffering: A proposal for a conceptual frame] (in Dutch). *Medisch Contact* 55: 1757–1759.
7. Kimsma, Gerrit K. 2003. Objectivering van de zorgvuldigheidseisen inzake het verzoek en het lijden: aanpak, valkuilen en verslaglegging [Objectifying the conditions of prudency with respect to a request and suffering: Approach, pitfalls and reporting]. In *Levensbeëindigend handelen van een arts op verzoek van een patient* [Life ending by a physician after a request from a patient], ed. Johan Legemaate and Robert Dillmann. Houten: Bohn Stafleu van Loghem.
8. Onwuteaka-Philipsen, Bregje, Didi M. W. Kriegsman, Gerrit van der Wal, Robert Dillmann, and Jacques ThM van Eijk. 1999. General practitioners' opinions on consultation of another physician in case of euthanasia. *European Journal of General Practice* 5: 137–142.
9. Onwuteaka-Philipsen, Bregje D., Gerrit van der Wal, and Lode Wigersma. 2000. Consultation and discussion with other physicians in cases of requests for euthanasia and assisted suicide refused by family physicians. *Cambridge Quarterly of Health Care Ethics* 9: 381–390.
10. Owuteaka-Philipsen, Bregje D., J. K. M. Gevers, Agnes van der Heide, J. J. M. van Delden, et al. 2007. *Evaluatie: Wet Toetsing Levensbeeindiging op verzoek en hulp bij zelfdoding* [Evaluation of the law on the Termination of Life on Request and Assisted Suicide (Review Procedures) Act] (in Dutch with an summary in English), 182. Den Haag: ZONMw.

12

Reviews after the Act

The Role and Work of Regional Euthanasia Review Committees

Gerrit K. Kimsma and Evert van Leeuwen

INTRODUCTION

Euthanasia is a crime in all countries of the world. Assistance in suicide is illegal in most countries. Some exceptions include Switzerland, Germany, and the states of Oregon and Washington in the United States – and then only under certain conditions. In the Netherlands, Belgium, and Luxemburg, both of these acts are still formally illegal unless a physician reports the intervention and the law-based "conditions of due care" are fulfilled. In the Netherlands, the decision has been made to separate the process of evaluation into a medical assessment by an independent physician *before* the act, and a semilegal assessment by a committee *afterwards*. This separation into two distinct interventions has evolved after several decades of debate.

Since 1998, and after three decades of strictly criminal proceedings, five regional committees have been formed to review cases retrospectively. The Dutch review procedure for cases of euthanasia and physician-assisted death (PAD) represents a shift from exclusively criminal proceedings to committee evaluations outside the formal legal structure. This procedure of decriminalization was canonized in 2002 in the Review Procedures for the Termination of Life on Request and Assisted Suicide and Amendment of the Criminal Code and the Burial and Cremation Act (Termination of Life on Request and Assisted Suicide [Review Procedure] Act; in Dutch: Wet Toetsing Levensbeeindiging op verzoek en hulp bij zelfdoding [WTL]). This shift reflects the legal attitude chosen in the previous euthanasia trials: to refrain from calling euthanasia murder, and to focus on the issue of careful medical procedures and treatment at the end of life, the so-called medical-ethical and medical-scientific norms, as described in Chapter 4 in this volume.

BACKGROUND

After the early 1970s, the legal authorities responded to reported cases of euthanasia with criminal procedures. Physicians were acquitted if they appealed to "force majeure" and could demonstrate that they had intervened on the basis of a conflict of duties – in this case, the duty to protect life versus the duty to alleviate suffering after a patient's explicit request. These criminal proceedings have now been replaced by a review of each case by a Euthanasia Review Committee (ERC) through a local medical officer, somewhat comparable to a medical coroner in the American system. ERCs must be seen as a means of achieving three intentions of Dutch politics and of the public in the area of euthanasia: to be *transparent*, meaning clarity and accountability; to be *careful,* following agreed-upon steps with due care in the final intervention; to be *reluctant* to have the law dominate discussions between patients and physicians on how and when to die.

Euthanasia Review Committees have been operative since November 1, 1998. According to the previous procedure, initiated in 1990, each case of euthanasia was considered an "unnatural death," was to be reported to a medical coroner, and was then taken up directly by the local prosecution. The prosecution studied the police-assembled facts of the case and reported a tentative judgment to a regional attorney general, who in turn presented it to a committee of five attorneys general, who then prepared an interim report. The state secretary of justice made the final decision to prosecute a physician.[1]

This rather cumbersome, time-consuming, and potentially threatening procedure was replaced by a system of ERCs. The ERC procedure is intended to do justice to the medical facts of a case and to place "the law at some distance." Nationwide, there are five ERCs that serve the five judicial regions of the Netherlands. They consist of three members (and three substitutes): a judicial expert who is the chair, a physician, and an ethicist. The ERCs are supported by government-paid legal council and staff.[2] From the start, the expectation was that the system would increase the number of reports by lowering physicians' resistance to reporting.[3]

The ERCs review reported cases of euthanasia and physician-assisted suicide, cases in which a patient has made a "competent" request and suffers unbearably, according to the Dutch definition. The reports are written by the physicians who perform the acts of euthanasia. The ERCs do not review cases considered "normal care," such as stopping life-sustaining treatment, treatment of pain that might result in death (double effect), or palliative sedation. Cases involving incompetent patients, including children, also fall outside the ERCs' areas of competence. A special committee was formed in 2006 to deal with cases involving children, including neonates, and with late abortions after 22–24 weeks of gestation. That committee, however, has only received a few reports since 2009.

Between 1998 and 2002, psychic suffering and psychiatric symptoms were considered to be outside the area of the ERCs' authorization. According to the new law on the termination of life, the 2002 WTL, requests from patients with psychiatric symptoms fall within the ERCs' area of expertise; the annual reports document several cases involving this group.[4] The WTL also changed the authority of the ERCs' decisions. Prior to 2002, all decisions were still subject to a legal evaluation by public prosecutors; after that date, ERC decisions that physicians had acted with due care and should not be prosecuted became final.[5] If physicians have not acted with due care, their cases are reported to the prosecution. The prosecution then investigates to determine if the lack of care warrants further criminal proceedings.

The committees assess whether the notifying physician has acted in accordance with all the statutory due-care criteria. These criteria, referred to in Article 293, paragraph 2 of the Criminal Code, are as follows. Physicians must

1. be satisfied that the patient's request is voluntary and well considered;
2. be satisfied that the patient's suffering is unbearable with no prospect of improvement;
3. inform the patient about his or her situation and prognosis;
4. come to the conclusion, together with the patient, that there are no reasonable alternatives available to the patient;
5. consult at least one other independent physician, who must see the patient and give a written opinion on whether the due-care criteria set out in sections a to d of the article have been fulfilled;
6. exercise due medical care and attention in terminating the patient's life or assisting in his or her suicide.

ERC PROCEDURES

The ERCs meet regularly, about every four weeks, in order to fulfill the requirement that primary decisions be handed down within six weeks of any act of euthanasia. Like most legal verdicts, their decisions are binary – either the physician proceeded carefully or "without due care." Cases that do not involve due care are forwarded to the criminal prosecutor and the Medical Inspectorate, a state medical review institution ("medical police") in order to check the quality of medical interventions.

The ERCs receive reports through municipal medical coroners, who are notified by physicians directly after any case of PAD that may have been an "unnatural death." They have no function in normal death cases. These coroners then make an on-site visit, check the facts of the physician's report of PAD, receive the relevant medical papers, and get in touch with the prosecution to receive the allowance for burial or cremation. Finally, they send these papers to the appropriate regional ERC.

The committee members prepare their cases at their homes or offices. They receive written case reports from the committee's legal secretary, anywhere between 30 and 50 cases for each meeting. This legal secretary is a lawyer with an administrative function to regulate the paperwork and present the cases in a standard format. Each case is reviewed separately at the meeting in the order of the date of reporting. A large part of the meeting focuses on unclear or problematic aspects of the cases that defy transparency. If a decision cannot be reached because of insufficient facts, a final conclusion is postponed until the reporting physician can provide more facts. If the information is still not sufficient to come to a conclusion, physicians are invited to appear personally in front of the committee for further questioning.

The style of discussion is always one of consensus; in case of a stalemate, the opinion of the chair is decisive. Since the ERCs are the final arbiters by law, most of the caseload is finalized by the ERCs. Of 20,623 cases heard between 1998 and 2008, 38 received the qualification "without due care" and were forwarded to the inspectorate for consideration of prosecution. None of these cases has led to a prosecution.

The ERCs proceed on the basis of

1. the case description by the legal secretary, seen as a sort of abstract of the case history and the events, including the PAD;
2. the physician's report, usually a completed model form;
3. the consultation report;
4. written living wills with a request;
5. medical communications between physicians and relevant parts of the medical record.

The case descriptions written by the secretaries are a compilation of information from these sources. The quality of the physicians' reports is not always satisfactory, but the material from diverse sources usually provides enough information for an assessment with respect to all of the conditions of "due care." The "completeness" of the information is researched by the Dutch government as part of its continuing evaluation of end-of-life practices.

In 2005, the government evaluated the WTL of 2002 by investigating the practice of euthanasia and other end-of-life decisions, the reporting, and the functioning of the ERCs. The focus of the ERC evaluation has been on the accumulated numbers from the 2005 reports to the ERCs, with special attention to the statutory due-care requirements that the committees must evaluate, such as the request, the suffering, the diseases and possible treatment alternatives, and the careful ending of life. The research shows considerable adherence to the norms and intentions of the law. In some cases, however, the descriptions of the reporting physicians have left unanswered questions. Consultations have usually added substance and completeness to the physicians' reports.

With respect to the *request*, for example, the investigation has found that it was in written form in 97% of the cases. The request was clearly voluntary in 95%, the physician's report was unclear in 3%, influence from family was observed in 1%, and the patient was not completely aware of his or her physical condition in 1%. Concerning the *hopelessness of suffering*, there were no explicit descriptions of hopeless suffering in 32% of the cases, even though the descriptions of the diseases, treatments, symptoms, and life expectancy were adequately informative on this point. The descriptions were adequate in the other 68% of cases. There were no curative options available in 23% of cases, no symptomatic treatments possible in 5%, neither of the two in 12%, and no specific description of a treatment mentioned in 24%, but given the diagnosis and the stage of the disease process, no questions remained.

With respect to the *unbearable nature of suffering*, 91% of the patients suffered from actual symptoms, and 7% suffered from the prospect of potential symptoms. More than a third suffered from *dependence, physical breakdown, or loss of dignity*. In summary, 99% of the patients endured some form of suffering and 20% also had prospective symptoms or problems.

FRAME OF THINKING/EVALUATION

ERCs focus on the total picture of each case history by looking at the actual files of patients, the history of requests, the ways in which physicians describe the presence of the conditions of the law, the consultant's report, and all other available medical papers. The completeness of the information and the convincing nature of the descriptions are relevant items for discussion at committee meetings. The consultants' reports are especially informative, in both the provision of data and its analysis. The reports of Support and Consultation Euthanasia Netherlands (SCEN) consultants are more complete than those of non-SCEN consultants (see Chapter 11).

The framework of analysis of the ERCs has been derived from jurisprudence over the past 35 years and can be summarized as *objectification, individualization, abstraction, and medical classification*.[6] Each term is connected to a specific landmark court case and the manner of thinking in that particular legal verdict, and serves as a conditional approach in the committees' evaluations.

Objectification is connected to the regional Leeuwarden Court's *Postma* case from 1973, and means that a physician must act according to specific norms that can be objectified. The conflict of duties, relieving suffering, and protecting life must be demonstrated in the description of the facts of a case. The first case brought to court in the Dutch euthanasia debate dealt with conflict of duties; the verdict concentrated on how physicians deal with terminal patients with unbearable suffering.

Individualization is based on the *Schoonheim* case from 1984. The term refers to the attention that is paid to the unique facts in each case, respecting the unpredictability of the process, development of symptoms, and loss of functions – including patients' interpretations. The case concerned the active ending of a woman's life. She was over 90 years old, suffered from several ailments, and experienced the further breakdown of her health and life in the future as unbearable. Individual facts, feelings, and expectations played a major part in the court decision. This individualization does not imply the absence of "strict" normative limits. Jurisprudence has drawn specific limits by allowing only physicians to be involved in euthanasia and PAD, denying acceptance of an unproven earlier request for euthanasia, and requiring a tougher consultation procedure in cases of psychiatric disease.

The condition of *abstraction* is based on the *Chabot* case from 1994. It means that the cause of that suffering, whether it is psychic or somatic, is not the essential factor in the assessment of suffering; rather, the essential factor is the seriousness of the suffering and how it is experienced by the patient. In this court case, the patient's assessment of her life and her life experiences convinced the High Council that she suffered unbearably without prospect for improvement. This decision has received criticism because it seemed to broaden the criteria for euthanasia to include deeply frustrating life events that cause suffering but that do not have a basis in a clear psychiatric illness, such as clinical depression. This expanded justification was limited, however, by the Dutch Supreme Court in the next euthanasia case, the *Brongersma* case, where a certain limit to the cause of unbearable suffering was "carved out."

The condition of *classification* is connected to the *Brongersma* case of 2002, in which the court limited the specification of the cause of suffering. The decision states that the suffering of a patient should have a basis in some medically classifiable somatic or psychiatric disease in order to justify a physician's involvement. Even though the category of "medical domain" is culturally dependent and, therefore, somewhat malleable, it nevertheless clearly excludes suffering on the basis of existential anguish or loss of meaning in life. Such causes are beyond what the Dutch Supreme Court found acceptable as justifications for euthanasia or PAD.

RESPONSES AND REACTIONS

The review of cases by five different committees in five different regions carries a risk of producing inconsistent decisions, and may cause inequality from a legal perspective. Given the weight of individual circumstances in each case, it is possible that committees differ in their conclusions regarding complex situations. To prevent potential inequalities, a procedure has been developed to "speak with one voice," at least in those cases in which the physicians are being judged as "not careful." Before a final judgment is made, such cases are presented to all members of all five committees. The final decision is collective.

Although the ERCs' focus is on evaluation, they also have an educational role.[7] Since legalized euthanasia and palliative care are relatively new phenomena, there is still much to learn. Committees may add commentary to their decisions. Even though most physicians are judged as "careful," there is sometimes a need to address a physician on particulars, such as completeness of information on suffering or details on the administration of drugs. Sometimes, it is important to correct false assumptions – for example, that all family members must agree before euthanasia can proceed. In a few cases, physicians are approached on behalf of a committee, mostly by a physician-member, and asked to provide more information on the facts that appear in the reports.

Committee members regularly give presentations for colleagues and other audiences in hospitals, schools, and community centers to inform the public about its function and its effects. The most important educational effect can be attributed to the public ERC annual reports, in which exceptional cases with specific details are published. These reports reflect developments and refinements in the application of the legal norms, and are available on the Internet at http://www.euthanasiecommissies.nl, including translations in English.

EFFECTS OF THE ERCS: ASSESSMENTS AND EVALUATION OF FUNCTION

Based on the information in the ERC annual reports, 20,623 cases were reviewed from November 1998 through December 2008.

Out of the many thousands of cases reviewed since 1998, only 38 have been characterized as being handled "without due care" and subsequently sent to the prosecution for legal review; no criminal investigations have followed. It thus seems fair to conclude that even though physician performance in these cases may not have been completely congruent with professional standards, the actions were not considered to be criminal. The Medical Inspectorate has reviewed many of these cases with the physicians, but there have been no further professional sanctions.

The average number of cases per year was 2,062, with a high of 2,322 cases in 2008 and a low of 1,815 cases in 2003. The average monthly numbers are 186, with numbers varying between 151 and 194 cases. There are no known reasons for the variation in numbers over the years.[8] There is some agreement that the numbers reported by family physicians tend to be complete, and the numbers of cases reported by specialists in hospitals are less so. The national surveys of 1990, 1995, 2000, and 2005 show an increase in reporting rates from 18% to 54% and 80%, respectively. There is no proof that the publication of the reports is directly responsible for this increase, although many hoped and predicted it would happen.

Most of the ERC cases are easy to assess: The cases are clear, the combined information is adequate, and the norms of the law are fulfilled, in spite of the inevitable vagueness of the notions of both a voluntary, well-considered request and unbearable and hopeless suffering. Each meeting produces a limited number of cases that require further analysis and discussion, more often because of a lack of adequate information than because the limits of the norms have been transgressed. Much attention is paid to the medical-ethical aspects of the cases, including possible therapies that should have been tried or at least proposed to the patient.

ERCs concentrate on the facts of the cases and then evaluate both procedural aspects, such as the presence of a consultation, and material conditions, such as the quality of the request and suffering. The material norms in particular are "open" and subject to interpretation. The flexibility and freedom to develop new interpretations was explicitly encouraged during the political debate in the Dutch Parliament. It should not be a surprise, then, that further distinctions of more subtle issues have been made over a period of 10 years.

The ERCs provide a much richer and more detailed picture of the process of decision making than the earlier judgments of criminal proceedings.[6] The judgments focus on individual cases and the totality of the disease, the treatments, the individual patients, patients' biographies, personal situations, and appreciation of present and future potential suffering. There is an eye for more detail and nuance. There are no "hard rules" that cannot be softened because of individual circumstances. The annual reports of the committees reflect certain shifts in the limits of "acceptable" suffering. Since 2006, the annual reports are available on the Internet in English, and it has become possible to read the decisions and arguments at http://www.euthanasietoetsingcommissie.nl/en/review-committees/annualreport/.

Over the past 10 years, more than a hundred case reports have been included in these annual reports. Attention is paid to the process of consultation and the role of SCEN consultants in 30 of these cases in detail. Sometimes, the focus is on timing. Consultations can be too early, with a risk for a repeat, or too late, making communication with the patient difficult due to progressive disease; in most cases, the time frame is still acceptable to the committees. Sometimes the speed of increased suffering makes a consultation impossible, but even that situation is acceptable to the ERCs. In rare cases, two physicians who were involved in a patient's end-of-life care have reported; only the one who applied the deadly means should have submitted a report. These items are essentially pedagogical and aim to increase the quality of consultations as the law intended.

The ERCs have also focused on the *treatment relationships* between the doctors who ended life and the extent to which they were the physicians in charge of those particular patients. The committees have not been lenient with physicians who were not continually in charge but ended the life of a family member due to familial motives of compassion or some other type of social relation.

With respect to *depression*, the general rule is that a patient with clinical depression is deemed incompetent and his or her request cannot be honored. In some cases under review, the ERC would analyze in detail whether there was a true clinical depression or a situation in which some symptoms were simply those of the disease itself (e.g., lack of energy) and the inevitability of impending death. On the basis of psychiatric evaluations and convincing descriptions from the reporting physicians, it was established that competence was not impaired and voluntariness was accepted in all cases.

Loss of consciousness or coma is another example of a complex evaluation. In general, the consensus is that comatose patients do not suffer and thus, by definition, do not qualify for euthanasia or PAD. Committees have evaluated several cases and concentrated on the presence of the signs of suffering in patients incapable of communication, and they have accepted a nuanced version of the relationship between (sub)coma and suffering. Thus, the essential element is a consensus on the presence of signs and symptoms of suffering before the loss of consciousness.

Cases of *early dementia, both in Alzheimer's disease and Lewy Body dementia*, are special with respect to acceptable euthanasia. The ERCs' position is that dementia serves as grounds for acceptable euthanasia only in exceptional cases. The cases that are described are striking in terms of how carefully the procedures have been followed, both with respect to the recognition of the individual's perception of suffering and the repeated psychiatric assessments of competence. A realistic fear about future suffering was recognized as actual suffering because the patient anticipated the impending reality of disintegration as a person, breakdown in all aspects of social and mental life, and loss of dignity – without other serious somatic symptoms. As discussed earlier (*Schoonheim* case of 1984), the Dutch Supreme Court accepted this justification of unbearable suffering only if it was grounded in a somatic disease. Esther Pans concludes that loss of dignity in a mental-social interpretation has so far received its most distinct acceptance in the context of (early) dementia.[6]

CONCLUSIONS

The Dutch euthanasia and PAD interventions do not lead to criminal procedures if the conditions of the law are followed. Physicians, who are the only ones entitled to be excused under the WTL, must report, and there are two moments of evaluation: a medical consultation prior to the act and a committee evaluation afterwards. The five regional committees complete these retrospective evaluations within the six weeks that the law requires. There is overall satisfaction with the functioning of the committees, which have published each decision on the Internet since 2006 and report each year to the secretaries of justice and health care and the Dutch Parliament. The ERCs' decisions have become final under the WTL. Over the years, the committees have shown some minor shifts in their evaluations of the "open norms" of a voluntary, well-considered request and of unbearable and hopeless suffering. In addition to the development on "material" norms, there have been clarifications on the other norms, for example, with regard to consultations and what it means to be the "physician in charge" within a treatment relationship.

From a legal perspective, the construction of ERCs is a new phenomenon. A multidisciplinary committee is allowed to decide that there will be no prosecution of a case that might be considered a special type of murder under criminal law. The committee efforts show that conscientious work in small teams can contribute to a well-functioning legal process.

References

1. Cuperus-Bosma, J. M. 1998. Regulering, toetsing en kwalitetisbewaking van levensbeeindigend handelen. De rol van het Openbaar Ministerie in de

meldingsprocedure euthanasie [Regulation, evaluation and quality control of life-ending interventions: The role of the public prosecution in the procedure to report euthanasia]. Thesis, Vrije Universiteit.

2. Regeling Regionale Toetsingscommissies Euthanasie (Regulation Regional Euthanasia Commissions). *Staatscourant* 1998, nr. 101.
3. Widdershoven, Guy. 1999. Euthanasia in the Netherlands: Some first experiences of evaluation committees. *The Hastings Center Report* 29: 47.
4. Euthanasia Review Committee (ERC). 2004. *Year Report 2003:* 16, case 5/2003, 17. Den Haag: Koninklijke De Swart.
5. Suyver, J. 2003. De positie van de toetsingscommissie onder de nieuwe euthanasiewet [The position of the ERC under the new euthanasia law]. *Tijdschr gezondheidsrecht* 4: 254–258.
6. Pans, Esther. 2006. *De normatieve grondslagen van het nederlandse euthanasierecht* [The normative foundations of the Dutch euthanasia jurisprudence]. Nijmegen: Wolf Legal Publishers.
7. Widdershoven, Guy. 2003. De werkwijze en ervaringen van de toetsingscommissies [The procedures and experiences of the evaluation committees]. In *Levensbeeindigend handelen van een arts op verzoek van een patient* [Life-ending interventions by a physician at the request of a patient], ed. J. Legemaate and R. J. M. Dillmann, 48–61. Houten/Antwerpen: BohnStafleu Van Loghem.
8. Klijn, Albert. 2003. De meldingsfrequentie euthanasie. Rekensom of beleidsevaluatie [The rate of reporting euthanasia: Calculation or policy evaluation]. In *Euthanasie: knelpunten in een voortgezette discussie* [Euthanasia: Bottlenecks in a continuing discussion]. 171–198. Kampen: Kok.

13

Palliative Care and Physician-Assisted Death

Dick Willems

What role did euthanasia policy play in the development of palliative care in the Netherlands – and, perhaps, vice versa? Is good palliative care, in whatever setting, compatible with physician-assisted death (PAD)? These are the central questions of this chapter.

It's been suggested, both within and outside of the Netherlands, that its liberal policies toward physician-assisted death were related to insufficient quality of care at the end of life. Doctors, this argument says, perform euthanasia because suffering patients do not receive appropriate care. Critics usually point to the lack of palliative care specialists and the scarcity of palliative care chairs in medical faculties in the Netherlands, as well as to the low numbers of hospice patients. Hence, the suggestion goes, the incidence of euthanasia would decline as soon as palliative care improved, simply because it would no longer be necessary to end the patient's life in order to end his or her suffering.

In this chapter, I will do three things. First, I will discuss the development of palliative care in the Netherlands during the last decade or so, drawing especially on information from the Ministry of Health, Welfare, and Sports. Second, I will discuss available evidence on whether this has led to a decrease in physician-assisted death. Third, then, I will raise the conceptual and moral question whether good care and euthanasia/assisted suicide are compatible, and argue that physician-assisted death may be an acceptable end to even the best palliative care.

END-OF-LIFE CARE IN THE NETHERLANDS

The provision of end-of-life care in the Netherlands underwent rapid change after 1995, and the range of care services for terminally ill patients expanded substantially. For example, in 1995 the Dutch government launched a program to support both the development of palliative care practices and the establishment of university-based knowledge centers in palliative care.[1] This program was motivated partly by the growing attention to palliative care worldwide, and partly by criticisms (both internal and external) that in the Netherlands, euthanasia was better organized than palliative care.

In the Netherlands, palliative care is not recognized as a medical specialty or subspecialty (as it is in the United States, England, and Ireland). The reason for this (sometimes contested) policy is too complex to explain in full here, but it is based on the idea that palliative care is needed in the last phase of many disease trajectories; it should not be seen as a separate form of care. Further, patients should receive palliative care from the doctors, or the teams, that have cared for them throughout their disease.[a] Dutch policies in palliative care thus rest on the principle that palliative care should normally be provided by health-care professionals (including family physicians, medical specialists, home-care workers and nursing home staff) who are part of the regular health-care system.[2] To provide high-quality palliative care, these non-specialists need a wide range of options for training and consultation – which is why the establishment of consultation services (operating from hospitals and nursing homes) became a policy aim.

The government identified a need for networks of palliative care providers throughout the Netherlands. By encouraging the development of networks nationwide, the government sought to further integrate hospice facilities into the regular health-care system and foster good cooperation and coordination among the different care providers. It also sought the optimal utilization of existing expertise with the ultimate goal of ensuring good-quality palliative care, to be demonstrated by a dovetailing of the demand for and supply of care, sufficient availability of care, and continuity and flexibility in the provision of care. The networks incorporate all of the institutions that provide palliative care in a region, town, or city – home care, residential homes, nursing homes, hospitals, and hospice facilities.

The palliative care networks are managed by the country's nine Comprehensive Cancer Centers (IKCs) (see http://www.ikcnet.nl/). The IKCs are long-standing regional organizations that advise, support, and train professionals (medical specialists, family physicians, nursing home doctors, nurses, and others) about care for cancer patients. Their increasing involvement in palliative care networks has meant that the IKCs have expanded beyond the domain of cancer into care for patients with other conditions.

Since 1996, there is the Network of Palliative Care for Terminal Patients Netherlands (NPTN), a national association of organizations and individuals involved in palliative care. Its main aim is the further development of palliative care for terminally ill patients. Besides the NPTN, there is a national support organization called Agora, which works mainly as an information exchange point for both care providers and users. Among other things, Agora provides information through a Web site (http://www.palliatief.nl).

[a] The drawback to this approach may be that it renders palliative care invisible, both in the health-care system and in education and research.

Currently, palliative care is provided in a variety of settings, by a variety of health-care professionals. Patients may receive palliative care from family doctors and home-care organizations in their own homes or in residential homes; in nursing homes, where care is provided by nursing home physicians; in hospitals; and in independent, professionally staffed hospices and volunteer-run hospices.

All of these providers (except home care by family doctors) may have specialized palliative care units. As a consequence, there are a relatively large number of options for nursing and care at home, and medical and nursing staffs in nursing homes and residential homes are becoming progressively better equipped to care for dying patients. Nonetheless, a striking feature of the situation in the Netherlands is that special facilities for terminally ill patients, such as hospices, have only appeared since the beginning of the 1990s, whereas neighboring countries had them earlier. This is probably explained by the generalist nature of much of Dutch health care and by the explicit policy aim to integrate palliative care into regular health care without turning it into a category of its own.

As a sequel to the 1995 stimulation program, and consistent with Council of Europe recommendations, the government has instituted the so-called Palliative Care Monitor.[3] This is a yearly questionnaire-based investigation (i.e., data based on self-reports), carried out by an independent research organization (Nivel – Netherlands Institute for Health Services Research). The monitor mainly describes organizational and financial aspects of palliative care: the number and size of palliative care teams and institutions, cooperation and networking, and budgets. The quality of the care delivered is not part of the investigation.

The most recent data show that from 2004 to 2006, the number of dedicated palliative care institutions rose by at least 40% and the number of dedicated palliative care beds in nursing homes, hospitals, and hospices by about 36%, to at least 844 beds. This means that the Netherlands has an average of 5.5 palliative care beds per 100,000 inhabitants – well within the standards set by the organization of health insurers (ZN) of 4 to 6 beds per 100,000. A separate NIVEL study recently showed that about one-third of terminally ill patients die at home, 27% in a hospital, 25% in a nursing home, and 15% elsewhere (including in residential homes).[4]

A recent study comparing different European countries showed that the Netherlands ranks sixth in number of palliative care beds per 100,000 inhabitants, very similar to England and Ireland.[5] Almost the same held with respect to the availability of specific palliative care resources, such as inpatient units, hospices, and (hospital) support teams. The same study counted the Netherlands among the three countries with, as the authors call it, "the most vital palliative care movements," measured by the number of scientific publications, the existence of a national association, and participation in palliative care congresses.

The following sectors contribute to palliative care in the Netherlands in several ways.

Home Care

The family physician is usually the main care provider for people who receive palliative care at home. In principle, everyone living in the Netherlands has a family physician. Most family physicians deal with only a few terminally ill patients per year; thus it's important that they (and other care providers) have sufficient opportunities for acquiring skills and for consultation in the area of palliative care. Specialty consulting teams and peer groups help fill those needs.

Physician-members of multidisciplinary consulting teams of specialists receive extensive training in palliative care in the two-year Core Training Program originally set up by the Dutch College of Family Physicians. Started in 2001, the core program now also involves medical specialists and nursing home physicians in addition to family doctors. Each "class" of around 50 physicians becomes certified palliative care consultants. Peer groups also provide advice and education. In each such group, 5 to 10 family physicians and a specialist consultant meet on a monthly or bimonthly basis to discuss their terminally ill patients. At the moment, there are about 50 such groups spread throughout the country.

When caring for terminally ill patients who remain at home, a family physician will often work closely with professional home-care workers (nurses, care workers, and helpers) from one of the approximately 120 home-care organizations in the Netherlands. Home care usually involves skilled nursing care, personal care, and domestic help. Some home-care organizations have teams of district nurses who have specialized in home-care technology, such as drips and medication pumps, which can be important in regard to terminally ill patients.

Residential Homes

There are approximately 1,400 residential homes in the Netherlands, with a total of approximately 113,000 beds. Such homes provide care for residents with less complex physical and psychosocial needs who are no longer able to live in their own homes. There are no precise figures about how many people receive palliative care from residential home staffs (primary care workers), but the number is likely to be substantial because in all cases, the residents are elderly and the policy is to care for these people until the end of their lives (to the extent possible).

There is an increasing trend for residential homes to admit terminally ill patients for short-term or respite care. These are primarily terminally ill patients who do not have complex care needs and who, for example, can no longer remain at home because family members are not available to provide care. Between them, in mid-2002 (the most recent year for which data are available) the 26 Dutch residential homes that had a hospice unit had a capacity of around 60 beds.

Nursing Homes

Palliative care receives particular attention in Dutch nursing homes. Physical and psychosocial care for people who need help during the last phase of their lives has traditionally been one of the core tasks of nursing home staff. There are approximately 330 nursing homes in the Netherlands, with around 57,600 beds and capacity for 4,600 outpatients (see http://www.nationaalkompas.nl). There are no precise data about how many residents of nursing homes receive palliative care, but their number is probably large.

In addition to providing palliative care to their own residents, like residential homes, growing numbers of nursing homes are also admitting terminally ill patients from outside for brief periods. In July 2002 there were 37 Dutch nursing homes with a hospice unit for short-term palliative care.[1] These units have a total capacity of about 152 beds.

Hospitals

Hospitals in the Netherlands (around 130 in total) provide palliative care as part of their care for those admitted and for outpatients. Many relevant specialists participate in palliative care consultation teams that support primary care workers in palliative care. Academic hospitals and specialist oncology clinics play an important role in the centers for the development of palliative care. Because hospitals in the Netherlands focus on acute and curative care, there are only a few dedicated hospice units in Dutch hospitals (three according to the government report on palliative care in 2006).[1]

Hospice

The Netherlands has relatively few independent hospices, all of them established after 1992, which is later than their counterparts in neighboring countries, such as the UK, Germany, and Belgium.[6] In 2002, there were 16 professionally staffed hospices, ranging in size from 4 to 10 beds, with a combined capacity of about 85 beds (see http://www.palliatief.nl). As of July 2002, all 21 of the volunteer-run hospices in the Netherlands were of small scale, from one to four beds. Their combined capacity was 61 beds. Currently, the number of Dutch people who die in an independent hospice is still relatively low (less than 1% of all deaths).[7]

Both professionally staffed and volunteer-run hospices strive to create a homelike environment.

Informal Care

In addition to professional care provided at home and elsewhere, informal care by family members and others is an important aspect of end-of-life care in the Netherlands. Research has shown that over a three-year period between 1997 and 1999, 6% of the Dutch population provided informal care to terminally ill people (see http://www.nationaalkompas.nl). This primarily involves domestic help, but also includes assistance in personal care and emotional support. Close relatives are usually very motivated to contribute to palliative care.

Finally, a lot of attention has been paid to quality improvement in palliative care. Guidelines have been published, among others by the IKCs mentioned previously, covering the complete area of palliative care, from the intricacies of pain and symptom management to the ways of dealing with existential crises and bereavement. All guidelines are available both in print and through the Web site at http://www.pallialine.nl.

DOES IMPROVED PALLIATIVE CARE LEAD TO A DECREASE IN PHYSICIAN-ASSISTED DEATH?

If palliative care has improved in the Netherlands, as is the case in the rest of Europe and the United States, does that have an impact on physician-assisted death? Between 1998 and 2006, two Dutch investigations took place into physician-assisted death in the Netherlands. One of the questions these investigations examined was whether a trend could be seen in the incidence of physician-assisted death that could be related to the developments in palliative care over the same period.

In the 2002 version of the nationwide study of medical decisions at the end of life, the relationship between symptoms and requests for euthanasia was investigated by comparing cancer patients who had not requested euthanasia with cancer patients who had died from euthanasia.[8] Some differences were found: Patients whose request for euthanasia had been granted seemed to suffer more from pain, nausea, vomiting, and/or coughing than patients who had not requested euthanasia. Researchers found that nausea and breathlessness were treated less frequently among patients who had requested euthanasia than among patients who had not. The total number of cases was very small, however, and the difference was not statistically significant. Neither physicians nor patients' surrogates who responded thought that patients who had euthanasia had received insufficient care.

In qualitative interviews in the 2002 study, physicians reported that their attitude toward euthanasia had changed under the influence of growing expertise in palliative care. For some, growing knowledge about palliative care was an important influence on their attitudes; one respondent reported that he had completely stopped performing euthanasia as a result of a better understanding of possibilities for palliative care. Others said that the influence was negligible or even totally absent. For example, one physician told the interviewer that he saw euthanasia and palliative care as totally different issues, the former being a pure expression of a person's autonomy, the latter a form of care that people may be needing at the end of their lives.

The quantitative part of the study showed that about 60% of physicians disagreed with the statement that adequate symptom control and care for the dying will undermine the justification for euthanasia in all cases, and only about 30% agreed with the statement saying that physicians in the Netherlands had insufficient expertise in palliative care to be able to find other possibilities than euthanasia.

Empirically, then, what few data are available indicate that the relationship between the quality of palliative care and the frequency of euthanasia in the Netherlands remains unclear. As in other countries, palliative care has rapidly developed in the Netherlands, while the frequency of euthanasia has remained relatively stable at around 2%. Even if a decrease in euthanasia due to innovations in palliative care remains possible, it is still improbable that better palliative care will make euthanasia entirely disappear. So the key philosophical and ethical question remains whether PAD and palliative care are mutually exclusive. To that question we now turn.

DOES GOOD PALLIATIVE CARE PRECLUDE PHYSICIAN-ASSISTED DEATH?

The definition of palliative care issued by the World Health Organization (WHO) in 2003 (and found on their Web site at http://www.who.int/cancer/palliative/definition/en/) is quite clear about the relationship between end-of-life care and physician-assisted death:

> Palliative care is an approach that improves the quality of life of patients and their families facing the problems associated with life-threatening illness, through the prevention and relief of suffering by means of early identification and impeccable assessment and treatment of pain and other problems, physical, psychosocial and spiritual. Palliative care
>
> - provides relief from pain and other distressing symptoms;
> - affirms life and regards dying as a normal process;
> - intends neither to hasten nor postpone death;
> - integrates the psychological and spiritual aspects of patient care;
> - offers a support system to help patients live as actively as possible until death;
> - offers a support system to help the family cope during the patient's illness and in their own bereavement;
> - uses a team approach to address the needs of patients and their families, including bereavement counseling, if indicated;
> - will enhance quality of life, and may also positively influence the course of illness;
> - is applicable early in the course of illness, in conjunction with other therapies that are intended to prolong life, such as chemotherapy or radiation therapy, and includes those investigations needed to better understand and manage distressing clinical complications.

The phrase "affirms life and regards dying as a normal process" says two things at the same time. First is that dying is a *process*, something slow, something that needs time. Performing euthanasia could prevent people from going through that process of dying – unless those who demand euthanasia have already gone through most of that process. Second is that dying is normal. Dying, the WHO says, is a normal thing that you need to accept. That does not make it an easy thing to do, even if one could think, as Dutch nursing home physician Bert Keizer wrote in a newspaper column some years ago, that everyone has done it up to now so it must not be difficult.

The "normal process" idea is associated with a concept of the *right time*. The phrase "intends neither to hasten nor postpone death" reaffirms that timing is crucial for the normalcy of death. The intention of palliative care should not be to change the timing of death. Respect the time for living and the time for dying. Again, this could indicate incompatibility with physician-assisted death. Yet one of the bigger problems associated with all the possibilities available nowadays to prolong peoples' lives is that it is increasingly unclear when that right moment is. So even if palliative care – for instance, high-quality pain management – is not *intended* for prolonging life, it often does so. One could consider this an (unexpected) form of double effect: Even though the WHO definition formally forbids any intention that the care provided should influence the moment of dying, such influence may well be inevitable. The philosophical question is whether hastening death as a consequence of care is compatible with that care.

One could argue that care is always concerned with helping people to live the life they want even at the very end, to flourish even when they are dying, and thus that care is contrary to stopping the life of a person. Care is conservative in a literal sense: It tends to want to keep what is there. So, even if physician-assisted death would be considered inevitable and therefore acceptable in some cases, and even if it can be done very carefully, it would not itself be part of care.

Double Effect

Dutch euthanasia policy has been criticized by those who say that good palliative care would make euthanasia unnecessary. The response from those in favor of Dutch policy has always had an ad hominem element: Supporters have tended to argue that critics have publicly vilified doctors involved in euthanasia, while themselves secretly using opioids and terminal sedation to achieve exactly the same effect. In fact, palliative care physicians have been accused of abusing the doctrine of double effect.

Sometimes, very ill patients may need considerable and rapidly increasing amounts of opioids. Though probably much less common than is generally thought,[9] there may be cases in which the considerable increase of such drugs contributes to the patient's death. This potential hastening of death stands in a continuum: It is not a sudden change of strategy, let alone something that looks like deliberately killing the patient. There are no clear borders between an adequate increase of the dosage of opioids and something beyond that.

This continuity between normal treatment and possibly life-shortening treatment may be what makes the use of potentially lethal dosages acceptable to many. Physicians, both in the Netherlands and elsewhere (e.g., the United States) find the intensification of pain and symptom treatment with a potential life-shortening effect more often acceptable than euthanasia.[10] Further, the intentions with which physicians increase dosages are not always crystal clear: Yes, the pain needed to be treated, but there may also have been a sincere hope that the patient could die soon(er).

In 1995, 2001, and 2005, Dutch physicians reported that they had given opioids in what they considered possibly lethal dosages to approximately one in six patients who died. The patients who died after receiving potentially lethal doses of opioids for pain differed from those who died as a result of euthanasia: 55% had cancer compared to 80% of those with cancer who had euthanasia. Data on the use of opioids with a possible life-shortening effect are derived from questionnaires and interview studies with physicians, and so the numbers crucially depend on the physicians' interpretation of their own actions. That raises the question of how good physicians are at distinguishing lethal from nonlethal dosages of morphine. Questionnaire data indicate that physicians tend to overestimate such effects rather than underestimate them.[11]

One might expect palliative care physicians to be less prone to thinking that they shortened a patient's life by increasing the morphine dosage. However, a study from Belgium showed that palliative care specialists more often than other physicians thought that increasing morphine dosages shortened the lives of their patients.[12]

ARE PALLIATIVE CARE AND PHYSICIAN-ASSISTED DEATH COMPATIBLE?

Several years ago, the Dutch minister of health at the time declared that in her view, euthanasia could be the dignified end of a period of excellent palliative care. Three situations are at least conceivable in which PAD and good palliative care are not mutually exclusive:

1. if there was a large symptom burden that could not be treated, or
2. if there was considerable symptom burden that could be treated but the patient did not want the treatment, or
3. if the request for euthanasia was not provoked by symptoms.

The first category is relatively simple but may be small. Especially if palliative sedation is conceived as a last-resort symptom-management strategy, and thus as good palliative care, then possibly no symptom is really intractable. However, the Dutch tend to regard sedation not simply as good palliative care. Looking at the discussions surrounding palliative sedation, one is tempted to think that it is regarded as something of a different category than, say, giving dexamethason for metastatic bone pain. So, simply to include palliative sedation in good palliative care seems a stratagem intended to take away the very possibility of intractable problems, and as a consequence, to exclude the justification for euthanasia given under 3.

Is physician-assisted death compatible with good palliative care in the sense of possibility 2, that is, when there are still treatment options available but the patient declines these options? This occurs, for instance, when a patient needs radiotherapy for metastatic pain but adamantly declines a visit to the hospital. One could say, in that case, that if physician-assisted death occurs, it is not performed in the context of optimal palliative care and, thus, not compatible with it. However, that would not be a very convincing line of reasoning, knowing that the wishes of the patient are considered to be paramount in palliative care.

Finally, some requests for PAD are not provoked by current suffering but by the wish to avoid approaching suffering: possibility 3. Even with excellent care and impeccable information about the possibilities of care should new suffering occur, some people may prefer to avoid such situations entirely and demand PAD. This may be because of fear, but also because of a sentiment of loss of dignity. It seems hard to maintain that in such cases, granting a request for physician-assisted death would be incompatible with good palliative care.

In conclusion, unless one rejects physician-assisted death in all cases (which, to be sure, is a perfectly tenable position), it hardly makes sense to say that palliative care and physician-assisted death are incompatible. Excellent palliative care and physician-assisted death may go together, both in practice and in principle.

References

1. Francke, Anneke L. 2003. *Palliative Care for Terminally Ill Patients in the Netherlands*. The Hague: Ministry of Health, Welfare and Sport.
2. Minister of Health. 2002. Definitief standpunt palliatieve zorg [Final position on palliative care]. Letter to the chair of the Second Chamber of the States General. The Hague, Ministry of Health, Welfare and Sport.
3. Mistiaen, P., L. Van Ruth, and Anneke L. Francke. 2006. *Monitor Palliatieve Zorg* [Palliative Care Monitor]. Utrecht: NIVEL: Netherlands Institute for Health Services Research.
4. Francke, Anneke L., L. F. J. van der Velden, L. Hingstman, Dick L. Willems. 2007. *Sterfte aan kanker en andere chronische aandoeningen* [Mortality from cancer and other chronic diseases]. Utrecht: NIVEL.
5. Centeno, Carlos, David Clark, Thomas Lynch, Javier Racafort, David Praill, Liliana De Lima, Anthony Greenwood, Luis A. Flores, Simon Brasch, and Amelia Giordano. 2007. Facts and indicators on palliative care development in 52 countries of the WHO European region: Results of an EAPC Task Force. *Palliative Medicine* 21:463–471.

6. Janssens, Rien, and Henk ten Have. 2001. Palliative care in the Netherlands. In *Palliative Care in Europe*, ed. Henk ten Have and Rien Janssens, 13–30. Amsterdam: IOS Press Ohmsha.
7. Francke, Anneke L., and Dick L. Willems. 2000. *Palliatieve zorg vandaag en morgen. Feiten, opvattingen en scenario's* [Palliative care today and tomorrow: Facts, opinions and scenarios]. Maarssen: Elsevier gezondheidszorg.
8. Onwuteaka-Philipsen, Bregje D., Agnes van der Heide, Dirk Koper, Ingeborg Keij-Deerenberg, Judith A. Rietjens, Mette L. Rurup, Astrid M. Vrakking, Jean Jacques Georges, Martien T. Muller, Gerrit van der Wal, and Paul van der Maas. 2003. Euthanasia and other end-of-life decisions in the Netherlands in 1990, 1995, and 2001. *The Lancet* 362: 395–399.
9. Thorns, Andrew, and Nigel Sykes. 2000. Opioid use in last week of life and implications for end-of-life decision-making. *The Lancet* 356: 398–399.
10. Willems, Dick L., Elisabeth R. Daniels, Gerrit van der Wal, Paul J. van der Maas, Ezekiel J. Emanuel. 2000. Attitudes and practices concerning the end of life: A comparison between physicians from the United States and from the Netherlands. *Archives of Internal Medicine* 160: 63–68.
11. Rurup, Mette, Christiaan A. Rhodius, Sander D. Borgsteede, Manon S. A. Boddaert, Astrid G. M. Keijser, H. Roeline W. Pasman, and Bregje D. Onwuteaka-Philipsen. 2010. The use of opioids at the end of life: The knowledge level of Dutch physicians as a potential barrier to effective pain management. *BMC Palliative Care* 9: 23.
12. Deliens, Luc, Freddy Mortier, Johan Bilsen, Marc Cosyns, Robert Vander Stichele, Johan Vanoverloop, and Koen Ingles. 2000. End-of-life decisions in medical practice in Flanders, Belgium: A nationwide survey. *The Lancet* 356: 1806–1811.

PART IV

LEARNING FROM THE PRACTICE

14

Unbearable Suffering and Advanced Dementia

The Moral Problems of Advance Directives for Euthanasia

Cees M. P. M. Hertogh

INTRODUCTION

Dementia as a motive for terminating life is a key theme in our rapidly aging Western society. Given the huge increase in the number of people who suffer from this disease or are confronted with dementia in their immediate environments, this is understandable. And where there is no adequate treatment or cure, the question of the possibilities of terminating life arises because people want to make sure that the autumn of their life is not darkened by dementia.

The debate on this subject appears very modern, but it has been conducted before. As early as the age of the Roman emperors, we find relevant reflections on dementia and on the attitude of the "wise man" toward an undignified old age in the works of the Stoic philosophers. To the Stoics, the right to end one's life in the manner one desires was a fundamental article of faith; if it was no longer possible to live in accordance with one's values as a rational and social being, one had to end that life. It is well known that various Stoics died by their own hand. Seneca, for instance, repeatedly expresses his respect for Cato, who threw himself onto his own sword to save his honor and freedom. Apart from such political motives, Seneca also considers the weariness of life (*taedium vitae*) that man can fall prey to in his old age to be a motive for suicide. But by "weariness of life" he refers not to the concept as it presently figures in the Dutch euthanasia debate but, rather, to dementia:

> Do not hear me with reluctance as if my statement applied directly to you, but weigh what I have to say. It is this: I shall not abandon old age, if old age preserves me intact for myself, and intact as regards the better part of myself; but if old age begins to shatter my mind, and to pull its various faculties to pieces, if it leaves me, not like, but only the breath of life, I shall rush out of a house that is crumbling and tottering.[1]

Similar considerations are found in Cicero (e.g., On old age [*De Senectute*]) and in emperor Marcus Aurelius's *Meditations*. The latter, however, is also aware of the self-determination dilemma to which the current debate on terminating life because of dementia is seeking a solution. In dementia, the emperor realizes,

> there will be no failure of functions like transpiration, nutrition, sense-impression, and desire; but the right employment of ourselves, precision in regard to the related elements of duty, analysis of the indications of sense, to know just whether the time is come to take leave of life, and all questions of the kind which specially require a trained judgement – these are extinguished before the rest.[a,2]

The modern way out of this dilemma is sought by various ethicists and Dutch policymakers in the instrument of a written advance directive in which the author requests euthanasia in case he or she falls victim to dementia.[b] For a patient who has become incompetent, this directive may replace the contemporaneous, well-considered personal request for euthanasia, which means that the first criterion of due care under Dutch euthanasia law is met. Today, the right to a well-considered suicide has therefore shifted to the right to a self-determined physician-assisted death that also includes the right to transfer responsibility for decisions about, and execution of, life-terminating action to others. But although policy permits euthanasia for incompetent people with dementia who have such an advance directive for euthanasia, this has so far been extremely rare in actual practice.[c,3]

In this contribution, I address the moral background of this discrepancy between the possibilities officially offered by the legal system and actual practice, which lags behind. This discrepancy is not desirable for any of the parties involved: Current legislation raises false expectations and imposes a heavy responsibility on surrogate decision makers. It also puts pressure on the doctor–patient relationship, a pressure that will only increase as the number of elderly patients who have an advance directive for euthanasia steadily grows with the aging of our population. The most recent study of euthanasia practice raises the question whether the current law, The Termination of Life on Request and Assisted Suicide (Review Procedures) Act, is sufficiently future-proof in light of this "aging pressure." In addition to "weariness of life," dementia will also remain on the moral and political agenda in the near future.[3]

[a] 2. Marcus Aurelius 1989, 16.

[b] Here I confine myself to a specific type of advance directive, namely, a written request for euthanasia (advance directive for euthanasia), drawn up when the author is competent and meant to take effect under more or less clearly specified situations of incompetence. Of course, advance directives in general may include a much more broader range of (written) instructions or desires, such as expressing preferences to forgo treatment, appoint someone to make medical decisions for the author in case of incompetence (durable power of attorney for health-care choices), etc.

[c] In the most recent end-of-life study, no cases of euthanasia for patients with advanced dementia and an advance directive for euthanasia were reported (see 3. Onwuteaka-Philipsen, et al., 2007).

THE PARADIGMATIC SITUATION

When Mrs. A came to live in our nursing home she had just turned ninety. The previous ten years she had lived in a sheltered accommodation, but that was no longer possible. As a result of Alzheimer's disease she has become increasingly forgetful and in need of care and assistance. She would start wandering and then be unable to find her way home. Washing and dressing herself had also become a problem. Mrs. A is unmarried and has only one niece – who is also elderly – whom she had appointed her surrogate in her advance directive for euthanasia. This directive states that she no longer wants to live if she starts to suffer from dementia. She had witnessed how her only sister had died from this disease and she wants to spare herself such an undignified end of life.

Mrs. A effortlessly adjusts to her new living environment. She is even doing better, relieved of the fear of loneliness and desperation she often fell victim to in her previous living environment. She is a person with a lot of humour, she likes to chat, and she takes part in all social activities. When, in the presence of her niece, we bring up the subject of the advance euthanasia directive – and put it in front of her for her to inspect – she examines it carefully and then responds resolutely, "You can throw that piece of paper away!" because "We all go when it is our time." She avoids a conversation about her cognitive condition. Of course she is a little forgetful, "but what do you expect when you get to my age? I even forget how old I am!"[d]

Mrs. A's case represents what I would like to refer to as "the paradigmatic situation" of a patient suffering from dementia who has an advance directive for euthanasia. She avoids questions about her loss of memory and she "normalizes" her cognitive problems as "to be expected" at an advanced age. Such behavior is characteristic of Alzheimer's disease and is described in many textbooks. A neuropsychological examination would probably indicate lack of insight about her disease (anosognosia) and problems with abstract thinking, which would partly explain how Mrs. A experiences and articulates her current situation. Her memory problems also play a role here, in that they make it difficult for her to compare present and past and, hence, prevent her both from realizing that her cognitive problems are gradually increasing and from worrying about that. In other words, she herself does not experience the progression that outsiders find so characteristic – and frightening – about this illness. Obviously, psychosocial factors also play a role here: To cope with the adaptive tasks her forgetfulness and dependence on others confront her with, she finds an explanation in "the normal problems of old age," and she accepts the help that is offered to her in the nursing home. The advance directive drawn up earlier is now rejected.

Taking a "precedent autonomy" view of advance directives, we should, however, consider Mrs. A's current views subordinate to the views she described in her advance directive because Mrs. A no longer has the capacity to see her life

[d] Case drawn from the author's personal medical practice.

as a coherent whole.[4] This is also in line with Dutch legislation regarding competence: As a result of her illness, Mrs. A. can no longer be deemed capable of revoking her advance directive. But this does not automatically mean that the directive should be followed. Mrs. A's current wish and active involvement in her situation preclude this and prevail over the advance directive. She may not be sufficiently competent to revoke her advance directive, but she is competent enough to suspend its execution. Furthermore, there is no suffering here; on the contrary, admittance into the nursing home, which in the past was a frightening prospect to her, has actually improved her well-being.

This type of case is frequently used as an argument against terminating life for a patient with dementia based on his or her advance directive.[e,5,6] The main arguments usually go as follows:

1. Lack of suffering – partly due to absence of awareness of illness, which means that the requirement of "unbearable and hopeless suffering" cannot be met. According to policy statements of the Royal Dutch Medical Association (KNMG) and the Dutch Organization of Nursing Home Physicians (NVVA), this is the main reason why the condition of advanced dementia as such does not meet the criteria for lawful euthanasia.
2. Discrepancy between the patient's present attitude or will – approving of his or her current life – and the earlier opinion laid down in the advance directive. On the one hand, the dilemma posed by this discrepancy rests on the gradual nature of the change in decisional capacity that characterizes disorders such as dementias. On the other hand, it also illustrates what is often referred to in quality-of-life research as "response shift," that is, the fact that people who are confronted with serious illnesses in their lives adapt to the changing conditions of their existence and change their preferences about (medical) care correspondingly. It is difficult, if not impossible, to determine how much adaptation as a "normal" psychosocial phenomenon and decreased competence as an expression of cognitive decline, respectively, contribute to this discrepancy. The dilemma, however, is an unmistakable moral fact for the physician as well as for the patient's surrogate. Even if they would judge the patient to be incompetent, the fact remains that this person with dementia expresses desires and preferences that deserve to be treated with respect. Therefore, neither physician nor family member can or will disqualify this person as a moral agent.[7,8]

VALIDITY OF THE STANDARD PARADIGM

But how valid is this paradigm? Although the terms *dementia* and *Alzheimer's disease* are often used interchangeably in vernacular speech and in the popular

[e] For example, in reports of expert committees of the Royal Dutch Medical Association and the Dutch Organization of Nursing Home Physicians.

media, it is clear that dementia is a heterogeneous illness that may have different causes and that is manifested in distinct symptom profiles. In this sense, the term *dementia* is somewhat comparable to the word *cancer*: It is a nonspecific, collective term, and one should beware misplaced generalizations. This also applies to the paradigmatic situation outlined here. In other words, there are numerous situations – also within the group of people who suffer from Alzheimer's disease – that will not conform to this paradigm.

In addition, research shows that people with dementia are frequently underdiagnosed and therefore undertreated for pain and other distressing symptoms.[9,10,11] These may be a consequence or complication of the dementia, but may also be related to chronic or intervening illnesses that exist separate from the neuropsychiatric disorder. One major reason for this underdiagnosis is the atypical presentation of complaints and the fact that communication is hampered as a result of the patient's cognitive problems. Evasive and agitated behavior, for example, may be a consequence or expression of unrecognized pain.[12] Prescribing psychiatric drugs in such a situation may lead to sedation, but not to adequate relief of symptoms.

Research into end-of-life care points in the same direction. Nursing home physicians who were interviewed about their experience with the death of a demented patient who had an advance directive for euthanasia indicated that prior to this death, patients frequently experienced distressing symptoms, such as shortness of breath, muscle spasms, contractures, confusion, pain, and anxiety.[13] When asked, these physicians interpreted these symptoms as "unbearable" and, in several cases, as "hopeless" as well. However, as we will show, the interviewers in this study used a rather biased and misleading interpretation of the term *unbearable suffering*, because this concept – as used in the law and in the ethical criteria for due care – presumes a mutual assessment by physician and patient, instead of a unilateral one by the physician. Thus, the symptoms reported in this study are more suggestive of failing palliative care or refractory symptoms.

These and similar findings indicate that there is much room for improvement in palliative care for people with dementia. It is therefore not appropriate to use them in a plea for euthanasia (as Rurup and colleagues seem to do),[13] inasmuch as termination of life can never be an alternative for inadequate palliative care. Nevertheless, in my opinion it is an illusion to claim that all suffering in and from dementia can be alleviated by intensifying symptom relief. Dementia remains a mysterious disease that can be accompanied by drastic, partly misunderstood, behavioral changes, and in which severe suffering is possible even in the absence of insight or awareness of illness. The following case illustrates this point:

Mrs. B has been suffering from Alzheimer's disease for a number of years. Because she needs more care than her daughter can provide, she must be admitted to a nursing home. The decision to place her mother there fills the daughter with guilt, all the more so because Mrs. B previously signed an advance directive in which she recorded her desire for euthanasia in case she would have to be admitted to a nursing home permanently or would become demented. Both situations have now occurred.

What makes it even more difficult for the daughter is that her mother is very unhappy in her new living environment. She has always taken a slightly gloomy view of life, but with the onset of the symptoms of dementia, her pessimism also increased, for which her general practitioner prescribed antidepressants. In the nursing home she is intensely sad and anxious. She longs for her own mother and her parental home and feels very much uprooted.

Initially the professional caregivers are able to comfort her, and when her daughter comes to visit she enjoys the contact. However, the situation gradually deteriorates and the sadness starts to prevail. All Mrs. B does is ask for her mother, and she is less and less receptive to the care and closeness of others. Antidepressants and other psychiatric drugs have no effect whatsoever. They only make her feel groggy, which makes eating and drinking more difficult. It is also more difficult for her daughter to get through to her mother. Moreover, Mrs. B frequently mistakes her for a stranger.

Care team, physician, and daughter feel helpless, and the question arises whether now is perhaps the moment to discuss the advance directive for euthanasia. Mrs. B's daughter has attempted to bring up the subject by gently trying to ask her mother whether she felt life was still worth living. But the conversation flags every time. Widening, fearful eyes and a penetrating call for mother are the result.[f]

No one will doubt that there is suffering here, suffering and also helplessness. The strong desire for parents and parental home is a well-known phenomenon that occurs frequently in the more advanced stages of Alzheimer's disease and other types of dementia. The psychology of dementia has provided various explanations, all of which share one common characteristic, that is, the fact that this longing is always linked to the need for safety and security and for something to hold onto, needs that are characteristic of dementia.[14,15] By putting themselves in the shoes of the person with dementia, caregivers often manage to meet these needs, but in all fairness they also regularly fail, no matter how hard everyone tries. The situation with Mrs. B is an example. The fact that it is impossible to fulfill her desire and the impotence of the care team and daughter are characteristic of what I have referred to elsewhere as the essential moral problem of the psychogeriatric care relationship, namely, the progressive loss of a shared world.[16] Sooner or later, the efforts to make and maintain contact founder on the unbridgeable gap between "our" world and the demented person's world. Herein lies the complexity, as well as the tragedy, of caring for people with dementia.

Care team, physician, and daughter stand empty-handed in the face of poignant and unsolvable suffering. This is an extremely painful situation, but the crucial question we must ask here is whether this suffering can also be termed "unbearable" in the sense of the Euthanasia Act? When answering this question, we must be aware that the designation "unbearable" in the second criterion for due care refers not primarily to the intensity or severity of the patients' suffering but to the opinion shared by doctor and patient that,

[f] Case drawn from the author's personal practice.

realistically, there is no alternative solution or way out of the situation other than medically assisted termination of life. In other words, the definition of the suffering as "unbearable" (the second criterion for due care) is the conclusion of a *dialogue* based on information (the third criterion) in which alternatives to terminating life have been weighed. Hence, the fourth due care criterion and the Explanatory Memorandum to the Euthanasia Act both expressly state that the physician *together with the patient* must have come to the conviction that the only way left to alleviate the patient's suffering is euthanasia or assisted suicide.

In the case of severe dementia, however, the loss of a shared world makes communication about the suffering at this level impossible. So there can be no mutuality and intersubjectivity – no reciprocity – and so meeting the unbearable suffering criterion becomes problematic. Thus, it is often said that the unbearableness of the suffering "cannot be verified," in such cases. But this formulation is inaccurate and passes over the essence of the matter, for we are not dealing here with hypotheses or diagnoses that have to be tested or verified. Every physician who has ever had to deal with euthanasia will agree that this ultimate form of relief of suffering is only possible in the context of a relationship of trust with the patient. In other words, it is morally impossible to actively end a patient's life without actual consent, without the conviction – practically up to the moment it is carried out – that this action meets the unmistakable wish of that patient.

An advance directive can never replace this necessary intersubjectivity. The execution of such a directive would confront physicians with a horrifying scenario, for then they would have to terminate the life of defenseless patients to whom they can no longer explain that this is what these now-demented persons wanted to happen in a long-forgotten past. Moreover, even if these persons can be deemed incompetent to make the actual decision, they can still resist the execution of the decision. In the situation of Mrs. B, this is a realistic expectation in view of her anxious and evasive attitude. There is no question that there is suffering here, but what holds us back – and must hold us back – is the defenseless power of human need and vulnerability. Despite obvious suffering, ending the patient's life out of respect for the advance directive is not an acceptable or humane path to tread. And in the absence of alternatives, all we can do is accept the insolubility of the suffering.

The loss of a common, shared world in dementia sharply brings out the extent to which the practice of euthanasia, from the first discussion to its eventually being carried out, rests on shared decision making. Moreover, the requirements of due care that have developed from practice are completely grafted onto the situation of a competent patient and a dialogue about that patient's suffering. These criteria for due care presume and support each other in such a manner that one cannot simply separate one criterion without affecting the coherence of the whole. Yet that is exactly what policymakers have done in Article 2, Paragraph 2, of the Euthanasia Act, which says that an advance directive can replace a patient's contemporaneous request, while "the other due care requirements have to be met *in a corresponding way*" (italics added), as the clever but cryptic legal formulation reads.

When it is impossible to consult with the patient, all that remains is a unilateral assessment of suffering by the physician, perhaps complemented with assessments by other caregivers and family members. This is insufficient and places too much responsibility on others. In this respect, there is no point in expanding the definition of unbearable suffering in the case of dementia, for example, by including in its scope the occurrence of symptoms like anxiety, depression, various forms of problematic behavior, and loss of control of one's environment. Such an expansion, suggested by Esther Pans[17], among others, does not change the lack of intersubjectivity and reciprocity or the moral dilemmas outlined earlier. The key problem is the criterion of unbearable suffering itself, as well as the fact that the practice of euthanasia and the rules governing it are thoroughly rooted in the context of end-of-life care for *competent* patients.

LOSS OF DIGNITY AS AN ALTERNATIVE?

In recent years, appreciation for the ethical dilemmas faced by physicians in this situation has increased among the protagonists of euthanasia for people with advanced dementia. They have not resigned themselves to the current situation, however. The Dutch Association for Voluntary Euthanasia (NVVE), for example, has been working toward the introduction of a new criterion as the normative measure for terminating life because of dementia, that is, the irreversible loss of personal dignity. Words of similar import are regularly found in existing advance directives for euthanasia as motives for euthanasia, for example, when these directives speak of lack of prospects for "return[ing] to a state of life that I [the author of the directive] consider reasonable and dignified." In addition, in the 1980s, the Dutch Supreme Court acknowledged that one's impending deterioration and the prospect of not being able to die in a dignified manner could be taken as forms of unbearable suffering. The Court rendered this decision in the *Schoonheim* case,[g] in retrospect the first "weariness-of-life" case. In the controversial assisted suicide case involving former Dutch senate member Brongersma in 2002, the same Supreme Court reversed this wide interpretation by pronouncing that the criterion of unbearable suffering must always have a medically classifiable origin.[h]

The NVVE now proposes to view suffering and dignity as two separate criteria, which in itself is an illuminating distinction. Both criteria are at present regularly mixed up, as the debate about the weariness-of-life motive shows. The NVVE postulates, however, that the criterion of dignity is also a valuable

[g] See Chapter 3 by Weyers and Chapter 4 by Pans..

[h] See Chapter 22 by Kimsma.

addition to the criterion of suffering as a justification for life-terminating action by physicians for people with dementia who have an advance directive. When physicians are unable to meet the requirement of unbearable suffering, as in advanced dementia, they might be convinced by the irreversible loss of personal dignity, provided that the patient has clearly and unequivocally defined what this means to him or her in an advance directive. Because this appears to be far from simple, the NVVE has also commissioned a comprehensive empirical study into the concept of personal dignity, in order to further clarify and operationalize the concept.[18]

In my opinion, these proposals are not very feasible and indeed are highly questionable. Their feasibility is limited because the dignity requirement forces physicians to step out of the medical domain and outside their acknowledged area of expertise, and not focus exclusively on the presence or absence of suffering. They are questionable because the moral justification for medical involvement in euthanasia is at issue. Without suffering, euthanasia can never be explained and justified as an act of mercy; yet the entire euthanasia practice as it has developed and taken shape in statutory due-care criteria in the Netherlands is based on just this: "Morally, the patient's suffering outweighs the patient's request.... If ever the physician abstains from judging the suffering, then he will disqualify/eliminate himself as a moral actor in the decision-making process. [Laat de arts dat oordeel los, dan schakelt hij zichzelf als morele actor in het hele beslissingsproces uit.]"[19]

Furthermore, if physicians had to assess the dignity of people with (advanced) dementia, it would necessarily be a unilateral exercise, just like the assessment of unbearable suffering in the present situation. For even though the patient may have defined in detail his or her own concept of dignity and what he or she sees as an irreversible loss of dignity, the advance directive cannot interpret itself. This is and will remain the responsibility of others – physicians and family members. It is up to them to determine whether and when this demented patient has indeed lost his or her dignity. This is no sinecure, and the ethical question I want to pose here is whether we – as potential authors of advance directives – have the right to burden our loved ones and caregivers with such a heavy responsibility.

A related ethical question is whether operationalizing what dignity and loss of dignity could entail might not negatively cross over into stigmatizing the people with dementia themselves, people who already have so very little to say and who are often weighed down by discrimination and stigmatization in our current "hypercognitive" society.[20] Were we to study how people with advance directives for euthanasia define personal dignity, we would not find it much different from the central values in this hypercognitive world, for those values are unlikely to be completely and incomparably personal and individual. We are already finding them in the way regular advance directives invoke self-sufficiency, autonomy, and independence. In other words, these so-called personal concepts of dignity will presumably fit in with the dominant Kantian version of human dignity in terms of rational self-control. Thus, what loss of personal dignity entails is, *mutatis mutandis,* easily inferred.

More relevant in my opinion and much more urgent from a moral perspective than such a redundant study with predictable results is critical reflection on this dominant characterization of human dignity, or dignity *tout court*. It has a long-standing tradition in our culture, one that goes back to the Enlightenment and has even older, Stoic roots. In this tradition, dignity is seen, to a considerable degree, as separate from need and vulnerability, which causes us to exclude and ignore important aspects and stages of our lives. Martha Nussbaum, whom I follow here, provides a keen diagnosis of this thinking about dignity when she writes:

> Need itself does not have dignity; it is only contingently linked to that which has dignity. This means that we do not think of the hunger of the body, its needs for shelter, for care in time of illness, and for love, as among the ingredients in its dignity. They are somewhat embarrassing facts about a being who also has dignity. This view subtly colors the way in which we will approach the task of giving relief to bodily need: we think of it as supporting a relatively undignified aspect of human life, in order that the dignified part should gain thereby. I believe that this is a distorted basis for thinking about the love and care we give children, the sick, and the elderly, issues that societies continually and increasingly must face, as the life span expands and many adults spend up to a third of their lives in a state that does not promise full mental and moral functioning. Some human beings, of course, live their whole lives in a state of radical mental dependency on others; good political thought must provide for, and show respect for, them too."[21]

I warmly support her plea for a fundamental reflection on dignity, for much is at stake here: our own moral functioning, the way in which we relate to others in our need, and our respect for people with cognitive impairments.

A DILEMMA WITH NO WAY OUT?

My goal here has been to clarify the moral background of the discrepancy between the formal possibilities of the law and practices in end-of-life care for people with dementia. I have attempted to demonstrate that this discrepancy goes to the ethical foundation of the way in which euthanasia is organized in the Netherlands, that is, as an exceptional type of assistance, entrusted to physicians, based on two fundamental ethical values: self-determination (of the patient) and mercifulness (as moral justification of the involvement of the physician). Take away one of these foundations and the carefully constructed edifice of euthanasia practice collapses. Physician-assisted death is not possible without a request, and it is not possible without suffering either. The problem of advance directives for euthanasia bears on this foundation in a special way because it reveals and clarifies a primordial condition essential to euthanasia, though not one directly expressed in the codified criteria for due care – namely, the value of reciprocity: for mercifulness cannot exist without responsive receptiveness.[i,22,23] Put metaphorically, the Samaritan can only be helpful if the wounded and robbed traveler to Jericho is ready to accept his assistance, not if the traveler rejects him, feels threatened by him, or does not understand him. Only the responsiveness of the other makes the Samaritan into a merciful giver, and this responsiveness cannot be replaced by a distant request on a piece of paper. What this assistance wants is consenting reciprocity at the moment it is given.

That is the essence of the moral problem presented here, and it cannot be solved within the boundaries of current laws, if it can be solved at all. Rather, this problem insists that we learn to better recognize this significance of reciprocity as a third moral pillar that supports the structure of the euthanasia practice, and that we accept the consequences.[j,24]

All of which leads us to a final question. If severe dementia does not meet the requirement of unbearable suffering, does that mean there can never be moral justification for life-terminating action for a patient with advanced dementia? If such a justification is to be found at all, it cannot be via the principle of dignity, but only and exclusively via the path of suffering. This is – I emphasize once again – the *only* legitimate reason for physicians to get involved in euthanasia or assisted suicide.

Various successive studies on the Dutch euthanasia practice have shown that, in very rare cases, physicians may end a person's life without there being an express request or an advance directive for euthanasia. Some of these cases have concerned people with dementia, but the reason for terminating life has not been related to dementia. The reason is nearly always a serious complication of another illness, for instance, pulmonary hemorrhage, shortness of breath that cannot be alleviated, or intractable seizures.[25] The number of cases like this is decreasing, very probably as a result of the increasing scale of palliative sedation. Physician organizations, such as the Dutch Association of Nursing Home Physicians and the Royal Dutch Medical Association, have formulated additional policy statements that leave room for euthanasia in a demented patient who has an advance directive requesting it, if the patient has suffering stemming from another medical source that cannot be relieved in any other way.[6,5] Here, again, termination of life is not based on suffering caused by dementia but on suffering arising from an intervening illness.

The NVVA, however, did not rule out that under very exceptional circumstances, an untreatable complication of the dementia – examples mentioned include severe self-mutilating behavior – can be a reason for life-terminating action.[6] The policy document in question speaks of "unacceptable suffering" and clarifies that although this judgment of unacceptability must be supported

[i] For philosophical backgrounds of the concept of reciprocity, see 22. Ricoeur 1992. For the concept of responsiveness, see 23. Tronto 1993.

[j] For more details and the presentation of a case illustrating the relevance of reciprocity as a value in the practice of euthanasia/assisted suicide, see 24. Hertogh 2009.

by an advance directive for euthanasia, it is based primarily on medical considerations. The situation must be one in which all regular possibilities of symptom relief fail, while the suffering is felt as if it were one's own. Only then does mercifulness overrule reciprocity.

There are, however, no descriptions of such desperate situations known from practice. Moreover, considerable progress has been made in the field of palliative care, especially in the form of palliative sedation, since this policy position was adopted in 1997. So the question is whether the term *unacceptable suffering* used in the NVVA document is now more or less covered by the term *refractory symptoms* used in the KNMG guideline for palliative sedation.[26] What both terms have in common is that they concern symptoms that cannot be controlled by selective, intensive symptom-specific interventions – even after consultation with other medical specialists. A second important similarity is the key role of professional judgment.

A difference may be found in the nature of the symptoms. The examples of refractory symptoms generally mentioned are pain, shortness of breath, nausea, anxiety, and delirium, but when we are talking about serious complications of dementia, we should perhaps also include very severe behavioral problems. However, this distinction is one of degree rather than principle. A difference that should be considered one of principle is the argument of time, which plays an important role in designating a symptom as refractory: The refractory nature of a symptom also consists of the limited remaining life expectancy, which means there simply is no time to apply other types of symptom relief. The description of the term *unacceptable suffering* lacks such a link with life expectancy, but there is a connection with the presence of an advance directive for euthanasia.

Despite these differences, I still think that it would be advisable to continue studying this gray area between palliative care and life-terminating action, both to examine whether a concept like unacceptable suffering is justified by reality and to further explore the possible applications of sedation in this special domain of palliative care. We owe this much at least to the increasing number of people with dementia and also to the growing group of elderly people who have an advance directive for euthanasia.

References

1. Seneca, L. A. [1883] 1967. *Ad Lucilium epistulae morales*. Ed. and trans. R. M. Gummere, 409. Cambridge, MA: Harvard University Press.
2. Marcus Aurelius. 1989. *The Meditations of Marcus Aurelius Antoninus and a Selection from the Letters of Marcus and Fronto*. Trans. A. S. L. Farquharson and R. B. Rutherford. New York: Oxford University Press: 16.
3. Onwuteaka-Philipsen, Bregje D., Joseph K. M. Gevers, Agnes van der Heide, et al. 2007. *Evaluatie Wet Toetsing Levensbeëindiging op verzoek en hulp bij zelfdoding* [Evaluation of The Termination of Life on Request and Assisted Suicide (Review Procedures) Act]. The Hague: ZonMw.

4. Dworkin, Ronald. 1986. Autonomy and the demented self. *Milbank Quarterly* 64: 4–16.
5. Royal Dutch Medical Association (KNMG). 1997. *Levensbeëindigend handelen bij wilsonbekwame patiënten* [Termination of life of incompetent patients]. Houten: Bohn Stafleu Van Loghum.
6. Dutch Association of Nursing Home Physicians (NVVA). 1997. *Medische zorg met beleid*. [Policy statement on end-of-life-care in demented patients in nursing homes]. Utrecht: NVVA.
7. Jaworska, Agnieszka. 1999. Respecting the margins of agency: Alzheimer's patients and the capacity to value. *Philosophy & Public Affairs* 28: 106–138.
8. Hertogh, Cees M. P. M., Marike E. de Boer, Rose-Marie Dröes, and Jan A. Eefsting. 2007. Would we rather lose our life than lose our self? Lessons from the Dutch debate on euthanasia for patients with dementia. *American Journal of Bioethics* 7: 48–56.
9. Mitchell, Susan L., Dan K. Kiely, and Mary Beth Hamel. 2004. Dying with advanced dementia in the nursing home. *Archives of Internal Medicine* 64: 321–326.
10. Frampton, Maria. 2003. Experience assessment and management of pain in people with dementia. *Age and Ageing* 32: 248–251.
11. Steen, Jenny T. van der, Marcel E. Ooms, Geritt van der Wal, and Miel W. Ribbe. 2002. Pneumonia: The demented patient's best friend? Discomfort after starting or withholding antibiotic treatment. *Journal of the American Geriatrics Society* 50: 1681–1688.
12. Achterberg, Wilco P., Anne Margriet Pot, Erik J. Scherder, Miel W. Ribbe. 2007. Pain in the nursing home: Assessment and treatment on different types of care wards. *Journal of Pain and Symptom Management* 34: 480–487.
13. Rurup, Mette L., Bregje D. Onwuteaka-Philipsen, Agnes van der Heide, Gerrit van der Wal, and Paul J. van der Maas. 2005. Physicians' experiences with demented patients with advance euthanasia directives in the Netherlands. *Journal of the American Geriatrics Society* 53: 1138–1144.
14. Miesen, Bère M. 1993. Alzheimer's disease, the phenomenon of parent fixation and Bowlby's attachment theory. *International Journal of Geriatric Psychiatry* 8: 147–153.
15. Cheston, Richard, and Mike P. Bender. 1999. *Understanding Dementia*. London: Jessica Kingsley.
16. Hertogh, Cees M. P. M., Anne-Mei The, Bère M. L. Miesen, and Jan A. Eefsting. 2004. Truth telling and truthfulness in the care for patients with advanced dementia: An ethnographic study in Dutch nursing homes. *Social Science & Medicine* 59: 1685–1693.
17. Pans, Esther. 2006. *De normatieve grondslagen van het recht* [The normative foundations of the right to euthanasia]. Amsterdam: Wolf Legal Publishers.
18. Dutch Association for Voluntary Euthanasia (NVVE). 2007. *Perspectieven op waardig sterven*. [Perspectives on dying with dignity]. Amsterdam: NVVE.
19. Dillmann, Robert J. M. 2003. Euthanasie: de morele legitimatie van de arts [Euthanasia: The moral legitimation of the physician]. In *Levensbeëindigend handelen door een arts*, ed. Johan Legemaate and Robert J. M. Dillman, 11–27. Houten/Diegem: Bohn Stafleu Van loghum.
20. Post, Stephen G. 2000. *The Moral Challenge of Dementia*. Baltimore: Johns Hopkins University Press.

21. Nussbaum, Martha C. 2001. *The Fragility of Goodness: Luck and Ethics in Greek Tragedy and Philosophy*. Cambridge: Cambridge University Press.
22. Ricoeur, Paul. 1992. *Oneself as Another*. Chicago: University of Chicago Press.
23. Tronto, Joan C. 1993. *Moral Boundaries: A Political Argument for an Ethic of Care*. New York: Routledge.
24. Hertogh, Cees M. P. M. 2009. The role of advance euthanasia directives as an aid to communication and shared decision-making in dementia. *Journal of Medical Ethics* 35 (2): 100–103.
25. Wal, Gerrit van der, Agnes van der Heide, Bregje D. Onwuteaka-Philipsen, and Paul J. van der Maas. 2003. *Medische besluitvorming aan het einde van het leven. De praktijk en toetsingsprocedure euthanasie* [Medical decision making at the end of life: Euthanasia practice and review procedures] Utrecht: De Tijdstroom.
26. KNMG. 2009. *Guidelines for Palliative Sedation*. Utrecht: Royal Dutch Medical Association (in Dutch).

15

Decision-Making Capacity in Patients Who Are in the Early Stage of Alzheimer's Disease and Who Request Physician-Assisted Suicide

Ron Berghmans

THE CASE OF HUGO CLAUS

In March 2008, the Flemish writer, poet, and artist Hugo Claus died at the age of 78. It had been known for a couple of years prior to his death that he suffered from Alzheimer's disease. Because of this affliction, Claus asked for and received euthanasia in the midst of his family and friends. The former Belgian Prime Minister Guy Verhofstadt was among those paying tributes to Claus, and said he imagined that the onset of Alzheimer's must have been "inevitable and unbearable torture" for someone "no longer able to knead his words into clear phrases, create the right expressions and metaphors." That was something that had "cost him no effort for over 60 years," Mr Verhofstadt said. "In each and every text and poem, he was an emotional beacon in our dark world. But I can live with the fact that he decided thus, because he left us as a great glowing star, right on time, just before he would have collapsed into a black hole."

INTRODUCTION

Many people fear the possibility of becoming demented, and some would – as Hugo Claus did – prefer an earlier death over having to progress into the final stages of Alzheimer's disease. One way to avoid the ravages of Alzheimer's is to stop eating and drinking[a,1] or to commit suicide. One may also wait until one catches a life-threatening illness and then refuse treatment (i.e., pneumonia as "the old man's friend"). Another possible route is to ask for assisted suicide or euthanasia, as in the case of Hugo Claus. Assisted suicide and euthanasia are

[a] The option to stop eating and drinking in the Dutch context has been coined as *versterven* ("starving"); recently the Dutch psychiatrist Boudewijn Chabot introduced the concept of "auto-euthanasia" to qualify all forms of life-shortening acts in which no physician is involved, but in which the person who wishes to die is at the same time in charge and in dialogue with one or more other intimate others.

legally available in only a few countries. In the Netherlands as well as Belgium, physician-assisted suicide is legally permissible if a number of specific conditions are met[2,3,4,5]; in the U.S. state of Oregon, terminally ill adults are allowed to obtain and use prescriptions from their physicians for self-administered, lethal medications;[6] in Switzerland, physician- as well as non-physician-assisted suicide is passively tolerated.[7]

Much controversy exists over the moral legitimacy of assistance in dying when this involves actively and deliberately shortening the life of the patient. This is particularly the case if patients do not (or do not only) suffer from somatic illnesses but (also) from mental disturbances, such as in the case of chronic mental illness or Alzheimer's disease or other neurological disorders.

Actually, in the Netherlands there is debate over the legitimacy of physician-assisted suicide and euthanasia for patients who have dementia.[8,9,10,11,12,13] In this debate, much attention is being paid to the role of advance directives if the patient suffering from Alzheimer's has lost the capacity to express wishes and make choices in a competent way.[14,15,10] In addition to the question whether it may be morally acceptable to actively (help to) terminate the life of an Alzheimer patient who lacks decision-making capacity as a result of the progression of the disease, there is debate over the moral and legal justifiability of physician-assisted suicide for patients in the early stages of dementia.

In this debate many important practical, ethical, legal, and societal issues are raised.[16,17,18,19,20,21,22] Here, the focus will be on the issue of decision-making capacity in relation to requests made by people who suffer from Alzheimer's disease or other dementias and who are in the early stage of the disease. For the sake of argument, the assumption is made that the prospect of the progression of Alzheimer's disease can be a morally legitimate reason to give assistance to persons who request active help in dying because they suffer unbearably or consider their life as being irreversibly devoid of dignity, if the following conditions (the so-called criteria of due care) are also met:

- The request is voluntarily made;
- The request expresses an enduring wish;
- The suffering is unbearable and without prospect of hope and relief;
- No reasonable alternative means exist to make life bearable; and
- The individual who expresses this wish is considered to have decision-making capacity.[23]

In this chapter. we will address the notion of decision-making capacity as a key threshold concept that allows or precludes physician-assisted suicide or euthanasia in Dutch law and practice, particularly as this notion applies to patients suffering from dementia in an early stage.

First, we will present a number of illustrative cases of physician-assisted suicide in patients with dementia. Then we address a number of theoretical questions concerning the concept of decision-making capacity, focusing on issues over which consensus exists in the literature.

In the second part of this chapter, we examine how decision-making capacity is construed in a number of cases reported in the Netherlands in which a patient who suffered from dementia requested and received physician-assisted suicide.

PHYSICIAN-ASSISTED SUICIDE IN DEMENTIA

A number of cases in which physician-assisted suicide was administered to a dementia patient have been reported more or less extensively in the annual reports of the Dutch Euthanasia Review Committees. We first describe a number of these cases for illustrative purposes. Then we address considerations relating to the issue of decision-making capacity (indicated in italics in the following case studies).

Illustrative Cases

A first case was published (and commented on) in the *Dutch Journal of Medicine* (NTVG).[24,25]

Case 1 involved a 71-year-old man who suffered from vascular dementia and, during a period of four years, had repeatedly requested physician-assisted suicide from his psychiatrist because he didn't want to await further progressive deterioration of his condition. It was clear to the psychiatrist that there was decline in mental functioning, but not to such a degree that the patient was unable to make a far-reaching and complicated decision. The procedure for physician-assisted suicide in the mental hospital required two conversations with the patient by a psychiatrist *who had not* before known him. This psychiatrist took the criteria of due care for euthanasia and physician-assisted suicide as guidance for the conversations and concluded that it was justified to answer the request positively because of the unbearable and hopeless nature of the patient's suffering and the patient's continuously present wish to end his life. Above that, in the perception of the psychiatrist the patient *was still able to consciously say good-bye.*

An independent nursing home physician unknown to the treating psychiatrist and the patient also concluded that the patient's wish was very well considered and present in an enduring sense for a long time. This physician took the view that during the conversation, the patient "certainly gave the impression of *being able to estimate his situation adequately. He knows what he chooses.*"

Finally, a professor of neurology consulted in the case confirmed the decision to provide physician-assisted suicide, and referred to the negative prognosis as indicated by neurological, neuropsychological, and imaging examinations. He confirmed that the course of the patient's illness made progressive deterioration probable. He also confirmed that a patient with multi-infarct dementia "certainly can be competent with regard to his will to end his life and *to overlook the consequences thereof.*"

The next two cases are from the annual reports of the Dutch Regional Euthanasia Review Committees that have been published since these committees started functioning in 1998, when substantial changes in the reporting procedure in cases of euthanasia and physician-assisted suicide were made.[26,27,28] The doctor now reports to one of five Regional Euthanasia Review Committees, each consisting of a lawyer (chair), a doctor and an ethicist. If the committee judges the doctor's behavior to have met the minimum requirements, it will advise against prosecution, and the prosecutorial authorities – while not formally bound to do so – will generally respect this advice. Cases that meet the minimum requirements but in which there has been some deviation from the "rules of careful practice" applicable to euthanasia and physician-assisted suicide will be dealt with informally or via medical disciplinary law. If in the view of the committee the doctor has seriously departed from the key requirements, the committee will advise the prosecutor to have a closer look at the case and possibly to bring a criminal prosecution.

It should be stressed that these cases contain descriptions in the annual reports of the Regional Euthanasia Review Committees and – because of their summarizing character – lack the richness of details of the real cases. The "real story" behind the cases thus cannot be other than partially told. In some respects, this may raise questions that remain unanswered, or that elicit criticism, which may be unjustified.

Case 2 (Year Report 2004, Case 3) was a male patient aged 65 who had suffered from Alzheimer's disease for three years. The concomitant depressive complaints were successfully treated pharmaceutically. In addition, the patient received day care in a nursing home. The patient suffered unbearably from the fact that he could in no way live independently anymore. Also he suffered seriously from *the insight into his future as a demented patient.* From the start of his illness, the patient clearly indicated to his physician that he did not want to go through the whole illness process. In the year preceding the termination of his life, the patient repeatedly requested physician-assisted suicide.

The physician referred the patient to a SCEN (Support and Consultation Euthanasia in the Netherlands) consultant. According to this consultant, the patient suffered unbearably from *being dependent on others, from awareness of his deterioration and loss of decorum, from loss of autonomy and self-respect, and from the knowledge of the worsening of his situation.* Although the consultant considered the patient's suffering to be "unimaginable" (*oninvoelbaar*), the consultant took the view that the awareness of deficits would decrease with the progression of illness and that the suffering would become less unbearable as time went by. Further, the consultant felt that the mental capacity of the patient could be questioned, as during the consultation the patient was *unable to follow reasoning.* Thus, despite the patient's consistent and enduring expression of a wish for termination of life, the consultant concluded that the criteria for due care were not fulfilled.

The physician subsequently consulted three other experts: a psychologist, a nursing home physician, and a geronto-psychiatrist. From these independent consultations it became clear that there was no sign of depression, that the patient wanted to *retain control over his life*, and that *he was aware that the progression of the illness would deprive him of this control.* The experts concluded separately that the patient was able to express a voluntary and well-considered request for termination of life and that he was *conscious of the consequences of this choice.* After this conclusion, the physician decided to honor the patient's request. The patient died as a result of assisted suicide.

In reviewing the case, the Regional Euthanasia Review Committee took the view that despite concerns about the patient's capacity raised by the consultant, the independent experts who were subsequently consulted concluded that the patient had mental capacity and was well able to express and argue his will.... The committee judged that the physician had acted in accord with the criteria for due care.

In *Case 3* (Year Report 2007, Case 3), Mrs. A, between 70 and 80 years of age, was diagnosed with early dementia (probably a mix of Alzheimer's disease with subcortical characteristics) at the end of 2004. A year before she had undergone neuropsychological testing because of memory complaints. The neurologist had concluded that she suffered from depression. Treatment of the depression, however, was not effective and eventually stopped. [The published case description gives no details about the treatment for depression.]

Mrs. A complained about fatigue, listlessness, tremor of the hands, forgetfulness, and loss of interest in different areas of life. She was examined by a clinical geriatrician to exclude a possible physical cause. No somatic cause could be identified, and ultimately the complaints were considered to be depressive in nature. The geriatrician took the view that there were no signs of a process of dementia. He recommended that the treating physician (in consultation with the neurologist) change the pharmaceutical treatment of the patient in order to improve her mood. By the end of 2004, the clinical geriatrician diagnosed early dementia and treatment was started. This had to be stopped because of troublesome side effects.

Immediately after being informed about this diagnosis – and several times thereafter – Mrs. A spoke with the treating physician about euthanasia. At the end of March 2005, she explicitly requested that the physician perform euthanasia. She expressed her wishes in a written advance directive. The physician consulted six colleagues in total: two general practitioners and four psychiatrists. The first consultant visited the patient in March 2005, the last consultant five days before the termination of life took place [in 2007]. The first four consultants (one general practitioner and three psychiatrists) took the view that the patient was suffering from a depressive illness and advised treatment of this disorder. Fully a year and a half later, the treating physician again consulted a fifth, independent, colleague GP who also was a SCEN physician. This consultant visited Mrs. A six weeks before the termination of her life.

Meanwhile, the patient was hospitalized in a nursing home and confined to a wheelchair. It appeared that she was suffering from Parkinson's disease. During the interview the consultant noticed that Mrs. A had *word-finding problems* – sometimes *she spoke unintelligibly*, and then she was understandable again. In the opinion of the consultant, her *thinking was logical.* Above that *she felt empathy for her family*. She could not remember everything well. However, she *showed that she remembered having discussed her euthanasia wish earlier* with a physician other than her GP. She expressed the view that her suffering was unbearable given the fact that she couldn't do what she wanted, such as her inability to express her thoughts in words and that she was totally dependent on others. Mrs. A told the consultant that she didn't consider herself a normal human being. Being asked what it meant for her if the euthanasia were not to take place, she answered that this would be a heavy blow.

According to this consultant, the patient's request was voluntary and well considered. In her advance directive, she had indicated that she didn't want to continue living if it meant being in a condition from which it would be unlikely or impossible to return to what she deemed a "reasonable and dignified state of life" (*een voor haar redelijke en waardige levensstaat*). According to the consultant, *she had moments of complete insight into her illness as well as moments in which she lacked such insight.* In the consultant's view, during these moments of *insight and realization* the patient was suffering unbearably. The consultant also was convinced that no other treatment options existed. She expressed doubts about the opinion of the consulting psychiatrists that the patient's depressive disorder ought to be treated. At the time these psychiatrists were consulted, the diagnosis of Parkinson's disease had not yet been made. Moreover, treatment for possible depression had not been effective. And although the consultant thought the euthanasia request imaginable (*invoelbaar*) and consistent, she nevertheless gave the advice to consult a psychiatrist or geriatrician once more in order to assess the mental capacity (*wilsbekwaamheid*) of Mrs. A. The mental capacity of Mrs. A had been doubted several times in the past.

The physician referred the patient to an independent psychiatrist as a sixth consultant. This consultant assessed the mental capacity of the patient 10 days before the termination of her life. According to the report of this psychiatrist, in spite of the evident dementia syndrome and word-finding problems, the patient could *describe clearly her condition and the meaning and implications of the diagnosis*. She *could indicate well the progression of the disease and the deterioration that would take place.* In the consultant's view, the patient was *clear about her wish for euthanasia* and was *able to see the consequences of that wish*. The sixth consultant further noted that in Mrs. A's case there existed a continuous *lijdensdruk*, literally, a continuous "pressure of suffering." ...

The committee judged that the physician in this case had acted in accordance with the criteria for due care.

Each of these cases illustrates the issue of competence or decision making with respect to the practice of physician-assisted suicide in the early stages of dementia. We will comment on this more extensively, but first wish to outline the issue of competence or decision-making capacity from a more theoretical perspective.

ASSESSMENT OF DECISION-MAKING CAPACITY: THEORY

Since the seminal article by Loren Roth, Alan Meisel, and Charles Lidz in 1977,[29] much scholarly and empirical work has been done on the conceptualization and practical assessment of competence or mental capacity, especially in psychiatry[30] and in the context of care for the elderly and patients with dementia[31].

What is competence? Competence is one of the elements of informed consent, the moral and legal principle that guides decision making with regard to both clinical medicine and clinical research.[32,33,34] Competence is generally conceived as an ability to make decisions or decision-making capacity.[33,35] There are a number of issues about which consensus exists.[36,37]

ISSUE 1. There is a general presumption of competence. This presumption implies that any adult person ought to be considered to have decision-making capacity unless there is evidence to the contrary.[37] This presumption applies equally to all groups of patients, that is, those suffering from somatic illnesses, as well as those who suffer from mental illnesses or neuropsychiatric disorders or who have a mental handicap. This presumption may be viewed as expressing a priori respect for the autonomy and dignity rights of persons. As such, these disorders and handicaps are not grounds for inferring incompetence. This means that the burden of proof lies with the health-care worker who takes the view that a patient lacks decision-making capacity.[38]

Here, a distinction is in place between this general assumption and the reasons that may elicit doubts about a person's competence, which may lead to an assessment of that person's decision-making capacity.

ISSUE 2. It is agreed that decision-making capacity is *task specific and decision relative*.[33] As already stated, decision-making capacity is not directly connected to specific disorders or diagnoses. Nor does a judgment about capacity imply a general disqualification of the person involved. Capacity is always related to a specific treatment or research decision. This means that patient A may lack capacity to make decision X, but at the same time may have capacity to make decision Y.[33]

The decision-relative character of decision-making capacity implies that more is asked of a patient when a complex decision is involved than for a less complex, more straightforward decision. In terms of understanding, complex decisions are more demanding. The wish for death that is implied in a request for physician-assisted suicide can hardly be considered a straightforward or simple decision, and in that perspective the decision-making capacity of a person asking for physician-assisted suicide will be evaluated differently from, for instance, the refusal of a treatment that is quite obvious and easy to understand.

Disagreement exists as to whether decision-making capacity ought further to be thought of in a *risk-relative sense*.[33,39] Risk relativity would imply that a more demanding standard is applied when the patient's decision involves greater risks.[40,41] This approach is based on the conviction that our concern for the patient's welfare requires us to demand a higher level of capacity for decisions pertaining to life and death than for decisions that may result in lesser harms.[42,43] Two major objections are raised against this approach.[44,45,46]

The strongest objection is that it supports an asymmetric view of capacity: An individual may at the same time have capacity to consent to treatment but lack capacity to refuse it. Many consider this implication counterintuitive, because it rejects the apparently intuitive "principle of symmetrical competence".[40] Proponents of a fixed standard who reject a risk-related approach pose the question: What level of capacity is necessary for an individual to make a certain decision? Proponents of a risk-related standard pose another question: What level of capacity is necessary for an individual to grant that individual decisional authority with regard to a specific choice? The first approach focuses on decisional capability, the second on decisional authority. The question regarding decisional *capability* refers to those capabilities that are considered necessary and/or sufficient for decision making. The question about decisional *authority* is about whether a person has the right to decide about a particular course of action. The latter perspective does not focus exclusively on individual capabilities, but incorporates risk as a relevant factor in deciding the level of decision-making capacity that is required.[47]

The second objection is that the risk-related approach conflates two issues: On the one hand, the question of whether or not an individual has capacity, and on the other hand, whether or not his or her choices should be respected or might be overruled on paternalistic grounds.[39, 41]

Those who argue against the risk-related approach maintain that a two-step model ought to be followed: first, the assessment of capacity, and second, the question of whether to overrule the decision of the individual. On this view, decisional capacity and decisional authority are separate questions. As already said, proponents of a risk-related approach see capacity and authority in a connected sense.

ISSUE 3. Consensus exists with regard to the *quality of the decision-making process* that ought to be decisive for a judgment about capacity. It is generally recognized that the *outcome* of the patient's decision making cannot be the basis for a judgment about capacity. Even if this outcome is considered unwise, irresponsible, or irrational by health-care workers or others, whether the decision should be considered a sign of capacity depends on the decision-making process as well as the values involved.

ISSUE 4. Agreement exists that decision-making capacity involves a *normative and evaluative judgment.*[48,33,49,43] Given the fact that a judgment about capacity has implications for the patient's rights, and given the fact that such a judgment involves an answer to the question of whether or not the patient's decision making is "good enough" to deserve respect by the health-care worker, values inherently are involved in such a judgment. Obviously, this is not to deny that descriptive aspects also are involved.

Standards and Criteria for Decision-Making Capacity

Different standards and criteria for the assessment of decision-making capacity have been proposed:[37,50]

1. According to one approach, mental competence involves the capacity to make any decision. If the patient is able to express a choice, he or she has capacity, regardless of the content of the decision. Here, the underlying conception of the moral principle of respect for autonomy is one

of respect for spontaneous behavior and preferences. In this approach, no attention is paid to the extent to which the behavior and preferences reflect comprehension of the situation in which the subject finds him- or herself. As a result, this approach is generally considered too liberal and insufficiently protective.

2. In another approach, decision-making capacity is conceived as making a rational decision. The corresponding criterion is the ability to make a good decision. This criterion hinges upon an evaluation of the outcome of the decision. However, the outcome of a decision is determined not only by a person's mental abilities but also by this person's values and lifestyle. Assessing capacity on the basis of the outcome of a decision runs the risk of ignoring or even condemning the subject's personal values. Therefore, this approach is in conflict with respect for autonomy and too protective.
3. A third approach, which attempts to avoid the disadvantages of the previous two approaches, focuses on the quality of the decision-making process that led the subject to his or her decision. The underlying concept of autonomy is one of well-considered decision making. As mentioned, there is emerging consensus that mental competence should be operationalized as decisional capacity, which is the ability to make an informed decision.

The third approach implies that at least some measure of understanding, reasoning, and appreciation of the situation at hand seems to be relevant in the context of assessing decision-making capacity.[51,52] This also should be the guide in cases in which a patient who has been diagnosed with Alzheimer's requests physician-assisted suicide.

ASSESSMENT OF DECISION-MAKING CAPACITY: PRACTICE

From the three illustrative cases discussed previously, it is possible to gain some insight into the considerations regarding decision-making capacity made in the practice of physician-assisted suicide for patients who have Alzheimer's. It should be underscored that this analysis cannot be more than preliminary because in the reported cases, no systematic attention is given to the topic of decision-making capacity, and for the greatest part, reference to this topic is made in rather general and abstract ways. Nevertheless, these cases contain information that illustrates the kind of points of attention considered relevant by those who are involved in the practice of physician-assisted suicide for patients with Alzheimer's: physicians, medical and other expert consultants, and Regional Euthanasia Review Committees.

On the basis of the case reports the following elements – which were italicized in the cases – can be distinguished:

1. Clear and consistent expression of the wish for euthanasia/assisted suicide;
2. Understanding of condition and diagnosis;

3. Insight into future consequences of Alzheimer's;
4. Being conscious of the consequences of the decision to obtain physician-assisted suicide;
5. Ability to reason or to follow/understand reasoning;
6. Logical thinking; and
7. Linguistic problems.

1. Clear and Consistent Expression of the Wish for Euthanasia/Assisted Suicide

In all cases, the patient expressed his or her wish for assistance in dying clearly and consistently. To have decision-making capacity seems to require at least the clear and consistent expression of a wish for euthanasia or physician-assisted suicide. This implies that there can be no doubt about the intention of the patient. It is a request for active termination of his or her life by the physician, and not a "cry for help" or an expression of demoralization or hopelessness.[53,54] In particular, the repetitive character of the death wish, as well as the fact that a time course is involved, are indications that there is a consistent wish to die.

2. Understanding of Condition and Diagnosis

It is obvious that patients ought to understand their condition and diagnosis. Some measure of understanding is necessary for them to be able to value and evaluate their situation and possible future. The question is how "deep" this understanding should be. This can be somewhere between two extremes: on one side, the understanding that "there is something wrong with me"; on the other side, having detailed knowledge and understanding of the nature and possible causes of dementia/Alzheimer's disease and the specific signs, complaints, and symptoms that are involved in having this condition. It seems reasonable to expect that the person involved has a general awareness of the condition he or she is suffering from ("awareness of illness"), without necessarily requiring that the patient express clear and full illness insight. In our three cases, the understanding of the patients was connected to an awareness of the future course of the dementia.

3. Insight into Future Consequences of Dementia

The prospect of a future of progressive deterioration and loss of control over one's life is the primary motivation for people with dementia who request physician-assisted suicide. In practice, as reflected in the three cases, in assessing the decision-making capacity of a patient who makes such a request, attention is paid to the patient's insight into the future consequences of dementia.

In Case 1, it was estimated that the patient was conscious about the consequences because he "knows what he chooses." In Case 2, the patient suffered from the awareness of deterioration and loss of decorum, from loss of autonomy and self-respect, and from the knowledge that his situation would continue to worsen. He also was aware that the progression of the illness would deprive him of this control. And in Case 3, the patient was assessed as being able to see the consequences of her wish for euthanasia because she "could indicate well the progression of the disease and the deterioration that would take place."

If insight into the future consequences of dementia is defective or lacking, then one may question the decision-making capacity. In the three cases, there is no mention of the way in which this insight is assessed. So one may ask: How should we assess insight into the future consequences of dementia?

The following reflections are relevant. It is obvious that having insight into one's future life and illness condition can never be complete – never be more than partial – as compared to the real experience. Imagining the future is notoriously difficult, as the future is not yet in existence. Gaining insight into the future consequences of dementia requires imagination.[55]

There will always be a difference between what may happen to a person with dementia from the perspective of the demented person as a "member" of the group of demented people (with an "average" expected illness course, and an average time until death, etc.) and from the perspective of *this* individual person with his or her particular and unique life and illness course and experience.

From a philosophical point of view, the problem of imagining future consequences of dementia becomes even more complex if we consider cases of dementia from the "other person" perspective. Philosophically, it may be argued that the demented person is another person than the nondemented person he or she was before, with radically different experiences, hopes, and expectations, and a wholly different "new" identity.[56,16,57] To imagine what it would be like to be another person requires me to imagine the logically impossible: What would I be like if I were no longer I? The break between the mentally normal and the mentally impaired self is alien to the experience of most human beings. These changes in personality, memory, intellectual abilities, needs, desires, and so on imply that the mentally impaired person is, in important ways, different from the person he or she once was.[56]

Insofar as the mental states of a person – in this case the "demented self" – deviate from what we are used to, the possibility for "'transpersonal introspection" becomes more problematic.[58] Anyway, our imagination is constrained by our own experiences, and these "color in" the conscious experiences we attribute to other people or creatures.[59,60]

With respect to the assessment of decision-making capacity, insight must be as realistic as possible and in line with what is reasonable to expect and predict with regard to one's future situation and condition so far as it concerns Alzheimer's. Part of the insight into the future consequences of dementia is that the individual is also aware of the possibilities that exist and are available for giving care and comfort to dementia patients. As a matter of fact, it should be recognized that dementia is an incurable condition. This, however, does not imply that "nothing can be done" to alleviate the suffering of dementia patients. For many secondary problems related to the dementia, treatment or palliative care may be provided.[61,62]

Above that, it is important to realize that although we cannot deny the impact of dementia and the experiences of loss resulting in multiple "negative" emotions in the patient, there are also indications that dementia sufferers do not undergo the disease passively and use both emotion-oriented and problem-oriented coping strategies to deal with its challenges.[63]

4. Being Conscious of the Consequences of the Decision to Obtain Physician-Assisted Suicide

Decision-making capacity in the context of physician-assisted suicide for patients with Alzheimer's requires that the patient be conscious of the consequences of the decision. This means that the person is aware that he or she will die as a result of lethal medicines that the physician gives to the patient. But it is not only the causal connection between lethal medicines and the resulting death of the person that matters here, but also other consequences involved in the decision to obtain physician-assisted suicide. As mentioned in Case 3, the patient felt empathy for her family. This refers to the broader consequences of the decision, in particular those that are other-regarding.

5. Ability to Reason or to Follow/Understand Reasoning

In Case 2, the first consultant questioned the patient's decisional capacity although a consistent wish for termination of life had existed and been expressed over a long period. This was because during the consultation, the patient was unable to follow and understand reasoning.

The ability to reason or to understand the reasoning of others presupposes that the cognitive impairments of the person involved are not (yet) too serious. Cognitive problems do not necessarily or continuously impair reasoning abilities or the potential to understand the reasoning of others. Clearly, if permanent defects in the reasoning abilities of the person exist, they can be taken as a critical sign that the capacity to decide about physician-assisted suicide is lacking.

6. Logical Thinking

In Case 3, Mrs. A's thinking was considered to be logical, although she sometimes could not express herself clearly. Logical thinking can be seen as an element of the ability to reason and to follow/understand reasoning. It is the formal aspect of it that involves basic logical rules regarding the truth and validity of linguistic utterances. In other words, the rules of logic are necessary for correct thinking.

Basic rules of logic involve, among other things, inductive reasoning, deductive reasoning, categorical syllogisms, and reasoning by analogy. Gross defects in the use of logic can be signs that a person lacks decision-making capacity, for instance, if cause and effect are reversed, or circular reasoning takes place – that is, an attempt to support a statement by simply repeating the statement in different or stronger terms.

7. Linguistic Problems

Linguistic problems that may play a role in the assessment of decision-making capacity involve word-finding problems and unintelligible speech, as in Case 3, where Mrs. A had problems finding the right words. She sometimes spoke unintelligibly but then expressed herself understandably again. The central question is whether such linguistic problems are expressions of impaired decision-making capacity. As such, problems with language do not automatically involve shortcomings in the ability to reason or to use logical thinking. Neither do linguistic shortcomings necessarily imply that the person is unconscious of his or her future perspective or unable to understand his or her present situation. As the novel and subsequent film *The Diving Bell and the Butterfly* poignantly show, in the most extreme cases – that is, of patients suffering from locked-in syndrome – even a total inability to express themselves linguistically need not prevent the persons from being able to evaluate their situation.

Other than in the case of somatic illness, with mental illness or dementia the illness itself may affect different mental faculties that are necessary for memory, information processing, understanding, reasoning, and decision making. This in turn may influence decision-making capacity in a restricting, negative sense. In the Dutch practice of physician-assisted suicide, the assessment of decision-making capacity in the early stage of dementia shows that different aspects need to be addressed. Alzheimer's disease, particularly in the early stages, does not necessarily impair decisional capacity for treatment decisions or decisions about participating in a clinical trial.[64,65] In the early stages of dementia, the mental impairments of patients are not necessarily so serious that they impair the capacity to decide about a request for physician-assisted suicide. In each and every individual case, an assessment of decisional capacity is a critical element of the decision-making process.

IN CONCLUSION

In the Netherlands, competence or decision-making capacity, though not the sole issue, is a crucial criterion in deciding whether or not physician-assisted suicide can be morally justified in the case of Alzheimer's disease and other dementias, because part of this moral justification refers to the principle of respect for autonomy.[66] Obviously, particularly in the early stages of dementia, patients and their caregiver(s) have psychological needs that must be addressed, and depression and demoralization may influence the way in which people try to cope with their situation.[67,54,53] The existence of such needs and problems, however, does not preclude physician-assisted suicide from ultimately becoming an acceptable option. In such cases, a responsible assessment of the decision-making capacity with regard to the request for physician-assisted suicide should take place.

Such an assessment should take into account not only cognitive capacities (information processing, understanding) but also noncognitive aspects, such as emotions.[68,36] As a decision about physician-assisted suicide involves an important interest of the person requesting it, a high standard of decisional capacity should be applied from a risk-related perspective. Appreciation and emotion are critical elements in the assessment of competence in patients with dementia who request physician-assisted suicide in the early stage of their disease.

The evaluation of competence or decision-making capacity is part of a dialogical process between patient and physician (and possibly other stakeholders). It is not so much the issue of "finding out" whether or not the patient is competent as it is of trying to create the conditions for good decision making and to "construct" competent decision making. Instead of focusing on independent choice, the focus is on decision making in relationship with the physician and others and on shared decision making.[47] This implies a shift from respecting individual choice to promoting and enhancing autonomy and competence.[69] The traditional cognition-based approach to decision-making capacity is in line with what has been framed as the independent choice model of medical decision making.[69] Neither from a practice perspective nor from a moral point of view can the independent choice model be considered adequate.

References

1. Chabot, Boudewijn E. 2007. *Auto-euthanasie. Verborgen stervenswegen in gesprek met naasten* [Auto-euthanasia: Hidden roads to death in dialogue with relatives]. Amsterdam: Uitgeverij Bert Bakker.
2. Haan, Jurriaan de. 2002. The new Dutch law on euthanasia. *Medical Law Review* 10: 57–75.
3. Cohen-Almagor, Raphael. 2004. *Euthanasia in the Netherlands: The Policy and Practice of Mercy Killing*. Dordrecht: Kluwer Academic.
4. Nys, Herman. 2005. Physician assisted suicide in Belgian law. *European Journal of Health Law* 12: 39–41.
5. Griffiths, John, Heleen Weijers, and Maurice Adams. 2008. *Euthanasia and Law in Europe*. Oxford: Hart.
6. Chin, Arthur E., Katrina Hedberg, Grant K. Higginson, and David W. Fleming. 1999. Legalized physician-assisted suicide in Oregon – the first year's experience. *New England Journal of Medicine* 345: 577–583.
7. Guillod, Oliver, and Aline Schmidt. 2005. Assisted suicide under Swiss law. *European Journal of Health Law* 12: 25–38.

8. KNMG (Royal Dutch Medical Association). 1997. *Medisch handelen rond het levenseinde bij wilsonbekwame patiënten (Commissie Aanvaardbaarheid Levensbeëindigend handelen)* [Medical action in regard to the end of life in incompetent patients (Commission on the Acceptability of Medical Behavior That Shortens Life)], in particular Chapter 7. Houten/Diegem: Bohn Stafleu Van Loghum.
9. Hertogh, Cees M. P. M., Marike E. de Boer, Rose-Marie Dröes, and Jan A. Eefsting. 2007. Would we rather lose our life than lose our self? Lessons from the Dutch debate on euthanasia for patients with dementia. *American Journal of Bioethics* 7: 48–56.
10. Hertogh, Cees M. P. M. 2009. The role of advance euthanasia directives as an aid to communication and shared decision-making in dementia. *Journal of Medical Ethics* 35: 100–103.
11. Luijn, H. van. 2008. Doden op verzoek bij (beginnende) dementie [Death on request in case of (early) dementia]. *NVBe Nieuwsbrief* 15: 9–11.
12. Health Council of the Netherlands. 2002. *Dementia*. The Hague: Health Council of the Netherlands, publication no. 2002/04E.
13. NVVE (Nederlandse Vereniging voor een Vrijwillig Levenseinde). 2008. *Perspectien op waardig sterven* [Perspectives on dying with dignity]. Amsterdam. Available at http://www.nvve.nl.
14. Widdershoven, Guy A. M., and Ron L. P. Berghmans. 2001. Advance directives in dementia care: From instructions to instruments. *Patient Education and Counseling* 44: 179–186.
15. Delden, Johannes. J. van. 2004. The unfeasibility of requests for euthanasia in advance directives. *Journal of Medical Ethics* 30: 447–451.
16. Dworkin, Ronald. 1993. *Life's Dominion: An Argument about Abortion and Euthanasia*. London: Harper Collins.
17. Dresser, Rebecca. 1995. Dworkin on dementia: Elegant theory, questionable practice. *Hastings Center Report* 22: 32–38.
18. Jaworska, Agnieszka. 1999. Respecting the margins of agency: Alzheimer's patients and the capacity to value. *Philosophy and Public Affairs* 28: 104–138.
19. Battin, Margaret Pabst. 1992. Euthanasia in Alzheimer's disease? In *Dementia and Aging: Ethics, Values, and Policy Choices*, ed. Robert H. Binstock, Stephen G. Post, and Peter J. Whitehouse, 118–137. Baltimore: The Johns Hopkins University Press.
20. Post, Stephen G. 1995. Dementia, assisted suicide, and euthanasia. In *The Moral Challenge of Alzheimer Disease*, ed. Stephen G. Post, 113–126. Baltimore: The Johns Hopkins University Press.
21. KNMG (Royal Dutch Medical Association). 1997. *Medisch handelen rond het levenseinde bij wilsonbekwame patiënten (Commissie Aanvaardbaarheid Levensbeëindigend handelen)* [Medical action in regard to the end of life in incompetent patients (Commission on the Acceptability of Medical Behavior That Shortens Life)], in particular Chapter 7. Houten/Diegem: Bohn Stafleu Van Loghum.
22. Gordijn, Bert. 2004. Alzheimer disease and euthanasia. In *Ethical Foundations of Palliative Care for Alzheimer Disease*, ed. Ruth B. Purtilo and Henk A. M. J. ten Have, 226–239. Baltimore: The Johns Hopkins University Press.
23. Griffiths, John, Alex Bood, and Heleen Weijers. 1998. *Euthanasia and Law in the Netherlands*. Amsterdam: Amsterdam University Press.

24. Meer, S. van der, R. C. A. De Veen, E. O. Noordthoorn, and H. F. Kraan. 1999. Hulp bij zelfdoding bij een patiënt met een organisch-psychiatrische stoornis [Assisted suicide in a patient with an organic-psychiatric illness]. *Nederlands Tijdschrift voor Geneeskunde* 143: 881–884.
25. Schudel, W. J. 1999. Kanttekeningen bij een casus over hulp bij zelfdoding bij een patiënt met een organisch-psychiatrische stoornis [Comment on a case of assisted suicide in a patient with an organic-psychiatric illness]. *Nederlands Tijdschrift voor Geneeskunde* 143: 884–886.
26. Widdershoven, Guy A. M. 1999. Euthanasia in the Netherlands: Some first experiences of evaluation committees. *Hastings Center Report* 29: 47–48.
27. Widdershoven, Guy A. M. 2004. Euthanasia in the Netherlands: Experiences in a review committee. *Medicine and Law* 23: 687–691.
28. Onwuteaka-Philipsen, Bregje D., Agnes van der Heide, Martien T. Muller, Metter Rurup, Judith A. C. Rietjens, Jean-Jacques Georges, Astrid M. Vrakking, Jacqueline M. Cuperus-Bosma, Gerrit van der Wal, and Paul J. van der Maas. 2005. Dutch experience of monitoring euthanasia. *British Medical Journal* 331: 691–693.
29. Roth, Loren H., Alan Meisel, and Charles W. Lidz. 1977. Tests of competency to consent to treatment. *American Journal of Psychiatry* 134: 279–284.
30. Okai, David, Gareth Owen, Hugh McGuire, Swaran Singh, Rachel Churchill, and Matthew Hotopf. 2007. Mental capacity in psychiatric patients. *British Journal of Psychiatry* 191: 291–297.
31. Marson, D. C. 1994. Determining the competency of Alzheimer patients to treatment and research. *Alzheimer Disease and Associated Disorders* 8: 5–18.
32. Faden, Ruth R., and Tom L. Beauchamp. 1986. *The History and Theory of Informed Consent*. New York: Oxford University Press.
33. Buchanan, Alan E., and Dan W. Brock. 1989. *Deciding for Others: The Ethics of Surrogate Decision-Making.* Cambridge: Cambridge University Press.
34. Youngner, Stuart J. 1998. Commentary on "Is Mr. Spock mentally competent?" *Philosophy, Psychiatry, & Psychology* 5: 89–92.
35. Brock, Dan W. 1993. *Life and Death: Philosophical Essays in Biomedical Ethics*. Cambridge: Cambridge University Press.
36. Berghmans, Ron L. P., Donna L. Dickenson, and Ruud H. J. Ter Meulen. 2004. Mental capacity: In search of alternative perspectives. *Health Care Analysis* 12: 251–263.
37. Welie, Sander P. K., and Ron L. P. Berghmans. 2006. Inclusion of patients with severe mental illness in clinical trials: Issues and recommendations surrounding informed consent. *CNS Drugs* 20: 20–83.
38. Weisstub, David N. 1990. *Mental Competency: Final Report*. Toronto: Queen's Printer for Ontario.
39. Culver, Charles, and Bernard Gert. 1990. The inadequacy of incompetence. *Milbank Quarterly* 68: 619–643.
40. Checkland, David. 2001. On risk and decisional capacity. *Journal of Medicine and Philosophy* 26: 35–59.
41. Buller, Tom. 2001. Competence and risk-relativity. *Bioethics* 15: 93–109.
42. Berghmans, Ron L. P. 2000. *Bekwaam genoeg? Wils(on)bekwaamheid in geneeskunde, gezondheidsrecht en gezondheidsethiek* [Sufficient capacity?

Decisional (in)capacity in medicine, health law, and health ethics]. Utrecht: Nederlandse Vereniging voor Bio-ethiek.

43. Berghmans, Ron L. P. 2001. Capacity and consent. *Current Opinion in Psychiatry* 14: 491–499.
44. Elliott, Carl. 1991. Competence as accountability. *Journal of Clinical Ethics* 2: 167–171.
45. Wicclair, Mark. 1991. Patient decision-making capacity and risk. *Bioethics* 5: 91–104.
46. Wilks, Ian. 1999. Asymmetrical competence. *Bioethics* 13: 154–159.
47. Brock, Dan W. 1991. Decision making competence and risk. *Bioethics* 5: 105–112.
48. Appelbaum, Paul S., and Loren H. Roth. 1982. Competency to consent to research: A psychiatric overview. *Archives of General Psychiatry* 39: 951–958.
49. Kopelman, Loretta M. 1990. On the evaluative nature of competency and capacity judgments. *International Journal of Law and Psychiatry* 13: 309–329.
50. Glass, Kathleen C. 1997. Refining definitions and devising instruments: Two decades of assessing mental competence. *International Journal of Law and Psychiatry* 20: 5–33.
51. Berghmans, Ron L. P. 2008. Informed consent and decision-making capacity in neuromodulation: Ethical considerations. *Neuromodulation: Technology at the Neural Interface* 11: 156–162.
52. Berghmans, Ron L. P., and Guy A. M. Widdershoven. 2009. Ethical perspectives on decision-making capacity and consent for treatment and research. In *Mental Illness, Medicine and Law*, ed. Martin Lyon Levine, 339–348. Aldershot: Ashgate International Library of Medicine, Ethics and Law.
53. Kissane, David W. 2004. The contribution of demoralization to end of life decisionmaking. *Hastings Center Report* 34: 21–31.
54. Kissane, David W., and Brian J. Kelly. 2000. Demoralization, depression and desire for death: Problems with the Dutch guidelines for euthanasia of the mentally ill. *Australian and New Zealand Journal of Psychiatry* 34: 325–333.
55. Elliott, Carl, and Britt Elliott. 1991. From the patient's point of view: Medical ethics and the moral imagination. *Journal of Medical Ethics* 17: 173–178.
56. Parfit, Derek. 1984. *Reasons and Persons*. Oxford: Oxford University Press.
57. Buchanan, Alan E. 1988. Advance directives and the personal identity problem. *Philosophy & Public Affairs* 17: 277–302.
58. Rhoden, Nancy K. 1988. Litigating life and death. *Harvard Law Review* 102: 375–446.
59. Nagel, Thomas. 1986. *The View from Nowhere*. New York: Oxford University Press.
60. Berghmans, Ron L. P. 2000. Advance directives and dementia. *Annals of the New York Academy of Sciences* 913: 105–110.
61. Have, Henk A. M. J. ten. 2004. Expanding the scope of palliative care. In *Ethical Foundations of Palliative Care for Alzheimer's Disease*, ed. Ruth B. Purtilo and Henk A. M. ten Have, 61–79. Baltimore: The Johns Hopkins University Press.
62. Powers, Bethel Ann, and Nancy M. Watson. 2008. Meaning and practice of palliative care for nursing home residents with dementia at the end of life. *American Journal of Alzheimer's Disease and Other Dementias* 23: 319–325.

63. Boer, Marike E. de, Cees M. P. H. Hertogh, Rose-Marie Dröes, Ingrid I. Riphagen, Cees Jonker, Jan A. Eesting. 2007. Suffering from dementia – the patient's perspective: A review of the literature. *International Psychogeriatrics* 19: 1021–1039.
64. Karlawish, J. H., D. J. Casarett, B. D. James, S. X. Xie, and S. Y. Kim. 2005. The ability of persons with Alzheimer's disease (AD) to make a decision about taking an AD treatment. *Neurology* 64: 1514–1519.
65. Karlawish, Jason H., Scott Y. Kim, David Knopman, Christopher H. van Dyck, Bryan D. James, and Daniel Marson. 2008. Interpreting the clinical significance of capacity scores for informed consent in Alzheimer's disease clinical trials. *American Journal of Geriatric Psychiatry* 16: 568–574.
66. Battin, Margaret Pabst. 1994. Euthanasia: The fundamental issues. In *The Least Worst Death: Essays in Bioethics on the End of Life*, ed. Margaret P. Battin, 101–129. New York: Oxford University Press.
67. Ganzini, Linda, and Melinda A Lee. 1997. Psychiatry and assisted suicide in the United States. *New England Journal of Medicine* 336: 1824–1826.
68. Charland, Louis C. 1998. Appreciation and emotion: Theoretical reflections on the MacArthur treatment competence study. *Kennedy Institute of Ethics Journal* 8: 359–376.
69. Quill, Timothy E., and Howard Brody. 1996. Physician recommendations and patient autonomy: Finding a balance between physician power and patient choice. *Annals of Internal Medicine* 125: 763–769.

16

Being "Weary of Life" as Cause for Seeking Euthanasia or Physician-Assisted Suicide

Mette Rurup

Life expectancy is increasing in industrialized countries, and in most Western countries 50% of the population can already expect to survive to the age of 80 years. Old age is often accompanied by disabilities and a reduced quality of life. Some elderly people consider this to be unacceptable and develop a wish to die. For those who think suicide too drastic a measure, their only alternative is to wait until time fulfills their wish to die.

In the Netherlands, however, where there is increasing openness about requesting assistance in dying from a physician, elderly people may consider this a third option. The availability of euthanasia and assisted suicide led to a debate about the ethics of these options for elderly people who wish to die but do not suffer from a severe physical or psychiatric disease – that is, for people who are "weary of life." Strict boundaries concerning which conditions would be considered severe and who would be considered "weary of life" were (and still are) conspicuously absent in such discussions.

This debate was further stimulated by the Brongersma case. Edward Brongersma was a very lonely, 86-year-old man who was physically declining and who did not want to deteriorate any further. He had had a wish to die for several years. He first asked his general practitioner for assistance with suicide in 1993 but was refused; in 1996, he had attempted suicide without assistance but failed. In 1998, Mr. Brongersma again asked his GP to assist in his suicide. After the GP assured himself that all criteria of due care were met, he assisted Mr. Brongersma with his suicide. Despite the fact that the criteria of due care seemed to have been met in light of previous case law (a well-considered and voluntary request, unbearable and hopeless suffering, no treatment alternatives, consultation with another physician, and reporting of the case to the authorities), the GP was prosecuted. The GP was acquitted at trial in 2000, but the prosecutor appealed and the physician was found guilty by the Court of Appeals (in 2001) and subsequently by the Supreme Court (2002), although no punishment was imposed. The Supreme Court judged that although the criteria of due care in itself had been observed, the euthanasia legislation was never intended for this type of case, basing this conclusion in part on ongoing discussions of euthanasia legislation in Parliament at the time. The Supreme Court judged that "requests for euthanasia or assisted suicide in which the suffering is not predominantly caused by a medically classifiable disease are not part of the medical domain in which a physician has the expertise to judge a request for euthanasia or assisted suicide."[1]

After the initial acquittal of the GP, the Royal Dutch Medical Association (KNMG) established a committee to determine the boundaries of the physician's role with respect to requests for euthanasia or assisted suicide by people who were "weary of life." The KNMG published its position in 2004, after the Supreme Court had ruled. Although the court had made clear that euthanasia or assisted suicide was not permissible on grounds that the person was tired of living, the KNMG committee concluded that the presence of a medically diagnosable disease should, in their opinion, *not* be a requirement for assistance in dying. The committee argued that although there were boundaries to the role of physicians, these should be more broadly defined than the Supreme Court had ruled in its Brongersma decision.

Because the case law has always followed the consensus among physicians in setting boundaries for euthanasia and assisted suicide, it is currently unknown what would happen if another physician were to report having assisted the suicide of someone who is tired of living. In spite of the position taken by the KNMG, the consensus appears to be that another conviction would be most likely. On the other hand, the classification of diseases is somewhat open–ended, and as discussed in the following, this leaves a small opening for lawful practice of euthanasia or assisted suicide for people who are weary of life, should more of the consequences of old age come to be classified as medically diagnosable conditions/diseases.

In this chapter, we describe the results of a study that was carried out in 2002, several months before the verdict of the Supreme Court in the *Brongersma* case was announced.[2,3] We interviewed 410 physicians with the aim of estimating the incidence of requests for euthanasia and assisted suicide in the absence of a severe (physical or psychiatric) disease, gaining general insight into the characteristics of the people who make such requests and their reasons for doing so, and learning more about how physicians – particularly GPs – deal with such requests. We also present three case descriptions drawn from the study to give the reader an impression of the people who request euthanasia or assisted suicide because they are tired of living.

We also reflect on the differences and similarities between people who request euthanasia because they are weary of life and those who request euthanasia and/or assisted suicide (EAS) who have a severe physical or psychiatric disease in order to better understand the category of being "weary of life." In addition, we examine two key criteria of due care for cases of weariness of life: unbearable suffering and the availability of reasonable alternatives to euthanasia and assisted suicide. Finally, we consider the likely future evolution of Dutch thinking and policy in this area.

RESULTS OF THE EMPIRICAL STUDY

Box 16.1.

In this study, commissioned by the minister of health, welfare, and sports and the minister of justice, euthanasia was defined as the administration of drugs with the explicit intention of ending the patient's life at his or her explicit request. Physician-assisted suicide was defined as the prescription or supply of drugs with the explicit intention to enable the patient to end his or her own life.

Design and Study Population

This study was carried out in 2002 as part of a large-scale study of medical decision making at the end of life and consisted of retrospective semistructured interviews with a random sample of nursing home physicians (NHPs) (n = 77), general practitioners (GPs) (n = 125), and clinical specialists (cardiologists, surgeons, and specialists in internal medicine, pulmonology, and neurology) (n = 208). To meet the criteria for inclusion in this study, these physicians had to be practicing in their registered specialty in the same nursing home, practice, or hospital for the past two years. Of the 482 physicians who met the selection criteria, 72 were unwilling to participate (15%), mostly due to a lack of time.

Measuring Instruments and Analysis

To enable the physicians to feel free to speak about potentially illegal acts, anonymity was guaranteed by the researchers. Moreover, the Ministry of Justice guaranteed that it would not initiate any judicial inquiries based on the information collected in this study.

The interviews, which averaged 1½–2 hours in duration, were conducted by physicians who had received specific training for this study. To enable us to estimate the number of requests for euthanasia and assisted suicide overall in the Netherlands, we asked NHPs, GPs, and clinical specialists to estimate the frequency with which they had received requests for euthanasia or assisted suicide from patients who had a physical disease, had a psychiatric disease, or were weary of life. Physicians knew beforehand what the subject of the interview would be.

Nursing home physicians and GPs were further asked about most recent requests for EAS in the absence of a severe disease.

(*continued*)

The interviewers explained our definition of EAS to each respondent as follows: "It does occur that patients do not want to continue living, whereas they do not have a severe physical or psychiatric disease. Sometimes this is referred to as suffering from life, being through with life, or being tired of living. It is possible that the patient has health problems – for example, a chronic illness or ailments of old age; it is also possible that the patient is healthy." After this explanation, the interviewer asked whether it had ever occurred that a patient who did not suffer from a physical or psychiatric disease had explicitly asked the respondent for euthanasia or assisted suicide. Whenever there was doubt about the definition of "severe disease," the interviewer provided further information, for example, that someone who had a clinical depression was considered to have a severe illness, whereas someone who only had depressive symptoms was not.

In addition, we asked only GPs to describe such a request in detail, on the assumption that their patients would more often meet our definition of not having a severe disease than would the patients of NHPs or clinical specialists. Those GPs who reported ever having granted such a request were asked to describe the most recently granted request (n = 4). Those who had not were asked to describe the most recent request not granted (n = 28). Of the 28 requests not granted, 3 were excluded from analysis because the patients appeared to have had a severe psychiatric disease.

The interviews consisted mainly of open-ended questions. Most questions did have prestructured answer categories, but these were not read out to respondents. These categories were given to the interviewers to bring nuance to answers that they might otherwise have missed. For some questions, respondents were shown the answer categories on cards – for example, with the question about important reasons for the request for euthanasia/assisted suicide – because for each of the reasons derived from previous research, we wanted to know whether it played an important role or not. Each question also allowed the respondent to describe the patient's individual situation in depth. During the interviews, physicians could check the medical records of cases they were discussing. However, due to the distinctiveness of requests for euthanasia or assisted suicide in the absence of severe disease, most physicians remembered these cases in detail.

To calculate estimates that were representative of the Netherlands as a whole, the numbers of (requests for) euthanasia and assisted suicide were weighted for the specialty of the physician and corrected for the 5% of the deaths attended by physicians other than the seven types studied.

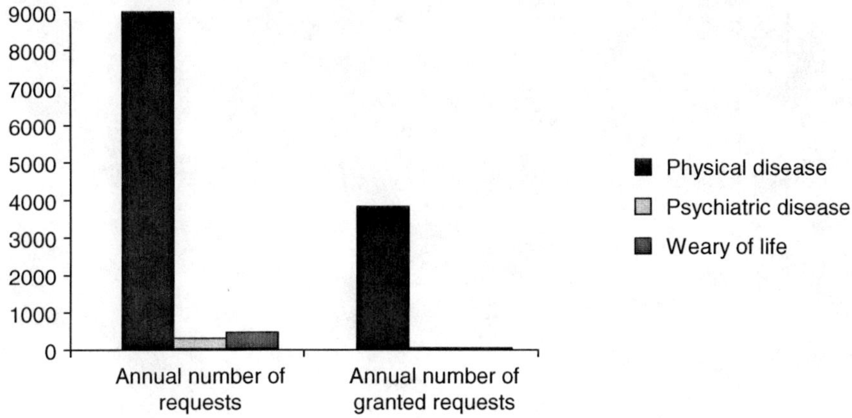

FIGURE 16.1.

Requests: Frequencies, Patient Characteristics, and Reasons

As Figure 16.1 shows, most people who request euthanasia or assisted suicide have a physical disease (most often, an advanced stage of cancer). Weariness of life is a relatively rare reason to request euthanasia or assisted suicide: We estimate that in the Netherlands each year, about 400 older people explicitly ask their physician for assistance in dying for this reason. Most of these people ask their GP, which is to be expected because the health care-system in the Netherlands is such that most older people know their general practitioner quite well, especially if they have chronic illnesses. This is not to say that older people do not also indicate to their general practitioner that they sometimes think life is not worth living anymore or say that life is not interesting anymore, but they do not explicitly ask for assistance in dying. About 30% of the GPs and NHPs we interviewed had at least once received an explicit request for euthanasia or assisted suicide from a patient who was not suffering from a severe physical or psychiatric disease.

Figure 16.1 also shows that requests from people who had a physical disease were granted in more than a third of cases, but requests from those who had a psychiatric disease or were "weary of life" were very rarely granted. Only 3% of the GPs and one of the NHPs reported having granted requests from people who were weary of life in the past; no physicians reported having granted such requests in the previous two years.

The average age of the people who requested euthanasia or assisted suicide because they were weary of life was 81 years at the time of their first request (Table 16.1). None of these people had a severe disease, but 79% had one or more nonsevere illnesses, such as stable status after cancer or a heart condition (11), visual or hearing impairment (7/5), decreased mobility (5), arthritis (3), and intestinal disorders (3). In spite of this, the physicians most frequently

TABLE 16.1. *Characteristics of People Who Requested Euthanasia or Physician-Assisted Suicide from Their General Practitioner in the Absence of a Severe Disease ($n = 29$)*

	n	%		*n*	%
Age at First Request (Years)			**Problems**[†,‡]		
60–69	3	10	**Physical**	6	22
70–79	9	31	(lack of appetite 7, sleeping disorder 6, pain 2)		
80–89	11	38	**Communicative**	6	22
90–97	6	21	(blind 7, deaf 5, unable to write 5)		
Gender			**Mobility**	6	22
male	13	45	(tiredness 9, dependent for ADL 7, unable to walk 5)		
female	16	55	**Mental**	11	41
Partner			(melancholy 12, unable to cope 11, depressed 10)		
yes	7	24	**Societal**	16	59
no	22	76	(lack of [leisure] activities 19, no valuable role in life 15, lack of social network 12)		
Children					
Good contact	12	41	**One or more nonsevere illnesses**		
Low quality/no contact	7	24	Yes	23	79
Unknown contact	2	7	No	6	21
No children	7	24	**Care evaluation**		
Unknown	1	3	Adequate	21	72
Health status			Inadequate	7	24
Good	9	31	Unknown	1	3
Reasonable	14	48	**Ever attempted suicide**		
Moderate	5	17	Yes	1	3
Poor	1	3	No	27	93
			Unknown	1	3

Under care of this GP for					
<1 year	1	3	**Competent to overlook own situation and adequately make decisions about it†**		
1–5 years	5	17			
>5 years	23	79	Yes	21	78
Personality traits			Not fully	6	22
Taken stock of life	25	86	**Received care†**		
Intellectual/educated	21	72	Umbrella care	15	56
Become isolated	17	59	Housekeeping	12	44
Difficulty with dependence	17	59	Residential home	7	26
Proud of own achievements in life	16	55	District nursing care	4	15
Difficulty with adjusting to old age	16	55	Spiritual care	3	11
Hopeless and despondent	13	45	Voluntary services	3	11
Difficulty with loss of standing	11	38	Home care	2	7
Difficulty with death of partner	8	28	Private nursing	1	4
Fear of loss of competence	8	28			
Simple-minded	6	21			
Financial problems	0	0			

Notes: Requests granted and not granted of $n = 29$.

† Two missing cases.

‡ For 33 items in five areas, the physician assessed on a scale from 1 to 5 the extent of the patient's problems at the time of the first explicit request for EAS. For example, the definition of physical problems was if the patient had considerable problems (score 4 or 5) with 2 or more items in that area. For each area, the 3 items that were most frequently assessed with a score of 4 or 5 are shown, together with the number of people who scored 4 or 5 on that item. In this way all problems were assessed.

TABLE 16.2. *Reasons for Requesting Euthanasia or Physician-Assisted Suicide in the Absence of a Severe Disease (n = 29)*

	All Reasons		Most Important Reason†	
	n	%	*n*	%
Through with life	16	55	9	32
Physical decline	16	55	4	14
Tired of living	14	48	1	4
No purpose in life	12	41	0	0
Melancholy/depressed	11	38	3	11
Loneliness	11	38	2	7
Dependence	9	31	1	4
Suffering from life	8	28	1	4
Deterioration/loss of dignity/loss of status	6	21	1	4
Not wanting to be a burden on family anymore	5	17	0	0
Pain	4	14	2	7
Cognitive decline	4	14	0	0
Death of a relative	3	10	2	7
Unable to live independently	3	10	0	0
Other	4	14	2	7

Notes: Requests granted and not granted of *n* = 29. More than one answer was possible.
† One missing case.

described their health status as reasonable and identified their problems as more often of a social or mental nature. In 72% of the cases, the physician stated that the patient was receiving adequate care.

The physicians reported that patients most often requested euthanasia or assisted suicide because of being "through with life" (55%), physical decline (55%), or being "tired of living" (48%) (Table 16.2).

Course of Action of the Physician and Course of Life of the Patient

Physicians refused requests for several reasons: The patient's suffering was not unbearable and hopeless (48%) and the patient did not suffer from a severe disease, and/or the patient's suffering was outside the realm of medicine (43%) (data not shown).

In 14 of 29 cases, the physician considered one or more types of treatment (Table 16.3). Four people refused all of the suggested treatments, while three people refused some of the suggested treatments but received one or more other treatments.

Ten people received one or more treatments. After receiving treatment, three of these people no longer wanted euthanasia/assisted suicide. Of these three, one was treated with antidepressant medication, the second received

TABLE 16.3. *Treatment Options and Withdrawal of Requests for Euthanasia or Physician-Assisted Suicide (n = 29)*

Treatment	Treatment Considered by the Physician†	Treatment Provided	Request Was Withdrawn or Became Less Explicit in Time
No	15‡	19‡	0
Yes	14	10	5
Anti-depressant medication	5	4	2
Psychiatric/psychological††	6	2	1
Psychosocial††	7	3	2
Analgesic medication	2	2	1
Other medical	4	3	2

Notes: Requests granted and not granted of *n* = 29.

† Possible treatment considered by the physician after the explicit request for EAS, which was not provided before the request.

‡ Four people refused all treatment, and so in 15 cases no treatment was considered and in 19 cases no treatment was provided.

†† Psychiatric/psychological treatment = treatment by a psychiatrist or a psychologist; psychosocial treatment = all other types of psychological or social support by the GP, social services, volunteers, etc.

psychosocial support, and the third was hospitalized and treated for shortness of breath and also received psychiatric and psychosocial support. Although these people were persuaded to moderate their request for euthanasia or assisted suicide, they still wanted to be able to end their life in due time if they so wished. Two individuals withdrew their requests completely, one case after treatment with painkillers and the other case after treatment of a medical problem in combination with antidepressant medication. The remaining five people maintained their explicit request for euthanasia/assisted suicide after they had received treatment; one of them went to another physician who granted the request.

Nineteen people who did not receive any treatment persisted in their request for euthanasia/assisted suicide, and in four cases the request was granted. Five people took their own lives after their request was denied; three hanged themselves and two died of self-starvation (one at the advice of the physician). The remaining 10 people persisted in their request for euthanasia/assisted suicide. At the time of the study, four had died of natural causes.

CASE REPORTS

The following three case descriptions below give an impression of the people who request EAS because they are weary of life.[2,3,4] Some characteristics have been altered to protect confidentiality. A detailed description of similar people has also been published.[5,6] In the first case:

An 81-year-old woman asked her GP if he had a pill for her to end her life. The GP had known her for a long time, and the question did not really surprise him. Since her husband died 15 years ago, she was living alone. Others around her had died and she was the last one of her generation alive in her family. She had good relationships with her three sons, even though she often complained that they did not spend enough time with her. She had a visual and hearing impairment and she had difficulty walking, but she was well taken care of in sheltered accommodation.

When her GP asked her why she wanted to end her life, she said that she was weary of life. She felt that she was physically declining, and she did not want to live to see her further deterioration. She had seen members of her family develop dementia and did not want that to happen to her. She had no prospects and felt lonely most of the time. She had balanced the pros and cons of her life and decided that she was better off dead. When her GP explained why he couldn't provide a pill, she seemed to accept the situation. After that they had several conversations concerning the subject. She seemed to accept her predicament, but she said regularly that she would rather be dead and that she hoped her GP would change his mind.

One consulting physician described a patient evaluated after a request for euthanasia/assisted suicide as follows:

A 91-year-old widow lives independently in sheltered accommodation. She has no physical or psychiatric disease, but her hearing and visual abilities have deteriorated and she walks with difficulty. She often doesn't feel well, is tired most of the time, and is not very active as a consequence. She seems to be alert and brisk, she looks well groomed, and her speech is clear and coherent. There are definitely no indications of any mood disorder. She has requested euthanasia many times in recent years because "she doesn't enjoy life anymore." This is mainly because of the loss of all meaningful contacts with her relatives and fellow residents.

Another consulting physician reported a third case:

A 92-year-old woman asked her physician to perform euthanasia many times in the past 10 years, but the physician never gave her a direct answer to this request. When asked why she has never insisted, she said that she was taught as a child not to complain about pain or other things, and that she has learned to make fun of situations in which one should really stick up for oneself.

When she was 82 she had surgery for a colon carcinoma. She was not expected to survive for more than two years after the surgery and could accept that "I had reached the age to go," she said. Unexpectedly, there have been no signs of cancer since the surgery.

She has had pains in her abdomen ever since the surgery. She finds it difficult to keep her balance and falls frequently, but was miraculously free from fractures until two months ago when she broke her left upper arm. Due to a serious macular degeneration she is unable to read, write, or watch television. Her husband and stepdaughter are both dead, and she never had any children of her own, due to infertility problems.

All her friends of her own age have died and she has become increasingly lonely. Several attempts have been made to alleviate her pain, but all the painkillers increase her dizziness. Every night she hopes that she will die in her sleep. She has considered and rejected suicide because she is afraid that her attempt will fail, and would only worsen her situation. She now hopes that her physician will seriously consider her request.

SUFFERING FROM WEARINESS OF LIFE: SIMILARITIES WITH SUFFERING FROM A PHYSICAL OR PSYCHIATRIC DIAGNOSES

As noted, it is estimated that each year 400 people in the Netherlands request euthanasia or assisted suicide because they are weary of life. But what does being weary of life mean? In the study reported here it was mostly defined as a negative; that is, "*not* suffering from a severe physical or psychiatric disease."

People who are weary of life appear to be a very heterogeneous group. Studies suggest that many people in this group suffer mainly from the physical ailments and social problems that are frequently encountered in older age.[3] Most seem to feel that they have no valuable role left to play. Circumstances such as the loss of a partner, increasing isolation due to the death of people around them, and physical frailty can make everyday life such a negative experience that it can turn being "weary of life" into a reason to actively wish to die and to request euthanasia or assistance in suicide from a physician.

People who are weary of life do not suffer from a severe psychiatric or physical disease, but that does not imply that they are in perfect physical and mental health either. Are there similarities between people who request euthanasia/assisted suicide because they are weary of life and those who do so because they have a severe physical or psychiatric illness?

Similarities with People Suffering from a Physical Illness

In fact, there may be more similarity across these two groups of patients then we generally appreciate. A common misunderstanding is that most people with cancer who request euthanasia or assisted suicide do so because they suffer from unbearable pain. Although this is true in many cases, a patient's reasons for requesting assistance in dying are usually much more complex and include things like loss of dignity, loss of meaning, loss of sense of self, and progressive physical decline. One study that developed a standard scale to measure symptoms (14 symptoms, adapted from the Edmonton Symptom Assessment System [ESAS]) found that the three most frequently occurring symptoms did not include pain or nausea but were "feeling bad," being tired, and being inactive.[7] It is interesting to note that when this same scale was used with 39 people who requested EAS because they were "weary of life" (people who did not have a severe medically diagnosable disease), the same three symptoms – feeling bad, being tired, and being inactive – were the most frequently occurring, each in more than half of those studied.[4] This implies that nonsevere diseases and old age can cause symptoms that are similar to those caused by severe diseases, as in fact the aforementioned third case suggests.

These results are interesting in light of the verdict of the Supreme Court in the *Brongersma* case[8] that euthanasia/assisted suicide is permissible only when the patient's suffering is primarily caused by a diagnosable disease, not "simply" being weary of life.[a] It seems that the distinction drawn by the court is not as obvious as it might have appeared. The court seems to have assumed that the task of physicians is limited to the treatment of medically diagnosable diseases, while the majority of the people who seek euthanasia or assisted suicide from their GPs have complaints that do not correspond to accepted medical diagnoses.

The notion of medically diagnosable diseases or conditions can itself be open-ended. As understanding of the consequences of aging – and even aging itself – increases and interventions are developed to address the negative consequences, aspects of aging are likely to be redefined as medical conditions that physicians can diagnose as such. (For a more comprehensive discussion of this subject, see Smith 2002 and related articles.)[9]

Most importantly, the aging process can lead to much greater suffering than many currently diagnosable diseases do. Most people would probably prefer to have a clinical diagnosis, such as measles or hay fever, than to suffer from consequences that are considered a "normal" part of the aging process, such as deterioration of mental and physical abilities or the inevitable death of loved ones. Most of these consequences obviously cannot be cured by physicians, but an increasing number actually can be treated – for example, hearing impairments, cataracts, or impotence.[10] As noted previously, the KNMG concluded that the legal demarcation set by the Supreme Court in the *Brongersma* case is not analogous to the complexity of medical practice.[11]

Similarities with People Suffering from a Psychiatric Illness: Depression

It could be said that all people who are weary of life and request euthanasia or assisted suicide suffer from at least one *depressive symptom*, since they all have a wish to die.[12] In the Netherlands, however, it is widely accepted that it is possible for a person to have a death wish without suffering from *clinical depression*. Of course, especially in other countries, not everybody agrees with this assessment; some say that anyone who has an explicit wish to die in the absence of a severe physical disease has a psychiatric disease.[13]

The truth depends largely on the definitions used. The classification of psychiatric diagnoses is much less stable than that of physical diagnoses because

[a] See also Chapter 3.

the knowledge in this field is much less advanced. The pathological processes behind even some of the most common psychiatric diseases, such as depression, are unknown, rendering the diagnosis liable to change as knowledge increases. Furthermore, the classification of what is a diagnosable psychiatric illness and what is "normal" has a cultural component. In this case, is it normal for older people who are nearing the end to develop a wish to die under certain circumstances? This question is a matter of debate.

THE CRITERIA OF DUE CARE IN CASES OF WEARINESS OF LIFE: UNBEARABLE SUFFERING AND OTHER REASONABLE SOLUTIONS

As discussed previously, the Supreme Court convicted the GP in the *Brongersma* case because the patient's suffering was not caused predominantly by a medically diagnosable disease. They did not convict the GP for failing to adhere to the criteria of due care. Two criteria are especially relevant in the situations we are considering: unbearable suffering, which (post-*Brongersma*) is sometimes erroneously mentioned as the reason euthanasia/assisted suicide is not permissible for patients who are weary of life, and the absence of other reasonable solutions, which is not specifically mentioned in the Supreme Court ruling but was the main issue in the appellate decision that preceded it.

One of the criteria of due care is that the physician is convinced that the patient experiences his or her suffering as unbearable.[b] The law does not specify which types of suffering are unbearable and which are not, because suffering is considered to be a subjective experience.[14] One might conclude that this is a simple criterion: If a patient chooses euthanasia or assisted suicide, he or she apparently experiences his or her suffering as unbearable, and so if a physician is convinced that the request for EAS is genuine and well considered, this criterion would always be met. But in practice, this criterion is considered to be one of the most difficult to judge, and it is the most debated among physicians as well as the authorities who must assess individual cases of euthanasia/assisted suicide.[7]

According to some, this complexity is caused by the fact that in practice, the criterion of unbearable suffering actually encompasses more than just the subjective experience of the person who requests euthanasia or assisted suicide; it also reflects societal attitudes about the limits of euthanasia/assisted suicide.[c] The courts never doubted that Brongersma experienced his suffering as unbearable, or that his GP had evaluated it carefully and had become convinced that this was the case.

The difficulty posed by another criterion of due care sometimes seems to be overlooked – that the physician and patient are both convinced that there is

[b] See Chapter 3.

[c] See Chapter 21 for a discussion of this subject.

no other reasonable solution for the patient's situation. This criterion requires the physician to investigate all possible options within the framework of medical palliative care and offer them to the patient.[14] If strictly adhered to, this criterion would be very demanding, as the number of options in palliative care is increasingly large. Moreover, the fulfillment of other criteria depend on meeting this one: The request can only be determined to be "well considered" if the patient is aware of his or her situation and prospects and of possible alternative solutions. Knowledge of alternatives is likewise required for determining whether or not the individual's suffering is hopeless. Although the patient can refuse alternative treatments without jeopardizing the legality of euthanasia/assisted suicide, knowledge of alternatives – if there are any – is essential.

Making these determinations may be demanding whenever someone requests euthanasia or assisted suicide, but is even more so when people request EAS because they are weary of life. Too little is known about the wish to die of people who do not have a severe disease, about how best to treat the psychological reasons that underlie such wishes, or about the likelihood that they will fade away, with or without intervention. On the one hand, one can simplify these difficult questions by assuming that by "another reasonable solution" the euthanasia legislation means an intervention that is currently available and at a reasonable cost. But to be confident enough to be *convinced* that there are no other reasonable solutions, one should at least have some evidence-based knowledge about the possibilities for interventions and the likelihood of such interventions to diminish death wishes, evidence that currently simply is not available.[15]

EXPECTATIONS FOR THE FUTURE

As we noted at the outset, most physicians in the Netherlands refuse requests for euthanasia or assisted suicide in the absence of a severe disease, mainly because they do not consider the suffering of these patients to be unbearable or hopeless. Among the physicians we interviewed, any requests had been granted more than two years previously. Thus, we have found no evidence in practice of a "slippery slope" of euthanasia/assisted suicide widening its scope to people who are not severely ill, even though the existence of a debate about assistance in dying for such individuals might, in itself, be considered an indication of a slippery slope.

For the immediate future, the verdict of the Supreme Court in the *Brongersma* case closed the door to legal euthanasia or assisted suicide for patients who are weary of life. However, to the extent that the consequences of old age may come to be classified as medically diagnosable (and treatable) conditions, the decisions have left a small opening for the more distant future.

Similarly, the KNMG has not foreclosed the possibility of a role for physicians in requests for euthanasia or assisted suicide from people who are weary of life. In its 2004 position paper, the KNMG indicated that the number of requests for euthanasia/assisted suicide from people weary of life is expected to increase in the future, for several reasons. The report suggested that it is likely people will become more outspoken, as well as more familiar with the concepts of autonomy. Further, as life expectancy increases, people will experience more physiological symptoms and limitations of old age, and they will consider the physician the right person to turn to with a request for euthanasia or assisted suicide. The KNMG acknowledged the complexity of medical practice in cases where people "suffer from life," but added that more clarification is necessary in order to decide whether or not this falls within the realm of medicine and, thus, whether physicians can or cannot consider granting requests for assistance in dying in such cases.

As the debate – and the evidence – currently stand, then, we cannot predict whether or not euthanasia and assisted suicide in the absence of a severe disease will be allowed in the Netherlands in the future. Both the legal and medical authorities have left room for a shift in either direction.

References

1. Dutch Supreme Court. *Nederlandse Jurisprudentie* 2003, nr. 167.
2. Rurup, Mette L., Martien T. Muller, Bregje D. Onwuteaka-Philipsen, Agnes van der Heide, Gerrit van der Wal, and Paul J. van der Maas. 2005. Requests for euthanasia or physician-assisted suicide from older persons who do not have a severe disease: An interview study. *Psychological Medicine* 35: 665–671.
3. Rurup, Mette L. 2005. Setting the stage for death: New themes in the euthanasia debate. Ph.D. diss., Vrije Universiteit, Amsterdam:
4. Rurup, Mette L., Bregje D. Onwuteaka-Philipsen, Marijke C. Jansen-van der Weide, and Gerrit van der Wal. 2005. When being "tired of living" plays an important role in a request for euthanasia or physician-assisted suicide: Patient characteristics and the physician's decision. *Health Policy* 74: 157–166.
5. Calman, Neil S. 2004. So tired of life. *Health Affairs* 23: 228–232.
6. De Burlet, H. M., and M. J. Hazenberg. 2003. "Tired of life": A reason to evaluate physical handicaps. *Nederlands Tijdschrift voor Geneeskunde* 147: 633–635 [in Dutch].
7. Wal, Gerrit van der, Agnes van der Heide, Bregje D. Onwuteaka-Philipsen, and Paul J. van der Maas. 2003. *Medical decision-making at the end of life*. Utrecht: Uitgeverij De Tijdstroom [in Dutch].
8. Dutch Supreme Court. 2002. *Nederlandse Jurisprudentie* 2003, nr. 167. December 24.
9. Smith, Richard. 2002. In search of "non-disease." *British Medical Journal* 324: 883–885.
10. Ebrahim, Shah. 2002. The medicalisation of old age should be encouraged. *British Medical Journal* 324: 861–863.
11. Dijkhuis, J. H., and Committee Members. 2004. In search of standards of conduct for physicians with regard to requests for assistance with life-termination from patients who are "suffering from life." Utrecht: KNMG [in Dutch].
12. American Psychiatric Association. 1994. *Diagnostic and Statistical Manual of Mental Disorders*. 4th ed. Washington, DC: American Psychiatric Association.

13. Linden, Michael, and Sven Barnow S. 1997. The wish to die in very old persons near the end of life: A psychiatric problem? Results from the Berlin Aging Study. *International Psychogeriatrics* 9: 291–307.
14. Explanatory memorandum on The Termination of Life on Request and Assisted Suicide (Review Procedures) Act [Memorie van toelichting bij het wetsvoorstel Wet Toetsing Levensbeëindiging op verzoek en hulp bij zelfdoding]. 1998–1999. Kamerstukken II, 26 691, nr. 3.
15. Rurup, Mette L. 2005. The role of the physician in requests for physician-assisted suicide in patients who are "suffering from life": The Dijkhuis Report commissioned by the Royal Dutch Medical Association. *Ned Tijdschr Geneeskd* 149: 2145–2147 [in Dutch].

17

Shared Obligations and "Medical Friendships" in Assisted Dying

Moral and Psychological Repercussions Reconsidered

Gerrit K. Kimsma and Chalmers C. Clark

INTRODUCTION

A crucial challenge to the practice of physician-assisted death (PAD) concerns the claimed negative impact such a practice would have on the doctor–patient relationship and trust in the medical profession generally. In this chapter, we focus on what is known about the impact of PAD on medical relationships in order to add an empirical dimension: We wish to evaluate concerns that PAD practice involves a "slippery slope" that will undermine the integrity of professional trust and medical relationships with patients. We argue that such claims present an inadequate picture of the broader range of psychological, moral, and emotional effects of PAD practice as practiced in the Netherlands and elsewhere. Preliminary data suggest that PAD can be congruent with a strong and healthy physician–patient relationship.[1]

When properly developed, acts of PAD reflect not only an ethically distinctive domain of medical care and practice but also one that can develop into a special but professionally "authentic" medical relationship that we term a "medical friendship." This relationship, in fact, is an ethically and psychologically requisite condition for carrying out PAD practice and one that helps impede the potential for depersonalizing tendencies that can affect care involving the treatment of dying patients. Not only can physicians ethically perform PAD, but the special nature of the physician–patient relationship dictates that they be the *only* ones who perform it. Finally, analysis of the Dutch experience indicates that in addition to the Dutch rules governing PAD, the alteration of the physician–patient relationship by a request for PAD can itself serve as an important "brake" preventing a slide down the slippery slope.

PHYSICIANS AND PAD

From the beginning of the twentieth century, a dominant opinion in international discussions was that allowing euthanasia will undermine the trust that society reposes in both practitioners and the medical profession generally.[2] Some argued that even if euthanasia were to be accepted by a society, physicians should not be the ones to perform it.[3] This argument seems self-contradictory. It implies that trust in the medical profession is requisite for a healthy society (something we agree with) while at the same time evidencing considerable concern about the fragility of that trust.[4] Ironically, such concerns about euthanasia are rarely accompanied by calls to deal with what seems to us should be the greater concern – society's mistrust of the system and the professionals who work in it. This exclusive focus on the superficial, rather than on the underlying problem, is true of many critics of euthanasia from countries where lack of trust in the health-care system is endemic. As Margo Trappenburg discusses in Chapter 6, trust in the health-care system was one of the factors that allowed PAD to develop in the Netherlands.

Practice in the Netherlands shows that involvement with dying patients is an emotional experience for physicians, patients, caretakers, and their families in great part because it necessitates a confrontation with death and the finality of life for all concerned. Indeed, the situation virtually forces contemplation of one's own mortality. There are strong indications that involvement in PAD reveals different conflicting emotions and psychological repercussions among those involved. In 1998, Dr. Howard Grossman, a Manhattan internist and plaintiff in an unsuccessful New York lawsuit that went all the way to the U.S. Supreme Court (*Vacco* v. *Quill*), came forward to say: "Anybody who has done it knows that it is a tremendous decision that you carry with you forever." [5] Unfortunately, it has taken quite some time before dimensions of physician response to PAD practice have gained sufficient attention, even in the Netherlands.

A physician–patient relationship changes in a fundamental way after a request for PAD has been expressed. Without this change, which involves greater intimacy, psychological involvement, and mutual respect, we do not believe that euthanasia should occur at all. These conditions are so important that it compels us to speak of a third, unofficial, requirement for PAD (after the two official material conditions: patient request and presence of unbearable suffering). That unofficial requirement concerns an internal struggle that takes place in the physician, resulting in adverse emotional and psychological effects. Such effects, we believe, need not be viewed as a negative sign or as an argument against crossing the line to help a patient end his or her life. This reaction may well signal an existential response, resulting from an authentic internal struggle in the physician, triggered by competing moral convictions over the duty of patient care, namely, the commitment to promote life, health, and well-being, and the competing duty to alleviate suffering.

EMPIRICAL DATA

Until fairly recently, the data on the impact of euthanasia on physicians and families was rather limited and often anecdotal.[6] The international literature seems to reflect a straightforward negative impact regarding PAD influence, rather than a balanced evaluation. However, that may not be much of a surprise if one considers the scarce data from countries without PAD policies.

In 2006, Kenneth Stevens, an Oregon anesthesiologist, published an analysis of medical and public reports regarding these effects. His conclusion is plain and clear: "[M]any doctors who have participated in euthanasia and/or PAS [physician-assisted suicide] are adversely affected emotionally and psychologically by their experiences."[7] He refers to many individual witnesses, to testimonies in legal and parliamentary investigations, and to a quantitative Dutch study. The practices involved include euthanasia, physician-assisted suicide, ending life without explicit patient request, and treatments with high doses of opioids (perceived as intentionally hastening death):

> In a 1995–1996 Dutch study, 405 Dutch doctors were interviewed regarding their feelings after their most recent case of PAD, in one of the categories considered by Stevens. The percentage of doctors expressing *feelings of discomfort* were: 75% following euthanasia, 58% following assisted suicide, 34% following ending life without an explicit request, and 18% for alleviation of pain with high doses of opioids. Fifty percent of the euthanasias and 40% of the assisted suicides were followed by "*burdensome feelings*" and 48% of the euthanasias and 49% of the assisted suicide cases were followed by *emotional discomfort*. The willingness to perform physician-assisted death again was 95% after euthanasia and 82% for life ending without an explicit request. Physicians sought support following 43% of the euthanasia cases and 16% of cases involving ending life without an explicit request.[8]

Given these statistics, it seems clear that for the bulk of Dutch physicians, PAD is not one of "the easier options," as Edmund Pellegrino claims.[9] The figures suggest that euthanasia causes the most destabilizing emotions of all the life-shortening interventions. Rather than seeing physician discomfort as either something to be avoided or a signal that PAD should not occur, we should see it as entirely appropriate to the gravity of the situation.

A close reading of the literature shows that physicians are not only negatively affected but also ambivalent about participation. Physicians report that even while they are committed to the availability of PAD, they often hope that an occasion for it will not occur in their practice. This hope is interpreted by some as revealing the inherent wrongness of PAD, providing proof enough that a conviction "not to go there" is morally sound. Anesthesiologist and PAD *proponent* Pieter Admiraal stated that "[y]ou will never get accustomed to killing somebody. We are not trained to kill. With euthanasia your nightmare comes true."[10] Rather than serving as a ground for rejecting PAD out of hand, Admiraal's dramatic words cause us to ask the questions: Why be in favor of it, why continue with it, if it has such repercussions? The answer may come as a surprise to ardent opponents of PAD: The emotional turmoil that such requests stimulate in physicians may keep them from developing attitudes of routinization and callousness in the practice.

We are convinced that the discomfort of Dutch physicians is a necessary social instinct that serves as a useful brake preventing PAD from sliding down a slippery slope. Dutch physicians are committed to their patients and perceive their role at the end of life as a conflict of duties that they must resolve with careful deliberation and personal involvement. That position is confirmed in our own research over the past 10 years and more. In 1994, we conducted interviews with family physicians and clinical oncologists who had published about their experiences with PAD, as well as with families/relatives who had lost one of their members that way (referred to us through colleagues or from our own practice). The central and unexpected finding of these interviews was the admission that after a request from a patient, physicians experienced anxieties, uncertainties, ambivalence, instability, sleeplessness, and sometimes an overall inability to function properly. But the stories also relate the development of deepened relationships and positive sensitivities emerging from a sense of felt purpose and resolve regarding the patient's wishes and the doctor's commitment to heed those wishes through the difficult journey ahead. This image of ambivalence and felt purpose and resolve was also observed in a qualitative survey of personal interviews with 15 physicians in 1997[11] and again with 30 family physicians (in the Amsterdam region) on their experiences and feelings about euthanasia practice in 2001.[12]

Qualitative interviews with 22 physicians in focus groups from other researchers, published in 2007, describe the emotions and reflections of physicians before, during, and after the process and act of euthanasia. The stories also show contradictory emotions, changes, and various stages of destabilization that often impeded their lives and daily routines. The physicians describe loneliness, but also feelings akin to being "morally heroic" by trusting patients and families. Feelings of guilt surface because of psychological associations with the actions of executioners in death penalty cases.[13] These associations are further aggravated by the fact that both practices employ highly similar methodologies.

There are other intense experiences, such as the final house call and the even more definitive action of injecting the deadly drugs or the handing over of a deadly cocktail or potion for the patient to drink. But there also arise feelings of relief and tender completion, especially when these sentiments are mirrored in the faces, words, and gestures of families. However, these situations sometimes result in cases of family pressure, manipulation, and even disrespect. But there is no escaping the strong feelings, the contradictory feelings, and feelings of resistance, and there is always a felt duty of nonabandonment of a patient in ultimate need.

When "natural death" preempts PAD, many of those involved, including attending physicians, experience relief. But for some physicians, "having been there" makes them decide never to do it again. While this is certainly true for some, the majority of physicians continue in the practice even while acknowledging significant emotional and psychological repercussions.

WHY THESE REPERCUSSIONS AND HOW ARE THEY TO BE EXPLAINED?

Physicians are both unanimous in their description of euthanasia practice as being incomparable to normal medical care and univocal in their narratives about their emotional experiences. When they enter into this practice, a need arises for a more personal relationship with patients. In euthanasia practice, there are elements of attention, interest, and the construction of relationships that go beyond the realization of normal care. That need, however, is not one-sided. Patients make it abundantly clear that there is, in fact, a mutuality of personal needs between doctor and patient that have yet to be fully understood or explored. For the doctor, the important thing seems to be that psychologically, a more personal relationship with a patient is a crucial aspect of the physician–patient relationship *for physicians* who assist in ending a patient's life. Similar though, perhaps, not as intense feelings arise in the intimate care of dying patients even when PAD is not on the table.

A personal relationship is needed for doctors to adequately identify with the special needs and demands of their seriously ill patients and to overcome strong emotional, psychological, and philosophical resistance to the extremity of what is demanded in the process of euthanasia. This process of identification is not unilateral but appears to be mutual. All, or nearly all, physicians we interviewed were clear that without this mutuality, ending a patient's life would be psychologically impossible or seriously ill-advised.[11] There are some public statements and at least one research study that corroborate our finding. The American physician Kenneth Vaux, in his 1988 commentary[14] on the anonymous "Debbie case,"[15] describes the phenomenon that he knew of well-respected physicians who had practiced euthanasia on colleagues and loved ones but not on their patients: "That physicians and nurses would request euthanasia of their colleagues or would assist their loved ones to have a more merciful death but would deny it to their patients says something about the moral nature of the act," says Vaux. It is, he concludes, above all, a "loving act." This difference in willingness to euthanize, depending on whether it concerns patients or relatives, was also described by a group of Italian neurologists in 1992.[16]

While these descriptions come from physicians and not from families, there are clear indications that the sense of deepened relationships is not a fantasy or attempt at self-justification. Research from American anthropologist Frances Norwood, working with family physicians, terminal patients, and families in Amsterdam, found that there are definite changes in relationships after a request for PAD. She found that the ongoing discussion about the inevitability of death and the option of PAD resulted in a deepening and strengthening of mutual bonds not only between physicians and patients but also among patients, family members, and friends.[17]

The need to relate to a person in well-developed interpersonal terms is reflected in the refusal of nursing home physicians to participate in ending lives of Alzheimer patients, even though the option of an advance directive allows the possibility in euthanasia law.[a] The formal argument to support their policy is grounded on the need to base the decision on the "actual will" of the patient, not the "past will" in the directive. According to recent Annual Reports of the Regional Euthanasia Evaluation Committees, the option for euthanasia is open only in cases of early Alzheimer patients. The patient must be capable of communicating, be competent, express a clear and enduring request, and be able to explain the unbearable nature of the suffering. Stated in another way, the patient must be able to engage the physician's empathy and understanding. The crucial ingredient is the possibility of a mutual relationship with a requesting patient, not merely the presence of an advance directive – no matter how much the patient may appear to others to "lack dignity."

UNDERSTANDING THE PARADOX: PSYCHOLOGICAL, MORAL, AND PHILOSOPHICAL DIMENSIONS

The emotional conflicts after a request for help to die primarily concern the physician's confrontation with his or her own mortality as well as that of the patient. In general, death is considered an absolute disruption of all we know and care about on the horizon of our lives. For caretakers who deal with dying patients, this issue is more complex since they have to confront death so frequently in their daily practice. At the same time, they are supposed to help their patients learn to cope with the finality of their lives. That process is both rational and unconscious. Sigmund Freud, the father of depth psychology, claimed that even though a human being is capable of understanding the finality of his or her death in a rational way, the unconscious appears to cling to the concept of personal immortality. That claim applies to us all – physicians, patients, families, and friends.

Abandonment of hopelessly dying patients is no longer acceptable medical practice. In ancient Greek medicine, things were different. When patients were dying, Greek physicians would withdraw from patient care under a claimed justification that medicine had nothing to offer and that nature should simply be allowed to take its course.[18] The acceptance of death by patients and the necessity of physician involvement have been studied and promoted broadly since the 1960s. Elizabeth Kübler-Ross, one of the pioneers of this movement, maintained that the process by which the patient reaches acceptance of death typically passes through phases of anger, bargaining, and denial (1969).[19] Ernest Becker, in *The Denial of Death* (1973), claims that the phenomenon of death is a powerful force that often shapes and structures neuroses from an early age.[20] And psychiatrist Avery Weisman, one of the few researchers who focused on the psychoemotive responses of physicians involved in caring for

[a] See Chapter 14 by Hertogh.

dying patients, makes a case for "compassionate objectivity" in the doctor–patient relationship.[21] None of these authors, however, details or describes the psychological coping mechanisms of physicians after a patient expresses a request for help to die. Since such practice was officially forbidden everywhere, it isn't surprising that a relevant literature is absent.

The psychological and philosophical conflicts that physicians experience when caring for dying patients verify the claims of unconscious resistance, fears, projections, and bargaining, as mentioned earlier. Howard Stein (1985), a student of Michael Balint, describes the confrontation with death and dying as an intense process that while rational and conscious at one level, also has an unconscious dimension that involves *transference* and *countertransference*.[22] These terms were originally used to characterize powerful attitudes and feelings that develop between psychotherapist and patient and are only partly conscious.[7] Today, it is widely accepted that transference and countertransference are at play in a wide variety of social interactions. Obviously, the potential for such psychological dimensions in doctor–patient relationships is likely to be strong.

As caretakers confront dying patients and their families, powerful unconscious thoughts and feelings are at work. These concern the origin of early desires to become physicians, personal and professional experiences with death, and the curative ethos of medicine itself. As the interviews show, dealing with dying patients presents a direct confrontation with the physician's own psychological constructs, images, fears, and fantasies.

Over time, caretakers have learned to deal with these fears and tend to keep a professional distance from the dying. However, when a patient expresses a request for PAD, the insulation of professional distance is disturbed and the physician is forced to identify more directly with the dying patient. Beyond the limits of his or her own fears, the physician needs to become convinced in a rational way that this suffering is bad enough to help end this particular patient's life. The recognition of the risks of this involvement is reflected in the legal requirement that a consultant become involved. It is no longer accepted in the Netherlands that physicians may assist in the death of family members or colleagues or close friends.

From a philosophical-ethical angle, the problem of helping someone to die seems to go against the grain of a universal and fundamental prohibition. This moral law is reflected, for example, in the resistance to the death penalty, abortion, and less often to service in the military. The command "thou shalt not kill" has deep roots in almost all cultures. However, the prohibition is not simply a self-evident moral truth. Our Christianity-rooted culture has reflected deeply and widely on the practicality of the absolute nature of this prohibition. An absolute prohibition conflicted squarely with the aspirations of Christianity to become the religion of the state, ever since Constantine the Great's conversion in 325. In order to become the official religion, the Church had to accept the killing of enemy soldiers. This option was not open to individuals, irrespective of their conflicts and situations. Individuals, according to Church father Augustine (354–430) were denied the right to kill a human being. The debate was ended after Thomas Aquinas (1224–1274) formulated the rule that only taking "innocent life" is immoral in all cases.[23]

Taking life in medicine thus seems to be part and parcel of a paradigmatic example of a fundamentally immoral action as generally conceived. Alan Buchanan has articulated this point in forceful terms:

> [C]ontroversies over the moral status of intentional killing reach far beyond medicine. The prohibition against intentional taking of human life is so deeply ingrained – so morally primal – that the killing of heinous criminals and aggressors in war is rejected by some persons of undoubted moral integrity. Indeed, even those who find capital punishment and the killing of aggressors acceptable usually do so with a sense of profound moral loss and feel obliged to articulate and refine moral justifications for such exceptions to the general prohibition. To take intentionally an innocent person's life may seem like the very paradigm of an immoral act. One is tempted to say: if anything is wrong, *that* is wrong.[24]

In spite of this "prohibitive paradigm," there have been, and are, a fairly large number of laypersons and physicians who support the option of ending the life of seriously ill people with incurable diseases who request such assistance.

In this ethical conflict between prohibition and acceptance, the arguments pro and con play an essential role. The fundamental principles against taking a life focus on the immorality of denying someone a sense of well-being, human dignity, the right to life, or perhaps something as broadly conceived as what Don Marquis calls a future of value.[25] Counterarguments thus are brought forward on two basic grounds. First, in the case of helping someone die, it is important to be clear that the illness itself has robbed persons of a future of well-being and that death is sometimes the least worst alternative. Second, principles of autonomy, when well formed, entail that having a right to life implies the option of waiving such a right. Well-realized freedom of choice is the essential part of the concept of autonomy that makes autonomy the fundamental argument to justify helping patients end their lives. A decision of this magnitude and finality must finally rest with the individual him- or herself. That central place is reflected in the Dutch definition of euthanasia: ending a person's life *at his or her request*. But, of course, there are strenuous objections to such reasoning. In the first instance, critics argue that ending lives, on the bases of such individual choice, raises the specter of a permissive system that holds the value of human life all too casually and might well slide down a slippery slope likely to succumb to a host of unsavory social and economic forces. A second argument can be found in response to the argument of compassion. That argument holds that assisted dying simply is not compatible with the meaning and role of doctoring. Indeed, some have said that the practice of euthanasia and assisted dying strikes at the very "soul of medicine." For these critics, the point can be expressed in the simple words: "doctors must not kill."[26]

In order to react to the unbearable and unrelievable suffering of a dying patient, however, those simple words cannot suffice. When confronted with such a dilemma, physicians historically have always faced the question of whether or not to engage in an intervention that defies such a fundamental prohibition. Given the enormity of such a circumstance, if a physician ultimately decides to assist a dying patient, *there must be an articulated relationship, between physician and patient, that makes it psychologically and morally possible to take that step.*

ENDING LIVES AND "MEDICAL FRIENDSHIPS"

In all models of the physician–patient relationship is a presupposition that there should be a balance between professional distance and patient involvement, a balance between heart and mind that maintains objectivity in judgment as based on medical protocol, along with sensitivity and care for the patient as a person. That is the underlying idea of all models of the physician–patient relationship, whether it concerns the technical-mechanical model, the paternalistic model, the model of equality, contract, conversation, or transparency. The difference in these models focuses on the measure and the methods by which physicians approach the wishes and needs of their patients.

As mentioned earlier, this balance is frequently challenged in providing care at the end of life. If there is a request for PAD, the challenge to the normal professional distance is even greater. The psychological confrontation with death, the need for a more personal relationship, and the awareness that one might have to end the life of a person are an assault on normal attitudes of "objectivity." The request involves sizable ethical risk and both personal and professional vulnerability. Such a challenge requires a distinctive balance among competence, compassion, and interpersonal mutuality. It is a risky path that physician and patient jointly enter, leading to one of the most intimate of all possible human experiences. That path is a process in which patients themselves must realize that they are challenging the moral and philosophical limits of what any person could ask of another. Physicians who are able to accede to such a request do so only after their own acceptance of the fact that the alternative amounts to an act of abandonment of the patient at a time of great medical and existential need. Indeed, it appears that patients usually understand quite well what their requests mean for physicians, and many actually await their doctor's arrival at the stage that the patient has already reached.

In our opinion, the model that best characterizes this relationship of respect and personal commitment is that of a distinctive form of care, concern, and indeed what might be called a "medical friendship." While the term *friendship* is not unambiguous within the context of the doctor–patient relationship, there is, however, more than ample reason for it to be fully justified. While some might consider a notion like "friendship" too thin and unfitting the professional doctor–patient relationship, we want to urge the reader to consider that meaning loss has frequently attended many key concepts from the classical tradition. One might note, for example, how the classical notion of "tragedy" has become popularly overused, or indeed the classical conception of "happiness" (Greek: *eudaimonia*). Our effort in developing this model of a medical friendship is focused more on a revival of the vitality and richness inherent in classical notions, rather than in neologism or contemporary populism. Indeed, the conception of friendship in a medical relationship has been encouraged by Ezekiel Emanuel and Linda Emanuel in their Deliberative Model, where "the physician acts as a teacher or friend, engaging the patient in dialogue on what course of action would be best."[27]

The model we find fitting to end-of-life intervention seems appropriate, especially using the classical Aristotelian model of friendship. According to Aristotle in his Nichomachean Ethics: "If friendship consists more in loving than in being loved ... it seems that loving is the distinctive virtue between friends."[28] He defines three forms of friendship: those based on pleasure, on utility, and on virtue. Key to a complete friendship is reciprocal love of shared virtue. The category of shared virtue seems to apply most naturally in medical situations at the end of life. In that situation, a physician carries out an intervention based on a sense of compassionate respect that has evolved over a period of time based on interpersonal adjustment.

In an earlier essay, we included a remark from a Dr. E of the Netherlands, who articulates just such a conception:

> In my practice the average number of PAD [cases] is twice every year, as it is in 50% of Dutch practices. An intensive interaction between physician and patient is very important. The process of coming to an interpersonal agreement is at the heart of a well-realized physician and patient relationship.... Euthanasia is the final stage of the intersubjective process. The patient informs the doctor about his or her complaints and the doctor informs the patient about the possibilities of medical treatment. It is a process with an equal position for both parties.[11]

Central to a virtue relationship is the assumption that such a friend would not ask the other to do that which does not accord with the shared virtue of the friendship. Requests that depart from shared virtue often turn the relationship into dimensions of utility, where one person uses the other as an instrument to realize his or her own goals, without respect for the other's circumstances, moral risk, virtue, and character. In such a case, if a patient spurns the interpersonal process, simply wanting the physician to perform a life-ending intervention, that patient acts unjustly toward the physician, disrespecting the extent of ethical and psychological hazard faced by the physician who has accepted entrance into such a process.

In another interview, reported in the same essay, we quoted Dr. A, also of the Netherlands. Dr. A was clear that the interpersonal relationship needs to be balanced with some emotional distance. He commented that "[w]hat I need in a close relationship with patients who ask me to help them end their life is a maximum of involvement with a certain emotional distance so that I can still exercise the necessary objectivity with full professional responsibility."[11] Dr. A also spoke of mutual respect required in the process. "It is important for you to make your own limits clear to the patient...I do not like it when the patient makes a party out of it," he said. "Some patients want to organize a party around their bed. I do not want to do euthanasia in an atmosphere like that." Dr. A also added that the situation is made difficult both if he does not like the patient or if the patient is a good friend: "I find the decision making process very difficult when I do not like the person at all. When I feel antipathy towards the patient ... I will ask my colleague to take over for me.... [O]n the other hand, when somebody is a personal friend ... I will ask my colleague as well."

In addition, longer observations over weeks or months, such as those from Norwood, with physicians, patients and families, describe how the development of professional, formal, distant relationships evolve toward relationships with greater moral mutuality. Physicians and patients usually take a long time to decide when a disease will have taken up enough of the patient's existence. That is a process of mutual decision making. The cognitive aspect of this process is the assessment of suffering based on symptoms and functional loss, especially in the context of the patient's biography. Norwood's analysis, as with ours, reveals that it is primarily the patient who initiates and carries the process forward.

Consequently, in our judgment and according to anecdotes of physicians regarding their own relationships with dying patients (both those who expressed a request to be helped to die and those whose life they actually ended), there is strong argument and developing empirical evidence to confirm the moral and medical value of the form of medical relationship we have termed a "medical friendship." It has been our claim that the key element to highlight in this relationship is a process of mutual development – as guided by respect for the distinctive situation of both patient and physician – and continually adjusted to account for a shared virtue.

AN IMPORTANT AFTERTHOUGHT

We are keenly aware of a potential counterclaim that what we describe in this chapter is more of an ideal than a reality for many or even most physicians who practice or could practice PAD. Some physicians may be uninterested in or incapable of forming the medical friendship we have described as necessary to PAD practice. We all know that in the day-to-day practice of medicine, pettiness, callousness, laziness, and neglect sometimes show their ugly faces. It could be argued that this must be no less true in PAD practice. Indeed, there are anecdotes about such occurrences in the Netherlands. Although our study and those of others have not identified such behavior, our own sample of interviews was small, and for that reason, the results cannot claim to be representative.

In our opinion, however, the inability or unwillingness of physicians to enter into the medical friendship is the exception rather than the rule. This may have to do with the fact that most of the practice of PAD involves family physicians who have chosen a relationship-oriented type of practice and spent a great deal of their training developing communication skills. However, our 1994 interviews did include hospital-based specialists. On the other hand, we identified these specialists because they had been willing to publish their experiences. And while it is true that in the more than a hundred cases for which one of us (Kimsma) served as a SCEN (Support and Consultation Euthanasia in the Netherlands) consultant in the past 11 years, there was not one case in which patients and families did not speak highly of their physicians, this finding too can be characterized as anecdotal.

It is possible that physicians ill-suited to PAD practice refuse to even consider requests for it or categorically find the patients disqualified (which itself could be considered unethical). On the other hand, it is certainly possible that some physicians practice PAD without the emotional and moral sensitivity that we have argued is necessary to restrain the practice. In any event, as Margo Trappenburg explains in Chapter 6, the Dutch population maintains tremendous trust in physicians and the health-care system, and it is worthy of note that the rate of PAD has not significantly increased over the past two decades. Certainly, Dutch groups opposed to PAD in principle have repeatedly voiced concern about abuse. However, these concerns have never been great enough to mobilize public opinion, the law, elected officials, the press, or organized medicine to call for drastic reform. On the contrary: The most rigorous debate today concerns calls for an expansion of the practice, rather than its limitation. And, here, medical friendship acts as a conservative force.

Even if there were proof that the inability of a few physicians to form a medical friendship has led to deviation from standard PAD practice, isolated examples of physician misbehavior have occurred throughout history, and no one has called for an end to medical practice.

References

1. Thomasma, David C., Thomasine Kimbrough-Kushner, Gerrit K. Kimsma, and Chris Carlucci-Ciesielski, eds. 1998. *Asking to Die: Inside the Dutch Euthanasia Debate*. Dordrecht: Kluwer Academic.
2. An early example can be found in an anonymous contribution in *The Spectator*, January 25, 1902, 134–135.
3. Teitelman, Michale. 1998. Not in the house: Arguments for a policy of excluding physician-assisted suicide from the practice of hospital medicine. In *Physician Assisted Suicide: Expanding the Debate*, ed. Margaret P. Battin, Rosamond Rhodes, and Anita Silvers, 203–223. New York: Routledge.
4. Sticker G. 1904. Das Recht der Aerzte zu töten [The right of physicians to kill]. In *Hochland, Monatschrift für alle Gebiete des Wissens, der Literatur und der Kunst*, I, Part II: 616–621.

5. Steinhauer, Jennifer. 1998. Was it mercy or murder? *New York Times*, October 17.
6. Reagan, Peter. 1999. Helen. *The Lancet* 353: 1265–1267.
7. Stevens, Kenneth R. 2006. Emotional and psychological effects of physician-assisted suicide and euthanasia on participating physicians. *Issues in Law & Medicine* 21: 187–201.
8. Haverkate, Ilinka, Agnes van der Heide, Bregje Onwuteaka-Philipsen, Paul J. van der Maas, and Gerrit van der Wal. 2001. The emotional impact on physicians of hastening the death of a patient. *Medical Journal of Australia* 175: 519–522.
9. Pellegrino, Edmund. 1998. The false promise of beneficent killing. In *Regulating How We Die: The Ethical, Medical and Legal Issues Surrounding Physician-Assisted Suicide*, ed. Linda L. Emanuel, 76. Cambridge, MA: Harvard University Press.
10. Gianelli, D. M. 1997. Dutch euthanasia expert critical of Oregon approach. *American Medical News*, September 15.
11. Clark, Chalmers C., and Gerrit K. Kimsma. 2004. "Medical friendships" in assisted dying. *Cambridge Quarterly of Health Care Ethics* 13: 61–67.
12. Obstein, K. L., Gerrit K. Kimsma, and T. Chambers. 2004. Practicing euthanasia: The perspective of physicians. *Journal of Clinical Ethics* 15: 223–232.
13. Van Marwijk, Harm, Ilinka Haverkate, Paul van Roven, and Anne-Mei The. 2007. The impact of euthanasia on primary care physicians in the Netherlands. *Palliative Medicine*. 21: 609–614.
14. Vaux, Kenneth. 1988. Commentary: Debbie's dying mercy killing and the good death. *Journal of the American Medical Association* 295: 2140–2141.
15. Anonymous. 1988. It's over Debbie. *Journal of the American Medical Association* 295: 272.
16. Crisci C., M. Guariglia, F. Gargano, and G. Caruso. 1992. Italian neurologists and euthanasia: A poll. *Italian Journal of Neurological Sciences* 13: 425–427.
17. Norwood, Frances. 2005. Euthanasia talk: Euthanasia discourse, general practice and end-of-life care in the Netherlands: The role of family in euthanasia decision making. Ph.D. diss., University of California San Francisco/Berkeley.
18. Lain Entralgo, Pedro. 1969. *Doctor and Patient*. London: World University Library.
19. Kübler-Ross, Elisabeth. 1969. *On Death and Dying*. New York: Simon and Schuster.
20. Becker, Ernest. 1973. *The Denial of Death*. New York: Simon and Schuster.
21. Weisman, Avery D. 1972. *On Dying and Denying*. New York: Behavioral Publications.
22. Stein, Howard. 1987. *The psychodynamics of medical practice: Unconscious factors in patient care*. Berkeley: University of California Press.
23. Rachels, James. 1986. *The End of Life*. Oxford: Oxford University Press.
24. Buchanan, Alan. 1996. Intending death: The structure of the problem and proposed solutions. In *Intending Death: The Ethics of Assisted Suicide and Euthanasia*, ed. Tom Beauchamp, 23–41. Upper Saddle River, NJ: Prentice-Hall.
25. Marquis, Don. 1989. Why abortion is immoral. *Journal of Philosophy* 86: 183–202.
26. Kass L., W. Gaylin, E. Pellegrino, and M. Siegler. 1988. "Doctors must not kill." *Journal of the American Medical Association* 259 (April 8): 2139–2140.

27. Emanuel, Ezekiel, and Linda Emanuel. 1989. Four models of the physician–patient relationship. In *Ethical Issues in Modern Medicine*, ed. John D. Arras and Bonnie Steinbock, 67–76. Mountain View, CA: Mayfield.
28. Aristotle. 1999. *Nichomachean Ethics*, Book Eight, VII:1159a9–60a9. Trans. with introduction and notes by Terence Irwin. Indianapolis: Hackett.

18

Depression, Euthanasia, and Assisted Suicide

Marije van der Lee

INTRODUCTION

Opposition to euthanasia and assisted suicide (EAS) stems partly from the perspective that a request for euthanasia is similar to a wish for suicide and that this is a symptom of underlying mental illness. Herbert Hendin, for example, states that there is no difference between a request for assisted suicide from a person with a medical illness and suicidal ideation stemming from a depression.[1] Others have agreed with Hendin.[2,3] Hendin further argues that "'normalizing' suicide as a medical option lays the groundwork for a society that turns euthanasia into a 'cure' for suicidal depression."[4] Euthanasia and physician-assisted suicide are hotly debated issues, and because arguments used in the discussion about legalization are often emotionally charged, the debate would benefit from evidence and rational argument. Using empirical data from studies in the Netherlands and the state of Oregon, I will argue that while there is a clear association between depression and a request for physician assisted death, they cannot be equated in all or even most cases. Next, I will discuss some of the dilemmas around depression and EAS and propose a way to deal with them.

Focus on Terminally Ill Oncology Patients

This chapter will be restricted to requests for EAS from terminally ill oncology patients in the Netherlands, from whom 80% of requests for EAS come[5,6,7,8]. It is estimated that EAS shortens life by less than one month in most of these cases[9]. In Oregon, where assisted suicide has been legal since 1994, one of the legal requirements is that the patient have a terminal illness that would, within reasonable medical judgment, cause death within six months. In the Netherlands, the Supreme Court ruled in 1994 that in exceptional cases, unbearable suffering and untreatable psychiatric illness without "physical" illness might be justifiable grounds for EAS. Likewise, the Belgian law allows EAS for mental suffering, without the presence of a terminal illness. Because these cases are rarely granted[10] and fall within a totally different scope, I will confine my remarks to requests for EAS from terminally ill oncology patients.

THE RELATION BETWEEN DEPRESSION AND EAS

The concern that depression causes patients to request EAS has prompted several studies about possibly related factors. Many of these studies have been carried out in countries where euthanasia is not legalized. While some studies have found no evidence for a relation between a wish for a hastened death and depression[11,12,13], others have indeed confirmed that a desire for a hastened death is associated with depression among terminally ill patients.[14,15,16,17,18,19,20,3,21,13]

The actual relationship between depression and requests for EAS can be openly and directly studied in a context in which euthanasia is legalized. So far there have been two such studies, one from Oregon and one from the Netherlands, where, respectively, assisted suicide and EAS are legal under strict criteria. The unambiguous conclusion drawn from these studies is that the majority of terminally ill patients in Oregon and the Netherlands who request physicians to assist in their death do not have depressive disorders. I will briefly describe the methodology and results of these studies, before discussing their results.

The Relation Between Depression and EAS Studied in the Netherlands

In the Netherlands, a prospective cohort study was conducted among consecutive cancer patients with an estimated life expectancy of three months or less who were admitted to an academic hospital[22] (see Figure 18.1 for a flow chart of this study). The aim was to investigate whether depression in terminally ill oncology patients is associated with the occurrence of explicit requests for EAS. In the Netherlands, euthanasia is practiced far more often than assisted suicide, and in this study all participants requested euthanasia.

Of the 198 who met the study criteria, 40 refused to participate and 18 were unable to complete the questionnaire. One hundred forty patients completed a questionnaire that included a screening instrument for depression: the Hospital Anxiety and Depression Scale (HADS). To diagnose "depressed mood," a cut-off score of 20 for the total scale on the HADS was used, as was advised in an earlier study[23].

A follow-up measurement was performed when a member of the cohort made an explicit and persistent request for euthanasia. The treating physician judged whether the patient's request was explicit and persistent. If so, the

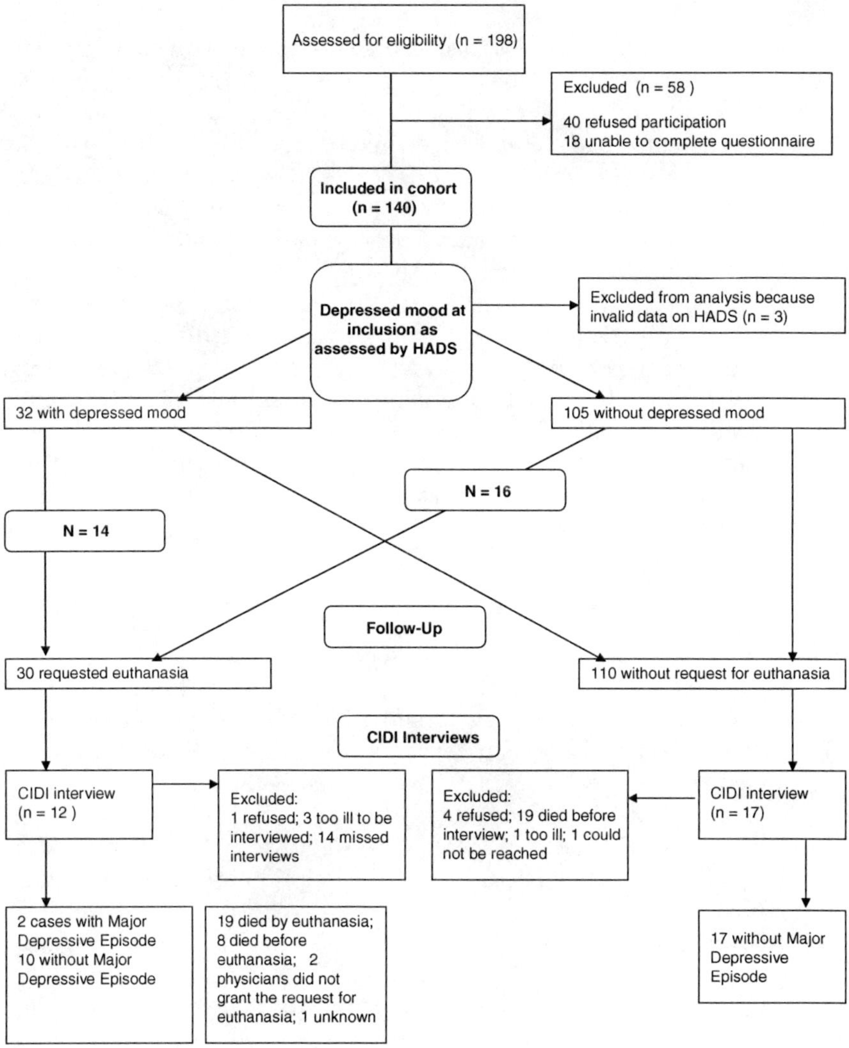

FIGURE 18.1. Flow chart study in 22. Van der Lee, et al., 2005.

standard procedure for handling requests was initiated; that is, an independent physician was consulted, and the researcher was notified of the request for euthanasia. Among these patients and among the random sample of the rest of the cohort (those who had not requested euthanasia), the presence of current and lifetime depressive episodes was assessed with the Composite International Diagnostic Interview (CIDI-auto)[24,25,26]. Two controls were sampled for each case of a request for euthanasia.

Results

Of all included patients, 32 (23%) had a depressed mood[a] at the time of inclusion, as assessed by the HADS (score > 20 points). Of these 32 patients, 14 (44%) requested euthanasia during follow-up (see the flow chart in Figure 18.1). Among the 105 patients without depressed mood at inclusion, 16 (15%) went on to request euthanasia (3 of the original 108 were excluded because of invalid data). The risk of a request for euthanasia for patients with depressed mood at inclusion in the study was 4.1 times higher than that of patients without it (95% confidence interval [CI] 2.0 to 8.5).

Of the 30 patients with a request for EAS, 12 had a follow-up interview for depression. Eight patients who requested euthanasia died before euthanasia could have been performed, and seven of them could not be interviewed in time (see Figure 18.1). Two Major Depressive Disorders (one with a mild recurrent episode, the other with a single severe episode) were diagnosed in these interviews. None of the 17 control patients (without a request for euthanasia) was diagnosed with a Major Depressive episode at the time of the interview.

The Relation Between Depression and EAS Studied in Oregon

In the state of Oregon, a cross-sectional survey was conducted to determine the prevalence of depression in Oregonians pursuing aid in dying[27]. The participants were 176 patients with a terminal illness (cancer or amyotrophic lateral sclerosis) who requested information about accessing aid in dying or made an explicit request for aid in dying to a physician. The Hospital Anxiety and Depression Scale was administered; patients with a score higher than 11 on the depression subscale were identified as depressed. In addition, the current mood-disorder section of the structured clinical Interview for American Psychiatric Association Diagnostic and Statistical Manual-IV Axis I disorders (SCID-I) was completed by a psychologist. This interview was audiotaped, and the tapes were reviewed by a psychiatrist who did not know whether or not the patient had requested EAS. An inclusive approach for diagnosing depression was used, so that all physical symptoms of depression were attributed to the depression diagnosis, even if they might have been a result of terminal illness. The criteria of suicidal ideation were attributed to a depressive disorder only if the patients endorsed suicidal thoughts or plans aside from requesting EAS. Cases of depression were defined as having a positive SCID

[a] The HADS is a screening instrument and cannot be used to diagnose a clinical depression or depressive disorder. It assesses depressed mood, and therefore I use the term *depressed mood* when I refer to the outcome of the questionnaire, and I reserve the terms (clinical or Major) *depression/depressive disorder* for the outcome of the clinical interview.

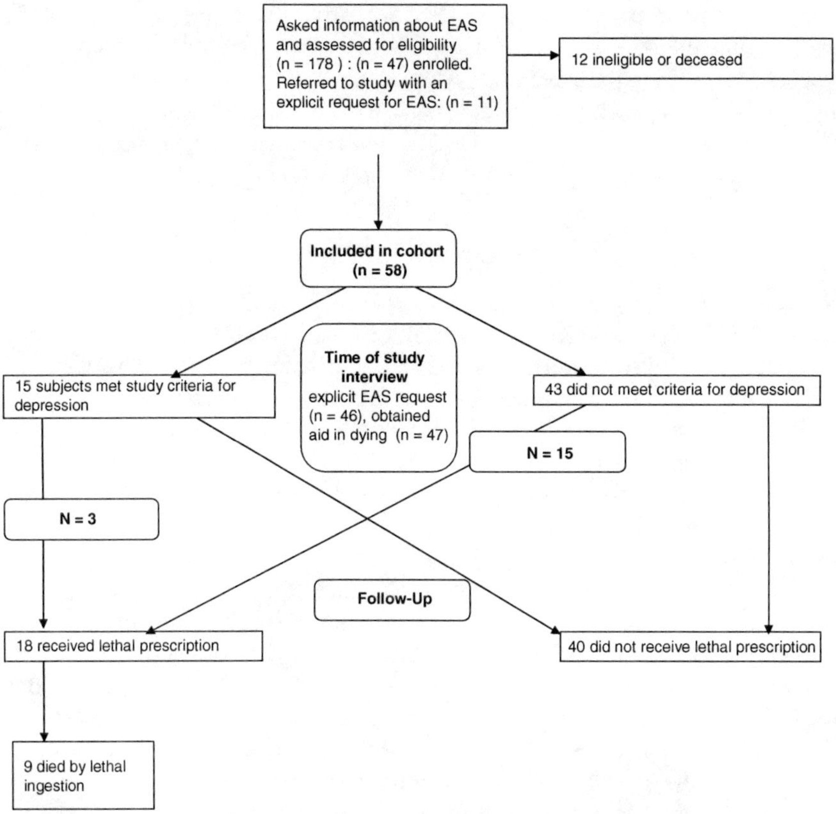

FIGURE 18.2. Flow chart study in 27. Ganzini, Goy, and Dobscha 2008.

and/or a HADS depression score equal to or higher than 11 on the depression subscale.[b]

Subjects rated their desire for death in the two weeks preceding the interview on an 11-point scale with end points labeled 0 = "I desire to live as long as possible" and 10 = "I have a strong desire to die soon."

Results

Of the 18 patients (17%) who received EAS, 3 met the aforementioned criteria for depression (see Figure 18.2 for a flow chart of this study). Fifteen subjects (26%) met the criteria for depression at inclusion. Seven of these

[b] In this study, the criteria for diagnosing depression are somewhat different from those in the study conducted in the Netherlands. I use the term (clinical) *depression* here as it is defined by the authors.

subjects did not attribute their pursuit of aid in dying to depression at all, while six felt that their request for EAS was somewhat or strongly influenced by depression. Among the 42 subjects who died by the end of the study, 18 (43%) received a lethal prescription and 9 (21%) used it and died by lethal ingestion. Remarkably, those who received a lethal prescription had a lower desire to die (as assessed with the 11-point scale) than those who did not.

DISCUSSION OF THE RESULTS FROM BOTH STUDIES

We can conclude from these two studies that the majority of terminally ill patients who make a serious, explicit, and persistent request for EAS do not have depressive disorders. Although the numbers are small, it seems that only a minority of patients who made a persistent, explicit request for EAS met the criteria for clinical depression.[27,28] This suggests that the prevalence of depressive disorders among patients requesting EAS is much lower than was expected from studies in jurisdictions where EAS is illegal. Furthermore, in jurisdictions where EAS is illegal, the relation between depression and "desire to die" as assessed with the questionnaire was often studied, but it was not known if desire to die was the same as a request for EAS. The Oregon study corroborates the assumption that desire to die is different from a serious, explicit, and persistent request for EAS, since the desire to die as assessed by the questionnaire was less in the group with a request. It is safe to conclude that suicidal ideation stemming from depression is not present every time there is a serious, explicit, and persistent request for EAS in the context of terminal medical illness. Thus, the assumption that every request for assisted death is a consequence of depression is false and not a valid argument for opposing legalization of EAS.

Other Dilemmas Concerning Depression and EAS

The results of these studies raise two important clinical and moral questions. First, what are the implications of the finding that there is a definite (though not universal) correlation between depressed mood and requests for EAS? Second, what can we say about the mental competence in decision making of the few patients with a depressive disorder who request EAS?

The design of both studies prevents us from drawing firm conclusions about causality. In the Dutch study, patients with a depressed mood were four times more likely to request EAS. In the Oregon study, one in four patients who seriously sought information about aid in dying had clinical depression, and about half of these patients (6/15) felt that depression somewhat or strongly influenced their interest in aid in dying. These findings force us to ask whether treating depressed mood or clinical depression might prevent some requests for EAS. If it could, we should organize systematic screening of patients who may request EAS.

Systematic Screening of Depression

Studies show that physicians often have difficulty recognizing depression in patients.[29,30] Screening can help both to identify depressed patients and to open communication between patient and physician about depression. Diagnosing depression in terminally ill patients is complex. Symptoms of depression, such as weight loss, insomnia, loss of energy, diminished ability to concentrate, and recurrent thoughts of death, may be due to the underlying disease or its treatment, rather than to depression. The Hospital Anxiety and Depression Scale is often used as a screening tool for depressive disorders in palliative oncology patients because it specifically excludes the somatic symptoms listed here. The HADS was found to predict the development of Major Depression in terminally ill cancer patients and is easy to administer.[31] Therefore, systematic screening for depressed mood is feasible.

Treatment of Depression

J. M. Wilson and Y. G. Jungner[32] have stated that we should only screen for disorders when treatment is available. A systematic review with a meta-analysis shows that psychotherapeutic (i.e., nonpharmalogical) interventions are useful for treating depressed mood in advanced-cancer patients.[33] Treatment should be offered to patients with depressed mood as early as possible in order to prevent the development of Major Depressive Disorders.[34,28] It is unknown whether treatment of Major Depression is successful in patients who have become terminally ill.[33] When screening starts after patients have expressed a request for EAS, at a point that is usually near death, there is also little time left for treatment, whether the patient dies with EAS or without it. Therefore, screening for depression should take place earlier, for example, in the period during which active life-prolonging treatment is stopped and a phase of symptom palliation begins. Treatment of depression is a worthy goal in and of itself, not only as a means for preventing physician-assisted suicide. This means that systematic screening should not focus solely on the few patients who request EAS, but on all palliative patients.

Depression and Competence

Although most of the patients requesting EAS are not depressed, some are. This begs the question: Are these patients competent to make this decision? Although the presence of mental illness including depression is not a de facto proof of incompetence,[35] we know that severe Major Depressive Disorders can have a negative impact on decision-making ability. This is the reason many physicians are reluctant to grant a request when they suspect that the patient has a depressive disorder. In the Netherlands, only one-third of all requests are carried out, and for 31% of the nongranted requests, depression is the reason given by physicians.[36] In a study of Oregon physicians, none of the 20% depressed patients received EAS.[37]

It has been suggested that psychiatric consultation should be part of the standard procedure for handling EAS requests as a means of guaranteeing competence. One study reported that only 6% of psychiatrists were very confident that in a single evaluation they could determine whether a psychiatric disorder was impairing judgment of a patient requesting EAS,[38] which demonstrates that standard consultation in a single evaluation is regarded as too complex. Some commentators have concluded that a psychiatrist should only be consulted in cases of doubt about the decision-making ability of the patient[39,40]. I agree that physicians should consult a psychiatrist only when they have doubts about a patient's decision-making ability. In the Netherlands, where an extensive system of family physicians (general practitioners) is responsible for 80% of EAS cases, the physician who receives the request has usually known the patient for some time, a situation that makes it easier to judge competence. The request for EAS must be persistent, and a physician who has discussed EAS on several occasions with the patient is in the best position to evaluate the consistency of the request. Thus, both patients and physicians have the responsibility to start communication about EAS as early as possible.

CONCLUSION

The claim that a request for euthanasia is always a symptom of underlying depression can be dismissed. The question of whether treatment of depression in terminally ill cancer patients would reduce the number of requests for euthanasia needs further investigation. I believe that it is important to systematically screen for depression and offer treatment of depression to *all* dying patients, preferably before the terminal phase starts. Since depression has a negative impact on medical symptoms and the quality of life of all patients and their families, it seems better not to restrict screening to those patients who express a request for EAS. Moreover, waiting to screen until near the end offers little time for treatment, even if it is indicated.

Early communication between patient and physician about a potential wish for EAS will help the physician judge the patient's competence when and if the request for EAS comes. When a physician has doubts about a patient's decision-making ability, a psychiatrist should be consulted.

References

1. Hendin, Herbert. 1999. Suicide, assisted suicide, and medical illness. *Journal of Clinical Psychiatry* 60: 46–50.
2. Block, S. D., and J. A. Billings. 1995. Patient requests for euthanasia and assisted suicide in terminal illness: The role of the psychiatrist. *Psychosomatics* 36: 445–457.
3. Kelly, Brian, Paul C. Burnett, Dan Pelusi, Shirlene Badger, Francis Varghese, and Margaret M. Robertson. 2003. Factors associated with the wish to hasten death: A study of patients with terminal illness. *Psychological Medicine* 33: 75–81.

4. Hendin, Herbert. 1995. Assisted suicide, euthanasia, and suicide prevention: The implications of the Dutch experience. *Suicide and Life Threatening Behavior* 25: 193–204.
5. Onwuteaka-Philipsen, Bregje D., Agnes van der Heide, Dirk Koper, Ingeborg Keij-Deerenberg, Judith A. Rietjens, Mette L. Rurup, Astrid M. Vrakking, Jean Jacques Georges, Martien T. Muller, Gerrit van der Wal, and Paul J. van der Maas. 2003. Euthanasia and other end-of-life decisions in the Netherlands in 1990, 1995, and 2001. *The Lancet* 362: 395–399.
6. Heide, Agnes van der, Bregje D. Onwuteaka-Philipsen, Mette L. Rurup, Hilde M. Buiting, Johannes J. M. van Delden, Johanna E. Hanssen-de Wolf, Anke G. J. M. Janssen, H. Roeline Pasman, Judith A. C. Rietjens, Cornelis J. M. Prins, Ingeborg M. Deerenberg, Joseph K. M. Gevers, Paul J. van der Maas, and Gerrit van der Wal. 2007. End-of-life practices in the Netherlands under the Euthanasia Act. *New England Journal of Medicine* 356: 1957–1965.
7. Maas, Paul J. van der, J. J. van Delden, L. Pijnenborg, and C. W. Looman. 1991. Euthanasia and other medical decisions concerning the end of life. *The Lancet* 338: 669–674.
8. Maas, Paul J. van der, Gerrit van der Wal, Ilinka Haverkate, Carmen L. M. de Graaff, John G. C. Kester, Bregje D. Onwuteaka Philipsen, Agnes van der Heide, Jacqueline M. Bosma, and Dick L. Willems. 1996. Euthanasia, physician-assisted suicide, and other medical practices involving the end of life in the Netherlands, 1990–1995. *New England Journal of Medicine* 335: 1699–1705.
9. Heide, Agnes van der, Luc Deliens, Karin Faisst, Tore Nilstun, Michael Norup, Eugenio Paci, Gerrit van der Wal, and Paul J. van der Maas. 2003. End-of-life decision-making in six European countries: Descriptive study. *The Lancet* 362: 345–350.
10. Groenewoud, Johanna H., Paul J. van der Maas, Gerrit van der Wal, Michiel W. Hengeveld, Alfons J. Tholen, Willem J. Schudel, and Agnes van der Heide. 1997. Physician-assisted death in psychiatric practice in the Netherlands. *New England Journal of Medicine* 336: 1795–1801.
11. Pacheco, Jaime, Paul J. Hershberger, Ronald J. Markert, and Geetika Kumar. 2003. A longitudinal study of attitudes toward physician-assisted suicide and euthanasia among patients with noncurable malignancy. *American Journal of Hospice and Palliative Medicine* 20: 99–104.
12. Suarez-Almazor, Maria E., Catherine Newman, John Hanson, and Eduardo Bruera. 2002. Attitudes of terminally ill cancer patients about euthanasia and assisted suicide: Predominance of psychosocial determinants and beliefs over symptom distress and subsequent survival. *Journal of Clinical Oncology* 20: 2134–2141.
13. Wilson, Keith G., John F. Scott, Ian D. Graham, Jean F. Kozak, Susan Chater, Raymond A. Viola, Barbara J. de Faye, Lynda A. Weaver, and Dorothyann Curran. 2000. Attitudes of terminally ill patients toward euthanasia and physician-assisted suicide. *Archives of Internal Medicine* 160: 2454–2460.
14. Breitbart, William, and Suzanne Krivo. 1998. Suicide. In *Psycho-oncology*, ed. Jimmie C. Holland, 541–546. New York: Oxford University Press.
15. Breitbart, William, Barry Rosenfeld, Hayley Pessin, Monique Kaim, Julie Funesti-Esch, Michele Galietta, Christian J. Nelson, and Robert Brescia. 2000. Depression, hopelessness, and desire for hastened death in terminally ill patients with cancer. *Journal of the American Medical Association* 284: 2907–2911.

16. Brown, J. H., P. Henteleff, S. Barakat, and C. J. Rowe. 1986. Is it normal for terminally ill patients to desire death? *American Journal of Psychiatry* 143: 208–211.
17. Chochinov, H. M., K. G. Wilson, M. Enns, N. Mowchun, S. Lander, M. Levitt, and J. J. Clinch. 1995. Desire for death in the terminally ill. *American Journal of Psychiatry* 152: 1185–1191.
18. Emanuel, Ezekiel J., Diane L. Fairclough, E. R. Daniels, and Brian C. Clarridge. 1996. Euthanasia and physician-assisted suicide: Attitudes and experiences of oncology patients, oncologists, and the public. *The Lancet* 347: 1805–1810.
19. Emanuel, Ezekiel J., Diane L. Fairclough, and Linda L. Emanuel. 2000. Attitudes and desires related to euthanasia and physician-assisted suicide among terminally ill patients and their caregivers. *Journal of the American Medical Association* 284: 2460–2468.
20. Jones, Jennifer M., Mary Anne Huggins, Anne C. Rydall, and Gary M. Rodin. 2003. Symptomatic distress, hopelessness, and the desire for hastened death in hospitalized cancer patients. *Journal of Psychosomatic Research* 55: 411–418.
21. Tiernan, E., P. Casey, C. O'Boyle, G. Birkbeck, M. Mangan, L. O'Siorain, and M. Kearney. 2002. Relations between desire for early death, depressive symptoms and antidepressant prescribing in terminally ill patients with cancer. *Journal of the Royal Society of Medicine* 95: 386–390.
22. Lee, Marije L. van der, Johanna G. van der Bom, Nikkie B. Swarte, A. Peter M. Heintz, Alexander de Graeff, and Jan van den Bout. 2005. Euthanasia and depression: A prospective cohort study among terminally ill cancer patients. *Journal of Clinical Oncology* 23: 6607–6612.
23. Le Fevre, P., J. Devereux, S. Smith, S. M. Lawrie, and M. Cornbleet. 1999. Screening for psychiatric illness in the palliative care inpatient setting: A comparison between the Hospital Anxiety and Depression Scale and the General Health Questionnaire-12. *Palliative Medicine* 13: 399–407.
24. Andrews G., and L. Peters. 1998. The psychometric properties of the Composite International Diagnostic Interview. *Social Psychiatry and Psychiatric Epidemiology* 33: 80–88.
25. Peters, L., and G. Andrews. 1995. Procedural validity of the computerized version of the Composite International Diagnostic Interview (CIDI-Auto) in the anxiety disorders. *Psychological Medicine* 25: 1269–1280.
26. Wittchen, H. U., L. N. Robins, L. B. Cottler, N. Sartorius, J. D. Burke, and D. Regier. 1991. Cross-cultural feasibility, reliability and sources of variance of the Composite International Diagnostic Interview (CIDI): The Multicentre WHO/ADAMHA Field Trials. *British Journal of Psychiatry* 159: 645–653.
27. Ganzini, Linda, Elizabeth R. Goy, and Steven K. Dobscha. 2008. The prevalence of depression and anxiety in patients requesting physician aid in dying. *British Medical Journal* 337. http://bmj.com/highwire/filestream/384131/field_highwire_article_pdf/0.pdf. doi:10.1136/bmj.a1682.
28. Lee, Marije L.van der. 2008. Depression and physician assisted dying. *British Medical Journal* 337. http://bmj.com/highwire/filestream/384131/field_highwire_article_pdf/0.pdf. doi:10.1136/bmj.a1558.
29. Balestrieri, Mattei, Giulia Bisoffi, Michele Tansella, Marilena Martucci, and David P. Goldberg. 2002. Identification of depression by medical and surgical general hospital physicians. *General Hospital Psychiatry* 24: 4–11.

30. Sollner, Wolfgang, A. DeVries, E. Steixner, P. Lukas, G. Sprinzl, G. Rumpold, and S. Maislinger. 2001. How successful are oncologists in identifying patient distress, perceived social support, and need for psychosocial counselling? *British Journal of Cancer* 84: 179–185.
31. Akechi, Tatsuo, Toru Okuyama, Yuriko Sugawara, Yasuo Shima, Toshiaki A. Furukawa, and Yosuke Uchitomi. 2006. Screening for depression in terminally ill cancer patients in Japan. *Journal of Pain and Symptom Management* 31: 5–12.
32. Wilson, J. M., and Y. G. Jungner. 1968. Principles and practice of mass screening for disease. Public Health Paper no. 34. World Health Organization, Geneva.
33. Akechi, T., T. Okuyama, J. Onishi, T. Morita, and T. A. Furukawa. 2008. Psychotherapy for depression among incurable cancer patients. *Cochrane Database Systematic Review*, April 16.
34. Akechi, Tatsuo, Toru Okuyama, Yuriko Sugawara, Tomohito Nakano, Yasuo Shima, and Yosuke Uchitomi. 2004. Major depression, adjustment disorders, and post-traumatic stress disorder in terminally ill cancer patients: Associated and predictive factors. *Journal of Clinical Oncology* 22: 1957–1965.
35. Sullivan, Mark D., and Stuart J. Youngner. 1994. Depression, competence, and the right to refuse lifesaving medical treatment. *American Journal of Psychiatry* 151: 971–978.
36. Haverkate, Ilinka, Bregje D. Onwuteaka-Philipsen, Agnes van der Heide, Piet J. Kostense, Gerrit van der Wal, and Paul J. van der Maas. 2000. Refused and granted requests for euthanasia and assisted suicide in the Netherlands: Interview study with structured questionnaire. *British Medical Journal* 321: 865–866.
37. Ganzini, Linda, Heidi D. Nelson, Terri A. Schmidt, Dale F. Kraemer, Molly A. Delorit, and Melinda A. Lee. 2000. Physicians' experiences with the Oregon Death with Dignity Act. *New England Journal of Medicine* 342: 557–563.
38. Ganzini, Linda, Darien S. Fenn, Melinda A. Lee, Ronald T. Heintz, and Joseph D. Bloom. 1996. Attitudes of Oregon psychiatrists toward physician-assisted suicide. *American Journal of Psychiatry* 153: 1469–1475.
39. Bannink, Marjolein, Arthur R. Van Gool, Agnes van der Heide, and Paul J. van der Maas. 2000. Psychiatric consultation and quality of decision making in euthanasia. *The Lancet* 356: 2067–2068.
40. Sullivan, Mark D., Linda Ganzini, and Stuart J. Youngner. 1998. Should psychiatrists serve as gatekeepers for physician-assisted suicide? *Hastings Center Report* 28: 24–31.

19

End-of-Life Decisions in Children and Newborns in the Netherlands

Pieter J. J. Sauer and A. A. Eduard Verhagen

INTRODUCTION

Modern technology and improved understanding of the pathophysiology of sick children, including newborn infants, have greatly increased their chances for survival. Forty years ago, approximately 10% of children diagnosed with acute leukemia survived, compared to more than 80% now. The survival of sick newborn infants has also increased enormously. Forty years ago, almost all infants weighing less than 1 kilogram did not survive; the survival of infants weighing between 750 and 1,000 grams is now around 80%. The higher survival rates, however, are accompanied by an increased number of children and newborn infants who survive with minor or major handicaps and/or sequelae.[1,2,3,4,5] There are two pertinent questions: Is the goal of modern medicine to achieve the greatest number of survivors? Or is the quality of life of those children and newborn infants who survive also important? In other words, must all treatment options be utilized for sick children and newborn infants, or should some children be allowed to die?

In this chapter, we will first describe a few cases to illustrate how these questions translate into dilemmas regarding end-of-life decision making in pediatric practice. Given that most discussions about end-of-life decisions involve newborn infants, we will focus predominantly on those infants in this chapter; some attention will also be given to older infants and children up to adolescence. Second, we describe how newborn infants in end-of-life situations can be categorized into three groups according to dimensions of physiology and intervention. Third, we reflect on the third and most controversial group of infants, whose extensive suffering cannot be relieved, and the option to deliberately end their lives as described in the "Groningen Protocol." We describe how the protocol followed the fundamental approach of medical and government reports in the Netherlands, which was acknowledged in court cases; that is, ending the life of a newborn who is enduring sustained suffering is legitimate if all requirements of due care are fulfilled. The Groningen

Protocol received intense media attention and criticisms that we will address in this chapter.

OLDER CHILDREN AND ADOLESCENTS

The burden of treatment should be balanced against the future quality of life in patients of all ages. Very intensive treatment that might prolong life for a span of only one to two months might not be considered appropriate. The same might be true when life expectancy is longer but the suffering is very severe and there are limited positive aspects of the person's life. These general ethical principles do not differ with respect to children and adult patients. The difference, of course, is in the ability of the patient to express a preference – that is, the younger the child, the less able he or she is to express his or her own opinion. Adult patients can balance treatment burdens versus benefits and make decisions. This is clearly impossible for a young child.

In most countries in Europe, a minor assumes full legal responsibility at the age of 18 years. The concept of a competent minor has been introduced in a number of countries, thereby giving responsibility to children starting at the age of 12 years. By that age, children are considered capable of expressing their own will clearly and of making decisions. Whether the consent of parents is also needed for individuals 12 to 18 years of age generally depends upon the type of decision. Parental consent is needed for end-of-life decisions. In the Netherlands, the child's opinion is also sought if he or she is younger than 12. Children with chronic diseases can be emotionally mature at 8 to 12 years. Even if the child and parents disagree, nothing can be done against the will of a child as long as he or she is approximately 8 years or older. Three examples illustrate these issues:

A child was born with cystic fibrosis, a congenital disease characterized by progressive damage of the lungs, liver, and pancreas. This child had been severely affected since birth. An operation was required directly after birth due to a bowel obstruction. From birth, the child suffered from malabsorption, insufficient growth, and many lung infections. By age 10, she had end-stage lung disease and was on continuous oxygen treatment. The only available treatment option was a lung transplant. When this option was discussed with the parents, they both agreed to let the child have the surgery. The child herself refused. She stated that "she had suffered enough and she did not want any more suffering." After further discussions, the transplant was not performed and the child died soon thereafter.

The second patient was diagnosed with acute lymphatic leukemia. At age 12, he had his second relapse; the only option involved very intensive treatment. The patient had already had intensive treatment during his previous relapse and decided he did not want it anymore. After some discussion, the parents agreed with his point of view and the child died without further treatment.

The third patient suffered since birth from epidermolysis bullosa, a skin disease in which the skin blisters after being touched. The child, now 14 years of age, experienced almost continuous severe pain. It is known that this disease will not improve. Indeed, the pain will continue and the skin will become so tight that the child will not be able to bend his fingers or open his mouth. Most of these children die of skin cancer at approximately 18 years of age. The boy, at 14, requested an active ending of his life. He felt that he had suffered enough and did not want to continue living. A child of 14 years of age is legally not able to ask for euthanasia. Still, all physicians involved felt that they could not let the suffering continue while this boy clearly indicated his wish to end his life. When the parents agreed, euthanasia was performed.

These cases illustrate that children, starting at age 8, as well as adults experience the same kinds of ethical dilemmas. Physicians must first obtain consent from children, beginning at age 8, and then parents for all treatment. After age 10, the child's opinion is of utmost importance and parents cannot simply overrule it. Ethical dilemmas involving children younger than 8 are comparable to those involving newborns.

END-OF-LIFE DECISIONS IN NEWBORN INFANTS

Discussions about end-of-life decisions in newborn infants in the Netherlands started around 1986. As a result of these deliberations, a working group of the Dutch Pediatric Association published the report "Doen of laten" (To treat or not to treat?) in 1992.[6] The report was accepted by all members of the Dutch Pediatric Association. Thereafter, two reports were issued by the Royal Dutch Federation of Physicians and a committee instituted by the Dutch government.[7,8] Basically, these last two reports endorsed the first report issued by the Pediatric Association.

All of these reports identified three groups of newborn infants for whom end-of-life decisions might be made. The first group includes infants with no chance to survive, even when all available options for treatment are used. The second group includes infants on life support who might survive but whose future outlook is so grim that continuation of treatment might not be indicated. The third group includes infants who are not dependent on life support but who are facing a life full of suffering that cannot be alleviated by any means. Active euthanasia should be considered in these last cases.

Discussions of end-of-life decisions are not restricted to the Netherlands. A study, published in 2000, compared end-of-life decisions for newborn infants in different European countries.[9] In 2005, after the publication of the so-called Groningen Protocol,[10] the discussions intensified and became more international. Currently, these discussions continue worldwide.[11,12,13,14,15,16,17,18,19] The protocol was viewed by several commentators as a radical new step down the supposed "slippery slope" from the Dutch system of euthanasia to Nazi practices.

CATEGORIES OF NEWBORN INFANTS FOR WHOM END-OF-LIFE DECISIONS MIGHT BE CONSIDERED

The first group (Group 1) includes newborn infants for whom death is imminent, even when all possible treatments are being applied. An example is this category is an infant born with underdeveloped lungs, often in combination with underdeveloped kidneys. It might be possible to keep such an infant alive for a few hours, but not much longer. Another group that is more controversial includes infants born with an extra chromosome 13 or 18. These infants have basically no psychomotor development, and at least 90% die in the first year of life due to congenital abnormalities. By consensus among Dutch neonatologists in the Netherlands, infants born with a gestational age under 24 weeks belong to Group 1.[20]

All Dutch neonatologists agree that treatment should not be initiated for infants in Group 1; if treatment has been initiated because the diagnosis is not yet clear, it should not be continued. These decisions are considered medical decisions and are to be taken by the responsible physician. While parents are, of course, informed extensively about the diagnosis and the prognosis, they cannot force the physician to continue treatment, which in these infants is considered futile. Given the fact that every intensive-care treatment imposes harm on the patient and that no survival can be expected, this treatment is not in the interest of the infant. All care should be taken to ensure that these infants do not suffer after stopping treatment. Legally, the patient dies from the illness and there are no legal consequences.

From an ethical point of view, the following comments can be made. At least in the Netherlands, it is up to the physician to decide whether a treatment is futile. The ethical issue involves defining *when* treatment becomes futile. There is no discussion when it is obvious that the child will die within hours despite all efforts. When the case involves a chromosomal abnormality, treatment is considered futile because there are no treatments to improve these infants' very severe cerebral abnormalities and life can only be extended by some months. In these cases, the short-term prognosis is more important than imminent death. When the case involves extreme prematurity, opinions might differ; it can be argued that treatment is futile in these infants and should not be started. The 1995 EPICure Study in Great Britain indicated that today, infants born at 23 weeks have a 20% chance to survive, as opposed to almost 0% 20 years ago.[21] Next to the very high chance of dying, there is the high risk of surviving with a severe handicap, almost 80% in this study.[22] While starting treatment in this group of children is considered futile in the Netherlands, the EPICure Study indicated that the issue is debated in other countries.

Group 2 includes patients who might survive with intensive-care treatment but will suffer from very severe neurodevelopmental and motor delays. It is questionable whether survival is really in the best interest of the infant in these cases. Will life for these infants become a burden rather than a pleasure? In the

Netherlands, the parents and physicians would discuss the appropriateness of continuing treatment. Treatment can be discontinued when both the parents and physicians are convinced that its continuation is not in the best interest of the child. A number of requirements must be met as safeguards in this decision. First, the prognosis must be as definite as possible. Additional investigations may be needed to better define the prognosis. Secondly, a decision should never be made by one physician; it must be shared by a team. The team should include nurses, social workers, and others. The role of the parents in these decisions is most important. The decision to stop treatment should never be made against the parents' wishes. If the parents ask that treatment be continued, it must be done. At the same time, however, the responsibility for the decision lies with the physician and not the parents. Parents should not feel that they must take the ultimate decision. This is a delicate, but very important, balance. Third, the infant must receive adequate medication so that he or she will not suffer when treatment is ultimately discontinued.

The decisions to end intensive-care treatment for patients in this group are, to a great extent, based on the patients' predicted quality of life. This raises a number of questions: Is it possible to predict the future quality of life? Since a child cannot express her or his will, can parents and physicians make this evaluation and, on that basis, make decisions? Are parents allowed to make these decisions?

The Dutch Pediatric Association indicated clearly in its first report in 1992[6] that making a prediction about future quality of life can be extremely difficult but should be done. If the future of the infant is not under consideration, treatment will be continued in all cases. The result will be that infants might survive with a very poor quality of life. The child might have to suffer all through adolescence until he or she is an adult and considered mature enough to ask for euthanasia. The official position of the association pediatricians was that this scenario was inhumane.

The Dutch Pediatric Association also indicated that quality of life cannot simply be calculated by adding points on different scales. Still, there are five items that should be taken into consideration when making any decision:

1. The degree of suffering pain, and discomfort in the present and what can be expected in the future;
2. The predicted ability or inability to be self-sufficient;
3. The predicted ability or inability to communicate in any way;
4. The expected hospital dependency; and
5. Duration of life expectancy.

In the Netherlands, the decision not to start or to stop treatment when the physician is convinced that treatment is not in the best interest of the patient is considered to be medical and falls within the scope of the physician's professional responsibility. Neither a patient nor the family can force a physician to start or continue a treatment that is considered to be against the patient's best interest. Nevertheless, when parents of a Group 2 patient want treatment to be continued, it will be continued. When treatment is stopped in Group 2 patients, there are no legal consequences. The patient's death is considered secondary to the underlying disease.

There are a number of ethical issues related to stopping treatment in these patients. First, can anyone really determine the child's best interest on the basis of future quality of life? Quality of life is so subjective that only the individual can decide whether it is acceptable. On the other hand, when no predictions and decisions are made, treatment will be continued in all infants, and a number of them will survive with severe handicaps and suffering. In the Netherlands, it is generally accepted that this cannot be the ultimate goal of medical treatment, that every medical treatment needs to be justified and the burden of treatment needs to be balanced against the outcome. A very bad outcome does not justify continuation of treatment. Parents and physicians need to make these decisions together. The parents are the legal guardians of the child and can be regarded as speaking in behalf of his or her best interests, and physicians have the expertise to predict the future quality of life as precisely as possible.

Group 3 includes infants who are not dependent upon intensive medical care but who have an extremely grim prognosis that involves extensive suffering. This is certainly the most controversial group of patients. These infants' lives might be ended by medication. In the Netherlands, the term *euthanasia* is restricted to actively ending the life of a patient upon explicit and repeated request. In the case of newborns, such an action is known as "deliberate ending of life." In the Netherlands, deliberate ending of life for infants has been performed mainly for those with extreme forms of meningomyelocele (neural tube defects) or very severe forms of skin diseases that involve great suffering. It has also been applied to infants who suffered greatly from other diseases, such as chromosomal abnormalities and very severe perinatal hypoxia.

In 1995, a Dutch obstetrician was acquitted of criminal charges for deliberately ending the life of a newborn infant born with extensive meningomyelocele.[23,24] On the basis of a description of the case and reports from medical and ethical experts, the judges concluded that the infant was suffering severely and had a predicted life that would be full of suffering, and that there was no means to relieve the suffering. Before making the decision, the obstetrician had consulted a number of experts, who all agreed. The parents also explicitly agreed with the decision. The procedure for administering the lethal medication was performed carefully, and the infant did not suffer additional pain from its effects.

A general practitioner was acquitted in 1996 for ending the life of an infant with trisomy 13.[24] The infant was suffering and had a very limited life expectancy, and the physicians were unable to end the suffering. On the basis of a number of expert opinions, including some from ethicists, the judges concluded that there was no other reasonable option and that the decision was justified.

Even though ending the life of a person in the Netherlands is qualified as murder, both physicians were found not guilty. An exception is made for euthanasia, as described in another chapter. In the case of a newborn, there is no request from the patient, and the parents do not have the legal right to decide for the infant in these matters. Therefore, even today, deliberately ending the life of an infant or child younger than 18 years of age, as well as that of an incompetent elderly person, is considered murder. The physician has the duty to report to the prosecutor any case involving the deliberate ending of the life of an incompetent person. The prosecutor will then start an inquiry, which usually ends in a court case where the physician has to defend him- or herself against the accusation of murder.

In the year 2000, we were confronted with two cases where parents persistently asked that the life of their child be deliberately ended. The first child was born with extreme perinatal asphyxia, and the second child suffered from an extreme form of skin disease. We consulted the prosecutor before making a decision. His response was straightforward: He completely understood the parents' intention and ours to end the children's lives, but told us that the case would be brought to court and that there would be an accusation of murder. Because no one involved in the cases felt comfortable about this approach, we worked together to design the Groningen Protocol.

THE GRONINGEN PROTOCOL

In 2002, we started a discussion with the prosecutor in Groningen regarding the deliberate ending of life in newborn infants, stipulating that this action might only be indicated in extreme cases. It was understood that the law prohibits these acts, and that physicians are conscientious, diligent persons who are not murderers. Prior to these discussions, each case of active euthanasia in newborn infants had resulted in a police investigation. Our aim was to prevent these investigations by agreeing on the necessary documentation needed by the prosecutor to make a decision.

We used data from earlier decisions made by the highest prosecutor in the Netherlands concerning when to prosecute a physician or when to dismiss a case.[25] On the basis of this information, we compiled a checklist of essential steps to take before making a decision and then presenting the case to the prosecutor.[10] The prosecutor promised that he would not start a police investigation when all information was available but would inform the physician within weeks about his decision regarding prosecution. Clearly, deliberately ending the life of a newborn infant is still murder and is not permitted. Under extreme conditions and when all requirements have been fulfilled, however, a case could be closed without prosecution or a verdict.

The requirements of the Groningen Protocol[10] are shown in Box 19.1:

Box 19.1. The Groningen Protocol for Euthanasia in Newborns

Requirements that Must be Fulfilled

The diagnosis and prognosis must be certain.
Hopeless and unbearable suffering must be present.
The diagnosis, prognosis, and unbearable suffering must be confirmed by at least one independent doctor.
Both parents must give informed consent.
The procedure must be performed in accordance with the accepted medical standard.

Information Needed to Support and Clarify the Decision about Euthanasia

DIAGNOSIS AND PROGNOSIS

Describe all relevant medical data and the results of diagnostic investigations used to establish the diagnosis.
List all the participants in the decision-making process, all opinions expressed, and the final consensus.
Describe how the prognosis regarding long-term health was assessed.
Describe how the degree of suffering and life expectancy were assessed.
Describe the availability of alternative treatments, alternative means of alleviating suffering, or both.
Describe treatments and the results of treatment preceding the decision about euthanasia.

Euthanasia Decision

Describe who initiated the discussion about possible euthanasia and at what moment.
List the considerations that prompted the decision.
List all the participants in the decision-making process, all opinions expressed, and the final consensus.
Describe the way in which the parents were informed and their opinions.

Consultation

Describe the physician or physicians who gave a second opinion (name and qualifications).

(*continued*)

List the results of the examinations and the recommendations made by the consulting physician or physicians.

Implementation

Describe the actual euthanasia procedure (time, place, participants, and administration of drugs).
Describe the reasons for the chosen method of euthanasia.

Steps Taken after Death

Describe the findings of the coroner.
Describe how the euthanasia was reported to the prosecuting authority.
Describe how the parents are being supported and counseled.
Describe the planned follow-up, including case review, post-mortem examination, and genetic counseling.

The idea of allowing a physician to end the life of a patient, especially when the patient cannot express his or her wishes, is very controversial. It can be argued that it is never acceptable and should not be the task of a physician. On the other hand, according to the Hippocratic Oath, a physician has the obligation to relieve suffering in patients. Suffering, including pain, can be so severe that it cannot be alleviated by any medication unless the patient is rendered unconscious. Even then, one can never be certain that there is no suffering. Everyone has different ideas about what to do in cases involving intense suffering.

In the Netherlands, active ending of life under these circumstances can be judged an acceptable parallel to the conditions of euthanasia. Death for these patients might be judged more humane than allowing them to stay alive. In other countries, ending the life of incompetent persons is considered unethical and a criminal offence. Of course, very strict safeguards are needed in the Netherlands. The parents have to agree explicitly with the decision. The suffering has to be extensive, both now and in the foreseeable future, and all other means of relieving suffering must have been tried. The prognosis has to be as definitive as possible, and at least two physicians have to independently agree about the decision. Finally, the patient should never suffer from the decision to end his or her life. When these requirements have been met, we feel that it is ethically and legally allowable to deliberately end the life, even in an incompetent person.

The Groningen Protocol has received intense criticism and the debate is ongoing. The slippery-slope argument is often raised against the Groningen

Protocol and the acceptance of a deliberate ending of life in newborns.[26,27] It is argued that this practice will lead to a failure of safeguards and erosion of norms, thereby allowing the termination of life without discussion. There is no hard evidence either for or against this prediction. It should be clear that the practice of deliberately ending the lives of newborns existed in the Netherlands, and who knows in how many other countries, long before the publication of the protocol. It was going on, at least partly, "under the table."[28,29] The protocol's main goal was to regulate and control that practice, making it transparent and subject to public review. The protocol allows doctors to be openly accountable for their decisions to all members of society. An opposing view might be that there are many bad things going on under the table in all societies, things that are so evil that we would not want to make them transparent and acceptable. In the Dutch society, however, there is a shared understanding that hastening death is not always the worst thing that can befall a human being, and that death is not synonymous with "evil." The Dutch go even further than other countries in their shared belief that even newborns have a fundamental interest in not prolonging a life that is, or will become, an intolerable burden.

Some critics of the Groningen Protocol worry that the requirement of "sustained suffering that cannot be relieved" seems far too subjective. [13,15,27] Others have argued in support of the protocol[14] by confirming that babies can certainly suffer from pain to an excruciating degree, as well as from other kinds of serious and irremediable conditions, such as total lifelong dependency, lack of any capacity for communication, or progressive paralysis resulting in total immobility.

There have been many misunderstandings about the protocol, including the assertion that it is aimed at babies with spina bifida.[30] In fact, spina bifida is not represented in the protocol as a condition associated with hopeless and sustained suffering. Other misunderstandings concern the role of the parents – for example, that they could be tempted to kill the baby so they don't have to care for it. This assumption strikes us as both unmotivated and meanspirited; it does not take seriously either children with disabilities or the parents who care for them. Publications describing the parents' role in end-of-life decisions do not support that assumption.[31,32,33,34,35] Moreover, parents in the Netherlands may request that their severely impaired babies' lives be terminated, but their request is not automatically granted. The final decision is always made by the medical team.

RECENT DATA CONCERNING END-OF-LIFE DECISIONS IN THE NETHERLANDS

In 2006, a committee of experts on deliberate termination of life in newborns (and on late termination of pregnancies) was appointed by the Dutch government, and the procedures for reporting such cases were changed.[36,37] This happened after members of the medical profession made repeated requests for more transparency and clarity about the review procedure for deliberate termination of life in newborns and about the criteria and requirements of due care.[38,39] According to the new regulations, physicians are required to report all cases of deliberate termination of a newborn's life to the public prosecutor, who in turn submits the report to the committee of experts.[40] The committee (consisting of a lawyer, an ethicist, and three physicians who specialize in neonatology) reviews the case and applies the criteria of due care to assess whether the physician acted accordingly.[41] The committee's recommendations are taken into account by the prosecuting authorities, who then decide whether charges will be brought against the physician.

The process of external review by the multidisciplinary committee of experts is already more transparent than it was in the past. Earlier, the prosecuting service reviewed the case without the help of medical experts and without public descriptions of the case, its considerations, or the final ruling. Now, as soon as the first cases are reported, the reviews by the multidisciplinary committee of experts contribute to the ongoing development and clarification of the standards regarding deliberate termination of life in newborns. This will encourage attending physicians to notify the authorities, which in turn will enhance transparency of medical practice and increase debate about what is going on.

Several years ago, we conducted a retrospective study in all 10 neonatal intensive care units in the Netherlands.[42] Since Dutch neonatal intensive care is concentrated in 10 centers, almost no newborn infant dies anywhere else. We reviewed all infants who died between October 2005 and September 2006, a total of 359 deaths. End-of-life decisions preceded death in 95% of cases; treatment was continued until death in only 5%. Fifty-eight percent of patients belonged to Group 1 – that is, no chance for the infant to survive; 42% were infants in neonatal intensive care with a very poor prognosis. Only one case was identified in which life was deliberately ended. In 92% of deaths in Group 2, the decision to end a life was based on the patient's future quality of life and mainly concerned future suffering. Parents were always involved in the decision-making process; consultation with other physicians occurred in 99% of cases.

It was remarkable that only one case was identified that involved the deliberate ending of life. This could be due to a lack of reporting of these cases, but it might also indicate that the deliberate ending of life has become a real exception. There are a number of reasons for that possibility. First, deliberate ending of life was mainly practised in infants with meningomyelocele. In the Netherlands, screening for congenital abnormalities during pregnancy was introduced for all pregnant women at the gestational age of 20 weeks. Meningomyelocele is one abnormality identified during this screening. The number of abortions after the twentieth week has increased since the screening was introduced, while the number of infants born with spina bifida has decreased. Other cases of very severe congenital abnormalities are also detected by the 20-week ultrasound, resulting in fewer infants with severe abnormalities at birth. It seems likely that this practice has limited the requests for the deliberate ending of life in newborns.

MEDICATION IN THE PERINATAL PERIOD

A striking issue discovered in our retrospective study was the use of medication during the period of dying. Analgesics and sedatives were administered to 224 of 340 newborns before the end-of- life decision, and to 292 newborns after the decision.[43] Moreover, the dose was increased in 204 of the 224 infants after the decision. Neuromuscular blockers were administered to 55 infants, either because they had been prescribed earlier for medical reasons or to prevent or to stop gasping after extubation. Giving neuromuscular blockers might be viewed as an act of active euthanasia; in all cases in this study, however, they were either prescribed earlier for medical reasons and it was considered unethical to stop in a dying phase, or given mainly on parental request to stop or prevent gasping. Sometimes parents are extremely upset when they see their child gasping. They feel that the infant is "fighting for life" and that we are not really helping the infant. Other parents explicitly stated that they wanted to prevent any gasping. It is unclear whether an infant is suffering when he or she is gasping. At the same time, it is unclear whether morphine and sedatives completely prevent any suffering in these infants. Therefore, in the Netherlands, neuromuscular blockers are used in conjunction with sedatives and painkillers to prevent and/or treat gasping. It is a way of helping the infants die in a humane manner.

Recently, palliative care has been proposed as an alternative for end-of-life decisions in newborns, including the deliberate ending of life. Although we do not want to question the importance and value of palliative care, we do not believe that it replaces the need to make decisions; neither is it a substitute for active euthanasia. Palliative care is basically the prevention of suffering in patients in the period before death.

There are important differences in the process of dying in adults and newborn infants. In newborn infants, the time between the decision to stop treatment and death might be longer than it is in adults. Secondly, an adult can indicate suffering, while in newborns it is more difficult to determine. Severe suffering can be observed, but more subtle suffering is difficult. Finally, in some cases the only way to adequately decrease suffering is to render the patient unconscious (terminal sedation). Terminal sedation in adults is an accepted medical practice in the Netherlands but is not an alternative to deliberate ending of life in newborns. By definition, terminal sedation requires an expected death within 14 days.[44] The timing of newborn deaths is often much more difficult to predict, mainly because adults suffer from very different illnesses (i.e., mostly end-stage cancer, vascular disease, or multiorgan failure).[45] In contrast, many of the cases of deliberate ending of life that were reported in the past concerned newborns with congenital malformations that caused discomfort and suffering; the infants, however, were expected to live for several weeks or months.[25] It is questionable whether keeping the infant sedated for many weeks to months, waiting for a certain death, is humane and qualifies as "good practice."

IS THE NETHERLANDS UNIQUE?

Are end-of-life decisions made more often in the Netherlands, or are they only discussed more? Studies from a number of countries, such as France and Belgium, indicate that end-of-life decisions are made in these countries almost as frequently as they are in the Netherlands.[46,47] We conducted a comparison among two centers in the United States (Chicago and Milwaukee), Montreal in Canada, and Groningen in the Netherlands.[48] Practices in Milwaukee and Montreal are very comparable to those in Groningen. It is only in Chicago that patients are never taken off the ventilator to let them die – not because of physicians who would not stop treatment but because of legal reasons.

We believe, therefore, that the approach in the Netherlands is not unique; what is unique is our open discussion regarding this issue. This difference is due partly to our feeling that we should not hide anything. Transparency prevents a slippery slope. It is important for parents to be able to discuss their feelings without being criticized when they question continuation of a treatment. Doctors want to be open to the public and transparent in their actions.

CONCLUSION

Discussions regarding end-of-life decisions in newborn infants and children started among pediatricians in the Netherlands more than 20 years ago. From the very beginning, these discussions were not restricted to physicians; society as a whole was involved. It is a generally accepted practice for physicians not to start or to stop treatment when the treatment is considered futile. On the other hand, parents cannot force a physician to start or continue treatment that is considered futile. In the case of a prediction of an extremely grim quality of life, treatment can be stopped when both parents and physicians agree that its continuation is not in the best interest of the child. Deliberate ending of life is considered justified when the child experiences extensive suffering, his or her life will be full of suffering, and the suffering cannot be alleviated by other means.

References

1. Hagen, Catherine Monrad, and Thor Willy Hansen. 2004. Deaths in a neonatal intensive care unit: A 10-year perspective. *Pediatric Critical Care Medicine* 5: 463–468.

2. Horbar, Jeffrey D., Gary J. Badger, Joseph H. Carpenter, Avroy A. Fanaroff, Sarah Kilapatrick, Meena LaCorte, Roderic Phibbs, and Roger F. Soll. 2002. Trends in mortality and morbidity for very low birth weight infants, 1991–1999. *Pediatrics* 110: 143–151.
3. Marlow, Neil, Dieter Wolke, Melanie A. Bracewell, and Muthanna Samara. 2005. Neurologic and developmental disability at six years of age after extremely preterm birth. *New England Journal of Medicine* 352: 9–19.
4. Singh, Jaideep, John Lantos, and William Meadow. 2004. End-of-life after birth: Death and dying in a neonatal intensive care unit. *Pediatrics* 114: 1620–1626.
5. Wilkinson, D. J., J. J. Fitzsimons, P. A. Dargaville, N. T. Campbell, P. M. Loughnan, P. N. McDougall, and J. F. Mills. 2006. Death in the neonatal intensive care unit: Changing patterns of end of life care over two decades. *Archives of Disease in Childhood:Fetal and Neonatal Edition* 91: F268–F271.
6. Nederlandse Vereniging voor Kindergeneeskunde. 1992. Doen of laten. Grenzen van het medisch handelen in de neonatologie [To treat or not to treat? Limits for life-sustaining treatment in neonatology]. Utrecht: Den Daas.
7. KNMG Commissie Aanvaardbaarheid Levensbeeindigend Handelen. 1997. Medisch handelen rond het levenseinde bij wilsonbekwame patiënten [Medical practice at the end of life in the case of non-competent patients]. Houten: Bohn Stafleu Van Loghem.
8. Verhagen, A. A. E. 1997. Overleggroep toetsing zorgvuldig medisch handelen rond het levenseinde bij pasgeborenen. Toetsing als spiegel van de medische praktijk [Assesment as mirror of medical practice]. Rijswijk: Ministerie van Volksgezondheid Welzijn en Sport.
9. Cuttini, Marina, M. Nadai, Monique Kaminski, G. Hansen, R. de Leeuw, Sylvie Lenoir, J. Persson, M. Rebagliato, M. Reid, U. de Vonderweid, H. G. Lenard, M. Orzalesi, and Rodolfo Saracci. 2000. End-of-life decisions in neonatal intensive care: Physicians' self-reported practices in seven European countries. *The Lancet* 355: 2112–2118.
10. Verhagen Eduard, and Pieter J. Sauer. 2005. The Groningen Protocol – euthanasia in severely ill newborns. *New England Journal of Medicine* 352: 959–962.
11. Manninen, Bertha A. 2006. A case for justified non-voluntary active euthanasia: Exploring the ethics of the Groningen Protocol. *Journal of Medical Ethics* 32: 643–651.
12. Kodish, Eric. 2008. Paediatric ethics: A repudiation of the Groningen Protocol. *The Lancet* 371: 892–893.
13. Kon, Alexander A. 2007. Neonatal euthanasia is unsupportable: The Groningen Protocol should be abandoned. *Theoretical Medicine and Bioethics* 28: 453–463.
14. Lindemann, Hilde, and Marian Verkerk. 2008. Ending the life of a newborn: The Groningen Protocol. *Hastings Center Report* 38: 42–51.
15. Chervenak, Frank A., Laurence B. McCullough, and Birgit Arabin. 2006. Why the Groningen Protocol should be rejected. *Hastings Center Report* 36: 30–33.
16. Vries, Martine C. de, and A. A. Eduard Verhagen. 2008. A case against something that is not the case: The Groningen Protocol and the moral principle of non-maleficence. *American Journal of Bioethics* 8: 29–31.
17. Jotkowitz, Alan B., and S. Glick. 2006. The Groningen Protocol: Another perspective. *Journal of Medical Ethics* 32: 157–158.

18. Catlin, Anite, and Renee Novakovich. 2008. The Groningen Protocol: What is it, how do the Dutch use it, and do we use it here? *Pediatric Nursing* 34: 247–251.
19. Gesundheit, Benjamin, Avraham Steinberg, Shraga Blazer, and Alan Jotkowitz. 2009. The Groningen Protocol – the Jewish perspective. *Neonatology* 96: 6–10.
20. Verloove-Vanhorick, S. 2006. Management of the neonate at the limits of viability: The Dutch viewpoint. *British Journal of Obstetrics and Gynaecology* 113 (Suppl. 3): 13–16.
21. Costeloe, Kate, Enid Hennessy, Alan T. Gibson, Neil Marlow, and Andrew R. Wilkinson. 2000. The EPICure Study: Outcomes to discharge from hospital for infants born at the threshold of viability. *Pediatrics* 106: 659–671.
22. Wood, Nicholas S., Neil Marlow, Kate Costeloe, Alan T. Gibson, and Andrew R. Wilkinson. 2000. Neurologic and developmental disability after extremely preterm birth: EPICure Study Group. *New England Journal of Medicine* 343: 378–384.
23. Gerechtshof Amsterdam [Amsterdam Appeal Court]. November 7, 1995. *Tijdschrift voor Gezondheidsrecht* [Dutch Journal of Health Law] 20: 30–36.
24. Gerechtshof Leeuwarden [Leeuwarden Appeal Court]. April 4, 1996. *Tijdschrift voor Gezondheidsrecht* [Dutch Journal of Health Law] 20: 284–291.
25. Verhagen, A. A. E., J. J. Sol, O. F. Brouwer, and P. J. Sauer. 2005. Actieve levensbeeindiging bij pasgeborenen in Nederland, analyse van alle meldingen van 1997/'04 [Deliberate termination of life in newborns in the Netherlands: Review of all 22 reported cases between 1997 and 2004]. *Nederlands tijdschrift voor geneeskunde* 149: 183–188.
26. Feudtner, Chris. 2005. Control of suffering on the slippery slope of care. *The Lancet*. 365: 1284–1286.
27. Kon, Alexander A. 2008. We cannot accurately predict the extent of an infant's future suffering: The Groningen Protocol is too dangerous to support. *American Journal of Bioethics* 8: 27–29.
28. Verhagen, A. A. E., M. A. van der Hoeven, J. B. van Goudoever, M. C. de Vries, A. Y. Schoutenvan-van Meeteren, and M. J. Albers. 2007. Uitzichtloos en ondraaglijk lijden en actieve levensbeeindiging bij pasgeborenen [Hopeless and unbearable suffering and deliberate ending of life of newborn infants]. *Nederlands tijdschrift voor geneeskunde* 151: 1474–1477.
29. Heide, Agnes van der, Paul J. van der Maas, Gerrit van der Wal, Carmen L. de Graaff, John G. C. Kester, Louis A. A. Kollee, Richard de Leeuw, and Robert A. Holl. 1997. Medical end-of-life decisions made for neonates and infants in the Netherlands. *The Lancet* 350: 251–255.
30. Jong, T. H. de. 2007. Deliberate termination of life of newborns with spina bifida, a critical reappraisal. *A Child's Nervous System* 24: 13–28.
31. Verhagen, A. A. Eduard, Mirjam de Vos, Jozef H. H. M. Dorscheidt, Bernadette Engels, Joep H. Hubben, and Pieter J. Sauer. 2009. Conflicts about end-of-life decisions in NICUs in the Netherlands. *Pediatrics* 124: e112–e119.
32. Heide, Agnes van der, Paul J. van der Maas, Gerrit van der Wal, Louis A. A. Kollee, Richard de Leeuw, and Robert A. Holl. 1998. The role of parents in end-of-life decisions in neonatology: Physicians' views and practices. *Pediatrics* 101: 413–418.

33. Jasper, Jill, William D. Clark, Gerardo Cabrera-Meza, Carol Lynn Berseth, and Caraciolo J. Fernandes. 2003. Whose child is it anyway? Resolving parent–physician conflict in the NICU setting. *American Journal of Perinatology* 20: 373–380.
34. Fetters, Michael D., Larry Churchill, and Marion Danis. 2001. Conflict resolution at the end of life. *Critical Care Medicine* 29: 921–925.
35. Prendergast, T. J. 1997. Resolving conflicts surrounding end-of-life care. *New Horizons* 5: 62–71.
36. De Minister van Justitie en de Staatssecretaris van Volksgezondheid Welzijn en Sport. 2006. Benoemingen commissie late zwangerschapsafbreking en levensbeëindiging bij pasgeborenen. *Staatscourant* 168: 20.
37. Dorscheidt, Jozef H. 2007. De centrale deskundigencommissie inzake levensbeëindiging bij pasgeborenen; enkele juridische reflecties. *Tijdschr Gezondheidszorg en Ethiek* (TGE) 3: 72–77.
38. Legemaate, J. 2005. *KNMG kennisdocument: de zorgverlening rond het levenseinde. Een literatuurstudie naar begripsomschrijvingen en zorgvuldigheidseisen.* Utrecht: KNMG.
39. Dutch Association for Pediatrics (NVK). Point of view: NVK on "Procedure active life-ending treatment newborns." Available at: http://www.nvk.pedianet.nl/index.htm?/standpunt_le.htm.
40. College van procureurs-generaal. 2007. Aanwijzing vervolgingsbeslissing levensbeëindiging niet op verzoek en late zwangerschapsafbreking. *Staatscourant* 46: 10.
41. De Minister van Justitie en de Staatssecretaris van Volksgezondheid Welzijn en Sport. 2007. Regeling centrale deskundigencommissie late zwangerschapsafbreking in een categorie 2-geval en levensbeëindiging bij pasgeborenen [Establishment of a central committe of experts for late term abortion in category 2 case and termination of life of newborn babies]. *Staatscourant* 51: 8–10.
42. Verhagen, A. A.Eduard. 2009. *End-of-life decisions in Dutch neonatal intensive care units*. Zuthphen: Paris Legal Publishers.
43. Verhagen, A. A. Eduard, Jozef H. Dorscheidt, Bernadette Engels, Joep H. Hubben, and Pieter J. Sauer. 2009. Analgesics, sedatives and neuromuscular blockers as part of end-of-life decisions in Dutch NICU's. *Archives of Disease in Childhood: Fetal and Neonatal Edition* 94: F434–F438.
44. Verkerk, Marian, Erik van Wijlick, Johan Legemaate, and Alexander de Graeff. 2007. A national guideline for palliative sedation in the Netherlands. *Journal of Pain and Symptom Management* 34: 666–670.
45. Heide, Agnes van der, Bregje D. Onwuteaka-Philipsen, Mette L. Rurup, Hilde M. Buiting, Johannes J. M. van Delden, Johanna E. Hanssen-de Wolf, Anke G. J. M. Janssen, H. Roeline W. Pasman, Judith A. C. Rietjens, Cornelis J. M. Prins, Ingeborg M. Deerenberg, Joseph K. M. Gevers, Paul van der Maas, and Gerrit van der Wal. 2007. End-of-life practices in the Netherlands under the Euthanasia Act. *New England Journal of Medicine* 356: 1957–1965.
46. Provoost, Veerle, Filip, Freddy Mortier, Johan Bilsen, Jose Ramet, Yvan Vandenplas, and Luc Deliens. 2005. Medical end-of-life decisions in neonates and infants in Flanders. *The Lancet*. 365: 1315–1320.

47. Larroque, B., G. Breart, M. Kaminski, M. Dehan, M. Andre, and A. Burguet et al. 2004. Survival of very preterm infants: Epipage, a population based cohort study. *Archives of Disease in Childhood* 89: F139–F1344.
48. Verhagen, A. A. Eduard, Annie Janvier, Steven R. Leuthner, B. Andrews, J. Lagatta, Arend F. Bos, and William Meadow. 2009. Categorizing neonatal deaths: A cross-cultural study in the USA, Canada and the Netherlands. *Journal of Pediatrics* 156: 33–37.

20

Hastening Death Through Voluntary Cessation of Eating and Drinking

A Survey

Boudewijn E. Chabot

INTRODUCTION

Voluntary refusal of food and fluid (VRFF) is and has always been a patient-directed option for hastening death. Patients may carry out this option on their own or, more ideally, as part of a palliative care plan. Several authors have discussed VRFF as an explicit alternative in countries or jurisdictions where euthanasia and physician-assisted suicide are forbidden.[1,2,3,4,5] Until recently, however, there have been no data documenting the frequency with which this option is chosen; the result is an important gap in knowledge about end-of-life decisions by competent patients.

A recent nationwide survey study in the Netherlands presented the first data about the frequency and characteristics of VRFF.[6,7] I will briefly review the methodology and results of that study. I will then present two cases and comment on the clinical, psychosocial, and ethical issues they illustrate. Finally, I will suggest a personalized approach to VRFF as an alternative to physician-assisted death (PAD) in the Dutch context.

THE STUDY

Research by Boudewijn Chabot and Arnold Goedhart[7] attempted to determine the frequency and circumstances under which VRFF is utilized in the Dutch population. We studied all cases of death in which VRFF was planned and completed by competent persons after discussions with proxies. A "proxy" was defined as any person (relative, friend, nurse, right-to-die activist, or others) who had been informed about the decision to hasten death using this particular method (see Chabot and Goedhart 2009 for methodological details on the definition, sample, and the frequency estimation).[7]

Out of a sample of 31,516 Dutch adults, 97 proxies reported on a death hastened by VRFF that they had witnessed as a confidant and that fit our research frame, definition, and strict exclusion criteria.[7] In particular, I excluded reports

TABLE 20.1. *Period with No Food or Drink and Disease Category (Cancer, Serious Disease, Not Serious)*

VRFF Duration	Cancer Disease (n = 39)	Serious Diagnosis (n = 31)	No Serious Diagnosis (n = 27)	Total (n = 97)
7–9 days	10	9	5*	24 (25%)
10–12 days	10	7	4	21 (22%)
13–15 days	8	4	10	22 (22%)
16–18 days	3	0	1	4 (4%)
19–30 days	8	4	3	15 (16 %)
31–60 days	0	6	2	8 (8%)
> 60 days	0	1	2	3 (3%)

Notes: No significant relationship between time it took to die and disease category (Mann Whitney z =1,19).

* Of these 5 cases, two deaths occurred after 7 days, one after 8 days, and two after 9 days.

on persons who died after fewer than 7 days of not eating or drinking because I suspected that either an underlying disease (cancer) or medication had substantially contributed to death in these cases. I considered dehydration a major contributing cause of death only in those cases in which death occurred after 7 or more days of not drinking – during which the patient was conscious and able to communicate for at least 4 days. Utilizing this last provision, I also excluded cases in which the VRFF decision was soon supplemented by continuous sedation, thereby precluding the patient's ability to confirm the decision to continue with this route to death.

Based on the 97 VRFF reported cases, we estimated the annual frequency of VRFF deaths to be 2.1% of the annual number of deaths in the Dutch population between 1999 and 2003. This appears to be about the same as the yearly frequency of physician-assisted death in 2001.[8]

Data on age, gender, social situation, and diseases were as follows: Eighty percent of the deceased were over 60 years of age, and most of them were women (60%). One in every three had a partner. Half of these deaths occurred at home, while the other half occurred in a nursing home or hospice. The diagnosis of cancer was reported in 40% of these deaths, and 32% had a serious somatic and/or psychiatric disease. While the remaining 28% had no serious disease known to the informants, most had one or more disabilities of old age (e.g., blindness, deafness, immobility, arthritic pain, etc.).

Death from VRFF can take anywhere from 7 days to two months. Death occurred within 7–15 days of complete cessation of all fluid intake in about 70% of patients; in the other 30%, it took 16–60 days because fluid intake had continued for some time after all food intake had stopped. Contrary to our expectations, we found no significant relationship between the time it took to die and disease category (see Table 20.1).

WHAT THE STUDY REVEALS

Because euthanasia is a legal option in the Netherlands, we expected most of the persons involved to have asked their physician for physician-assisted death.[7] It turned out, however, that only half had asked for PAD and were turned down, 40% had not asked for it, and 10% of the informants answered "unknown." These refusals by doctors are less surprising than one might think because asking for PAD does not automatically lead to receiving it. As Roeline Pasman documents in Chapter 9, Dutch studies report that about two out of every three explicit and repeated requests for PAD were either refused, withdrawn, or undecided.[9,10] The most frequent reasons for the refusal cited by study informants were the following: "The doctor said the patient was not yet terminal" (21%); "The suffering was neither hopeless nor unbearable" (26%); "religious reasons" (20%); "The doctor was afraid of judicial consequences" (17%).

We were surprised that apparently there had not been a request for PAD in about 40% of the VRFF cases.[7] Informants frequently told us that the patient thought the request for PAD would not be negotiable because he or she "didn't have cancer." Some Dutch patients are apparently aware of the legal conditions of due care and do not request PAD when they realize that they "don't have a chance."

Chabot and Goedhart asked the informants whether VRFF had been a first choice in order to find out whether the deceased considered this route a dignified death; 64% answered "yes," 30% said "no," and 6% answered "unknown." The more straightforward question "Would the deceased have considered this hastened death a dignified one?" was answered in the affirmative by 74%, negative by 17%, and unknown by 8%.[7] When the question was rephrased to reflect the informant's opinion about dignity, the percentages remained the same. At least two out of every three VRFF deaths was reportedly a "dignified death," which came as somewhat of a surprise considering other findings. Research in Oregon has shown that hospice nurses generally rate the quality of dying by voluntary refusal of food and fluid as "good."[11] Since hardly any of the 97 VRFF cases died in a hospice, I expected the level of palliative care for these patients to be lower than for the patients in the Oregon study. Even though the level of care may have been lower, at least two out of three informants reported a positive assessment, and that finding remains puzzling.

Therefore, we hypothesized that in cases where a request for PAD had been turned down (e.g., the case of Mrs G, the next section), the informant would find a "VRFF death" less dignified than in cases without a request (e.g., Mrs B). However, the data did not confirm this hypothesis. This finding calls for further qualitative research to provide insight into what respondents mean by attributing "dignity" to dying. In general, there is agreement that the term *dignity* is not very specific, and there seem to be a number of possible meanings attached to it.[12] Nora Jacobson[13] distinguishes social dignity from human dignity, and calls it an ambiguous and multivalent concept. With respect to the findings, I suspect that the high percentage of informants (74%) who reported on the "dignity of VRFF death" reflects an assessment, in retrospect, of a "right choice" that was justified and deserves to be respected now that the person is no longer alive. Another interpretation may be that these responses cover up feelings of loss, guilt, or other painful emotions in connection with these deaths. The bottom line is, however, that I simply do not know what is meant by the assessment of a death via VRFF as "dignified."

I tried to find out why these self-chosen VRFF deaths, which require great effort and at least basic palliative care, do not appear in the death statistics – despite their unexpectedly high prevalence of 2.1% in the Netherlands.[6] I asked the proxies which doctor had come to do the postmortem and, in a separate question, whether the police or a coroner had been involved. To my surprise, a coroner performed the postmortem in only 4 of the 97 VRFF deaths. The case was processed as an "unnatural death through suicide" in only 2 of the 4 cases. Apparently, a death by VRFF is only rarely perceived as a suicide – possibly because it is the result of an omission (specifically not eating and drinking), rather than an act. In many cases of VRFF, it is difficult for the doctor who does the postmortem to assess dehydration as a major cause of death. Another reason why these deaths are not labeled as "suicides" may be that the long interval (one or two weeks) between stopping the intake of food and water and the time of death blurs a causal relationship. Moreover, there are many reasons why relatives prefer not to inform the post-mortem doctor of what went on before death. There may also be considerations on the part of physicians – that is, a doctor doing the postmortem may want to spare relatives a "suicide" label.[14,15]

TWO CASES

I illustrate the differences in possible courses of events in VRFF deaths with two case histories, which differ because of the relationship with the general practitioner. Loving children were present in both cases.

The first case was prepared and carried out at home with the support of the general practitioner (GP):

Mrs B, an 86-year-old widow, was the mother of two supportive children and had several grown-up grandchildren. She felt that her life was drawing to a close since she had suffered from a few transient ischemic attacks. She was afraid that these might be precursors of a partial paralysis or aphasia that would result in a nursing home admission, ending her independent status at home. She did not want to burden her GP with a request for PAD. Over many weeks, she discussed with him in detail the possibility of ending her life by stopping eating and drinking. The GP considered her to be completely competent and without any signs of depression. One day she informed her children that she had decided to hasten her death and ignored their protests. She refused all food that was offered to her and gradually reduced her fluid intake over 10 days. The children organized day and night care and took turns looking after her and sleeping at her bedside. She made little use of the sleeping tablets and sedatives that her GP had given her for sleep or anxiety. After she stopped all fluid intake (which was offered to her twice a day), she became weaker and slept many hours; she remained capable of communicating with her children. Her GP did not prescribe any morphine. She became unconscious 10 days after she had completely stopped drinking (20 days after she stopped all food intake), and she passed away in her sleep after another 24 hours. Her daughter remarked, "This has been a worthwhile time in our lives because we were all able to care for her and make her dying bearable. It was important for her and for our peace of mind that the doctor visited every day and gave us so much of his time."

In the second case, an impulsive decision to hasten death by VRFF was made and carried out in spite of resistance from the GP:

One year before her death, Mrs G (age 83) moved from her own house into a chronic care facility. Hemorrhages in the white matter of the brain had caused a strong tremor, one spastic arm, and difficulties with walking, swallowing, and talking. She had one son and a daughter-in-law with whom she had a positive relationship. As her symptoms increased, she became socially isolated in the facility and decided to ask her GP for a physician-assisted death. He flatly refused to help in hastening her death. Two days later, Mrs G refused all food and drink, a decision that had not been discussed with anyone. Her son knew her as a strong-willed personality and worried about her statement "I will have the willpower to continue with this method of hastening my death," as this was a method that she herself had called "degrading." The GP deemed her to be capable of making this decision and not at all depressed. The nurses put a glass of water next to her, but after the first night she never took a sip of it. Beginning on the second day, the GP prescribed 500 mg of paracetamol/acetaminophen six times daily because of severe low back pain, a dosage that was doubled on day 4. She developed blisters and scabs around her mouth on day 7 due to deficient mouth care, and an awful stench came from the mouth secondary to fungal infections. On day 10, the GP prescribed a morphine plaster (fentanyl 25). She became comatose and died on day 11 in the presence of her relatives. Her daughter-in-law said, "Over the last week she was in a disgraceful state. The last days some nurses were coming out of her room in tears."

COMMENTARY

Neither of these patients was in the terminal phase of an illness. Both might have lived for several years. They were fully competent and well informed about how their diseases might progress. Both decided to take death into their own hands and discussed this decision with their children. Mrs G stopped eating and drinking at the same time, and only received paracetamol as palliation. Mrs B stopped eating first and stopped drinking completely after about 10 days. A nurse showed her children how to apply meticulous mouth care. Mrs B. received sleeping tablets and anxiolytic medication, which she rarely used. No morphine was given and she remained lucid until 24 hours before death. Both patients were offered a glass of water at least twice a day; by refusing the water, they showed their relatives that they really wanted to die.

These and other cases demonstrate that consuming no more than about 50 cc of fluid for mouth care results after about seven days in a profound weakness that resembles the last phase of a fatal illness – without pain or breathing difficulties. Up to a few days before death, patients are often lucid, but talking may become impossible because of the dry mouth and weakness. Delirium is a major complication that can be suppressed with a low dose of an antipsychotic. Continued abstinence from drinking causes the concentration of sodium and potassium in the blood to change, and is probably the eventual cause of death after the patient has slipped into a coma. The flow of potassium ions through the membrane of heart cells will cause ventricular fibrillation, resulting in instant death.[16]

Clinical and Psychological Aspects of VRFF

Sometimes elderly or sick people in and outside the Netherlands deliberately hasten their deaths by voluntary refusal of food and fluid while receiving optimal palliative care. [17,3,16] VRFF is regarded by some Dutch patients as an "emergency exit" in case a physician turns down a persistent request for a physician-assisted death. Others consider VRFF as more "natural" and, therefore, more acceptable than physician-assisted dying – that is, because of religious reasons. It requires strenuous efforts to stop drinking and reflects a strong desire to control the process of dying. It makes the process much easier when someone is well informed about the course it may normally take, what problems may occur, and how these can be avoided. Consultation with family members and a commitment by a physician to provide adequate palliative care are important before someone decides on this method of ending life. Psychological or spiritual comfort from relatives and nursing staff is as indispensable as day-to-day care. However, not all doctors in the Netherlands have the necessary experience or know that VRFF can lead to a dignified death. Similarly, they do not seem to know how to supervise and palliate such a death. Some refuse to assist because of the standard moral associations with "suicide".[18,19]

Chabot[16] summarized several physiological mechanisms that explain why VRFF can be tolerated reasonably well by elderly persons as long as adequate mouth care is provided. Many people who have experienced temporary fasting know that the feeling of hunger disappears after a few days and is often replaced by a sense of well-being. When the intake of sugar or other carbohydrates ceases completely, the body may produce a morphine-like substance (endorphin) that has a positive effect on mood. Another effect of strict fasting is that the body produces ketone bodies when fatty acids are broken down, and these seem to have an analgesic effect.[20,21]

The feeling of thirst seems to be caused predominantly by dehydration of the mucous membranes of the mouth, not by the sodium concentration in the blood.[22] If the mouth can be kept lubricated, it appears that the feeling of thirst can be tolerated in elderly persons.[23,4,16] That observation has been confirmed in hospice-based terminal palliative care. [24,17] The kidneys will stop producing urine after about a week in the absence of fluid intake, and metabolic waste products are no longer removed from the blood. Many patients become drowsy when their kidneys are no longer able to excrete urea, but do not usually find this drowsiness unpleasant. Once drinking has ceased, the patient will only ingest fluid through regular refreshment of the mouth. Half a glass of water (about 50 cc) a day is sufficient for this, and is ingested by moistening the mouth regularly with an atomized water spray (three puffs contain 2 cc) and sucking crushed ice (5 cc) wrapped in gauze a few times a day.[16] Mouth care with saliva substitutes and treatment to prevent fungal infections can be provided by a nurse with the help of primary caretakers, preferably under the supervision of a GP or a doctor who has been trained in the provision of end-of-life palliative care.

Abstaining from food and water can be too difficult for some people. The advantage of this method for a self-directed death, as opposed to PAD, is that a person can change his or her mind at any time, which is not unusual during the first few days. Approximately one in every six people in Oregon who consciously refused to drink in order to hasten death while receiving excellent palliative care changed his or her mind and started eating and drinking again; this was often due to pressure by a member of the family who did not agree with the decision to end life.[11]

The moral and psychological situation of children or confidants is complicated. Qualitative research[25] has shown that opposition from family members is quite common when someone wants to die by VRFF. They can be overwhelmed by anger, helplessness, and other emotions. Some cannot bear to watch the course of events. They will either withdraw from the discussions or, more often, be excluded by the person who has made the decision. Those who wish to remain in contact until the end often must force themselves to continue to show tact and respect.

The decision to stop all food and fluid is usually made amid intense emotional struggles with relatives. Informants speak of many conflicting sentiments; for example, loyalty to the person with a deeply felt wish to die clashes with an internal opposition to losing that person. This emotional conflict can last a long time. Some relatives seem to be less troubled by this ambivalence because they feel that they would make the same decision in the same situation. Informants were remarkably reticent about their internal and external struggles with the person who died, even years later. They seemed fearful of doing an injustice to the memory of someone who had "taken matters into their own hands." This emotional conflict is perhaps the reason why they allow only a veiled glimpse into their struggles. These struggles testify to feelings of being rejected when someone chooses to end his or her life despite all efforts to help that person continue living a meaningful life.

Providing Information on VRFF: A Personal Approach

An important question that I have struggled with over the years concerns the tension between physicians' moral duties toward competent patients who deliberately choose death through VRFF and the legal prohibition against assisting in suicide.[19] Moral duties precede issues of legalization. However, developments around PAD, both in the Netherlands and the United States, "have encouraged us to frame virtually all moral questions as ones of legalization."[a,26] This focus on legal solutions for moral problems prevents us from dwelling on "the moral justification of individual acts of hastening death." In my opinion, this has an undesirable effect on the trust relationship between patients and physicians. I agree with Tom Beauchamp and maintain that the key moral issue here is the liberty to choose and the justification (if any) for limiting that liberty.[b,26]

In my opinion, respect for this liberty in situations where elderly or very ill people opt for VRFF means that physicians should inform patients and help guide the process toward a death with dignity. The practice of VRFF forces the Dutch medical profession to confront new issues around a process of dying in which the patient is the central figure, and not the physician. Physicians should feel morally justified in complying with requests for information. In the context of VRFF, this means that my focus is on the process of informing patients completely and adequately in order to support their ability to make an informed choice. A physician who gives a competent patient incomplete or inaccurate information about VRFF severely limits that patient's liberty to choose. Physicians and patients exercise that liberty in various ways, but it is essential to provide correct information on the VRFF option and the problems that are likely to occur.

Almost all patients with terminal illnesses and elderly disabled persons lack information about how they can hasten their own deaths in a dignified manner. Surprisingly, only some seem to have a real interest in being informed. Also, Dutch physicians rarely provide information on VRFF to patients whose requests for PAD have been turned down because the conditions of due care have not been met. Some are ignorant about this option for a humane death. Others find it inconsistent to turn down a request for PAD and then inform the patient about how to end his or her own life while being attended by relatives. Still others are uncertain and inexperienced about the type of palliative care measures involved after fluid intake has stopped, for example, how to respond if the patient wants to be sedated into unconsciousness shortly after refraining from drinking so as not to suffer from thirst.

I have interviewed many physicians and relatives over the past 10 years who had cared for someone who died after stopping all eating and drinking.

[a] 26. Beauchamp 2004, 118.
[b] 26. Beauchamp 2004, 128.

Contrary to my earlier convictions, during the period of research I gradually became convinced that a death by VRFF can be a humane, though certainly arduous, route to death for elderly patients. The patient and his or her caretakers must, however, be well informed and convinced that there is no other alternative. In addition, proportionate palliative care must be offered in response to the symptoms and complaints that occur. While it really is a last resort,[3] it is an option that is available to every competent person who knows that death will come soon.

In situations where the legal conditions of due care for PAD are not satisfied, I have decided that it is within my professional duty to provide information on the process of VRFF to any competent patient who asks for a hastened death with dignity. I also feel obligated to provide this information for patients who do not explicitly ask about VRFF but show an interest in how they might die a good or dignified death.

While discussing VRFF with patients, questions about palliation inevitably surface. Thirst, for example, does not cause "unbearable suffering" as long as mouth care is optimal. Thus, stopping food and liquid does not generally require continuous sedation. On the contrary, the patient's intermittent consciousness is essential for reaffirming the decision to hasten death. It is only after 5–7 days without eating and drinking that there may be symptoms that justify some palliation (e.g., a low dose of midazolam administered subcutaneously through a pump four to six times a day). This will put the patient to sleep during some daytime hours, but not continuously. Communication remains possible at certain intervals. After about 7 days without drinking, there may be irreversible damage to some organs, thereby justifying an increased midazolam dose. If discomfort still appears to be present, some morphine might be added (e.g., 2.5 mg subcutaneously two to four times a day or a 12.5 mg fentanyl plaster); this amount will not be the cause of death.

It is important to realize that these palliative measures are intended for patients in the Netherlands who do not qualify for legally possible PAD, but nevertheless want to remain in control over their own approaching deaths. Several sociologists[27,28,29] have argued that the contemporary fascination of very old persons or very ill patients with the right timing of death is a consequence of the problem created by modern medicine. As more people live longer in a more or less sedated state with, for example, end-stage cancer or cognitive impairments, more will die a social death weeks, months, or even years before their biological death. Some of them strive to bring their social death closer in time to their biological death by VRFF. By making their social and biological deaths coincide in time, they hope to be remembered by their loved ones as the people they were before they became too weak or too confused to communicate. It is, therefore, unlikely that Dutch citizens are the only ones who try to control the timing of their death by VRFF.

References

1. Bernat, James L., Bernard Gert, and Peter R. Mogielnicki. 1993. Patient refusal of hydration and nutrition: An alternative to physician-assisted suicide or active euthanasia. *Archives of Internal Medicine* 153: 2723–2728.
2. Quill, Timothy E., Bernard Lo, and Dan W. Brock. 1997. Palliative options of last resort: A comparison of voluntary stopping eating and drinking, terminal sedation, physician-assisted suicide, and voluntary active euthanasia. *Journal of the American Medical Association* 278: 2099–2104.
3. Brock, Dan W. Physician-assisted suicide as a last resort option at the end of life. 2004. In *Physician-Assisted Dying: The Case for Palliative Care and Patient Choice*, ed. Timothy E. Quill and Margaret P. Battin, 130–149. Baltimore: The John Hopkins University Press.
4. Terman, Stanley A. 2007. *The Best Way to Say Goodbye: A Legal Peaceful Choice at the End of Life*. Carlsbad, CA : Life Transitions Publications.
5. Warnock, M., and E. MacDonald. 2008. *Easeful Death: Is There a Case for Assisted Dying?* Oxford: Oxford University Press.
6. Chabot, Boudewijn E. 2007. Auto-euthanasia: Hidden dying trajectories in conversation with proxies. Ph.D. diss., University of Amsterdam, Uitgeverij Bert Bakker (in Dutch).
7. Chabot, Boudewijn E., and Arnold Goedhart. 2009. A survey of self-directed dying attended by proxies in the Dutch population. *Social Science & Medicine* 68: 1745–1751.
8. Onwuteaka-Philipsen, Bregje D., Agnes van der Heide, Dirk Koper, Ingeborg Keij-Deerenberg, Judith A. C. Rietjens, Mette L. Rurup, Astrid M. Vrakkin, Jean Jacques Georges, Martien T. Muller, Gerrit van der Wal, and Paul J. van der Maas. 2003. Euthanasia and other end-of-life decisions in the Netherlands in 1990, 1995 and 2001. *The Lancet* 362: 355–359.
9. Jansen-van der Weijde, Marijke C., Bregje D. Onwuteaka-Philipsen, and Gerrit van der Wal. 2005. Granted, undecided, withdrawn, and refused requests for euthanasia and physician-assisted suicide. *Archives of Internal Medicine* 165: 1698–1704.
10. Heide, Agnes van der, Bregje D. Onwuteaka-Philipsen, Mette L. Rurup, Hilde M. Buiting, Johannes J. M. van Delden, Johanna E. Hanssen-de Wolf, Anke G. J. M. Janssen, H. Roeline W. Pasman, Judith A. C. Rietjens, Cornelis J. M. Prins, Ingeborg M. Deerenberg, Joseph K. M. Gevers, Paul J. van der Maas, and Gerrit van der Wal. 2007. End-of-life practices in the Netherlands under the Euthanasia Act. *New England Journal of Medicine* 356: 1957–1965.
11. Harvath, Theresa A., Lois L. Miller, Kathryn A. Smith, Lisa D. Clark, Ann Jackson, and Linda Ganzini. 2006. Dilemmas encountered by hospice workers when patients wish to hasten death. *Journal of Hospice and Palliative Nursing* 8: 200–209.
12. Chochinov, Harvey M., Thomas Hack, Susan McClement, Linda Kristjanson, and Mike Harlos. 2002. Dignity in the terminally ill: An empirical model. *Social Science & Medicine* 54: 433–443.
13. Jacobson, Nora. 2007. Dignity and health: A review. *Social Science & Medicine* 64: 292–302.

14. Maxwell Atkinson, John. 1978. *Discovering Suicide: Studies in the Social Organization of Sudden Death*. London: Macmillan.
15. Das, C. 2004. Death certificates and doctors: Rules and reality. Ph.D. diss., Vrije Universiteit Amsterdam (in Dutch).
16. Chabot, Boudewijn, and Christian Walther. 2010. *Exit at the End of Life: Self-Determined Dying by Voluntary Refusal of Eating and Drinking*. Munich: Reinhardt Verlag (in German).
17. Ganzini, Linda, Elizabeth R. Goy, Lois L. Miller, Theresa A. Harvath, Ann Jackson, and Molly A. Delorit. 2003. Nurses' experiences with hospice patients who refuse food and fluids to hasten death. *New England Journal of Medicine* 349:359–365.
18. Jansen, Lynn A. 2004. No safe harbor: The principle of complicity and the practice of voluntary stopping of eating and drinking. *Journal of Medicine and Philosophy* 29:61–73.
19. Schwartz, Judith. 2007. Exploring the option of voluntarily stopping eating and drinking within the context of a suffering patient's request for a hastened death. *Journal of Palliative Medicine* 10: 1288–1297.
20. Owen, O. E., S. Caprio, G. A. Reichard, Jr., M. A. Mozzoli, G. Boden, and R. S. Owen. 1983. Ketosis of starvation: A revisit and new perspectives. *Clinics in Endocrinology and Metabolism* 12:357–379.
21. Hamm, Robert J., Janet S. Knisely, Ann Watson, Bruce G. Lyeth, and D. F. B. Bossut. 1985. Hormonal mediation of the analgesia produced by food deprivation. *Physiology and Behavior* 35: 879–882.
22. Vullo-Navich, Kimberly, Shirley Smith, Maria Andrews, Alan M. Levine, James F. Tischler, and Jeanne M. Veglia. 1998. Comfort and incidence of abnormal serum sodium, BUN, creatinine and osmolality in dehydration of terminal illness. *American Journal of Hospice and Palliative Care* 15: 770–784.
23. Phillips, P. A., B. J. Rolls, J. G. Ledingham, M. L. Forsling, J. J. Morton, M. J. Crowe, and L. Wollner. 1984. Reduced thirst after water deprivation in healthy elderly men. *New England Journal of Medicine* 311: 753–759.
24. McCann, Robert M., William J. Hall, and Annmarie Groth-Juncker. 1994. Comfort care for terminally ill patients: The appropriate use of nutrition and hydration. *Journal of the American Medical Association* 272: 1263–1266.
25. Chabot, Boudewijn E. 2001. *Dying-Labour*. Nijmegen: SUN (in Dutch).
26. Beauchamp, Tom L. 2004. When hastened death is neither killing nor letting die. In *The Case for Palliative Care and Patient Choice*, ed. Timothy E. Quill and Margaret P. Battin. Baltimore: The Johns Hopkins University Press.
27. Walter, Tony. 1994. *The Revival of Death*. London: Routledge.
28. Seale, Clive, and Sjaak van der Geest. 2004. Good and bad death. *Social Science & Medicine* 58:883–887.
29. Kellehear, Allan. 2007. *A Social History of Dying*. Cambridge: Cambridge University Press.

PART V

THE CHALLENGE OF UNBEARABLE SUFFERING

21

The Subjectivity of Suffering and the Normativity of Unbearableness

Henri Wijsbek

INTRODUCTION

The most fundamental of the six criteria of due care that must be met for lawful euthanasia in the Netherlands is arguably that the physician must be satisfied that the patient's suffering is unbearable, with no prospect of improvement.[a,1,2] It is also the most difficult criterion to establish; or, rather, the determination of unbearableness is. The absence of any prospect of improvement can generally be determined straightforwardly; it simply means that the condition underlying the suffering is incurable according to accepted medical standards and that there is no reasonable prospect of alleviating the symptoms. Unbearableness, on the other hand, is one of the most intractable elements in the practice and regulation of Dutch euthanasia.[b] In view of the fundamental role of this criterion and the practical difficulties it tends to cause, it is surprising to find that the literature on this topic is virtually all but nonexistent.

As far as I can see, the only way to make the practice more tractable and transparent is to analyze the concept of unbearable suffering. As M. R. Bennett and P. M. S. Hacker remarked in the course of discussing the intelligibility of ascribing psychological attributes to the brain: "One cannot look for the poles of the Earth until one knows what a pole is – that is, what the expression 'pole' means, and also what counts as finding a pole of the Earth. Otherwise, like Winnie-the-Pooh, one might embark on an expedition to the East Pole."[3,c] Likewise, physicians cannot ascertain that their patients are suffering unbearably unless they know what unbearable suffering is – that is, what the concept "unbearable suffering" means. In this chapter, I shall first draw on

[a] Govert den Hartogh argues convincingly that relief of suffering is the fundamental justifying ground for euthanasia in the Netherlands, and so does Esther Pans. See 1. den Hartogh 2007 and 2. Pans 2006, as well as her Chapter 4 in this volume.

[b] This is mentioned almost every year in the Regional Review Committees' Annual Reports.

[c] 3. Bennett and Hacker 2003, 71.

Eric Cassell's seminal work as well as on some Dutch sources to explicate the meaning of "suffering." I will then examine the common assumption that the practical difficulties of the criterion of unbearable suffering are caused by the fact that suffering is subjective. Finally, I turn to the meaning of "unbearable," since I believe that its implications for the practice of euthanasia have been improperly neglected.

CASSELL ON SUFFERING

The American physician Eric Cassell begins his groundbreaking 1991 book *The Nature of Suffering and the Goals of Medicine* with a bold claim. The claim is premised on the attractive view that "[t]he test of a system of medicine should be its adequacy in the face of suffering" (p. vii)[4] Fifteen years earlier, the medical historian Thomas McKeown had formulated the goal of medicine in a similar, broadly humanistic way: "To assist us to come into the world and comfortably out of it, and during life to protect the well and care for the sick and disabled."[5,d]

Cassell's bold claim was, and still is, that medicine fails the test because suffering is not adequately conceptualized and understood. As long as medicine confines its attention to physiology, suffering will remain a mystery. Understanding suffering requires that the traditional dichotomies between mind and body, subjective and objective, be abandoned. Instead of directing all its attention to diseases, which "are specific entities characterized by disturbances in structure or function of any part, organ, or system of the body," medicine should concern itself with illness, "the set of disordered functions, body sensations, and feelings by which persons know themselves to be unwell (1991, p. 49)." In Cassell's view, the distinction between disease and symptoms, on the one hand, and illness and suffering, on the other, is crucial for a proper understanding of suffering because suffering is distinct from what initiates it.

Recent research has vindicated the view that there is not any direct correspondence between the seriousness of the symptoms that elicit a sensation and the quality of the sensation itself.[e,6] Some pains, like those of childbirth, can be extremely severe and yet endured, even considered uplifting, because they supervene on a meaningful, nonthreatening process. In contrast, people may suffer considerably from apparently little pain when the source is unknown or potentially harmful. One of Cassell's patients once told him that she had initially believed that the pain in her leg was sciatica and that she could control it with small doses of codeine, but when she discovered that it was due to the spread of a malignant disease, she had to take much greater amounts of medication for relief. In addition to the perceived meaning of pain, the impossibility

[d] 5. McKeown 1976, 192.

[e] Patrick Wall presents some dramatic cases to illustrate the impact that meaning has on the experiencing of pain (see 6. Wall 1999, Chapter 1).

of controlling it is often reported to give rise to suffering, both when it is so severe that it is virtually overwhelming and when it continues for a long time. But the meaning a patient attributes to a symptom is the most important factor influencing the quality of the sensation. This is the reason that Cassell claims that "[s]uffering is ultimately a personal matter – something whose presence and extent can only be known to the sufferer" (1991, p. 35).

By the same token, disease and illness are not directly related either. People can have a chronic disease – diabetes or hypertension, for instance – without perceiving themselves as ill or suffering; and chronic illness can occur in the absence of a disease. A bodily appearance radically deviating from a conventionally accepted norm is not a disease, but it may nonetheless bring illness and indeed severe suffering in its wake.

The need for individual information distinguishes clinical practice from medical science. Science deals with general processes and objective facts, practice with particular patients and their subjective experiences. Cassell notes that "objective" and "subjective" have special connotations in medicine and that it is essential for medical practice to understand what these terms mean for physicians. A thermometer can be used to measure the temperature of the patient's body, and the reading on the thermometer is an objective measure of the elevation of body temperature. No matter who reads the thermometer, the outcome will be the same for all observers. On the other hand, the feeling of feverishness is subjective because a feeling can only be experienced by the subject – the patient having the experience. But "subjective" also has the further connotation of "idiosyncratic" – unique to this subject. The patient who has the fever has ideas about its meanings that result from his or her particular biography. Consequently, suffering is subjective in two different senses: It is an experience tied to the particular person who has the experience, and only that person is in a position to know the quality of that experience.

Suffering, then, is not something persons just get, in the way that they may get a disease like meningitis or measles. Symptoms such as pain, shortness of breath, weakness, nausea, loss of interest, diarrhea, and so on are not brute facts of nature that simply *cause* suffering; rather, they may be *converted* into suffering by the specific meaning a person attaches to them. But bodily symptoms like these are not the only possible source of suffering; suffering can also arise from the loss of opportunities and functions essential for leading a satisfying life. Bodies may malfunction, but only persons can suffer.

The concept of a "person," then, bears a lot of weight in Cassell's account of suffering. A person, on his understanding, is an irreducible unity composed of several aspects. Roughly speaking, a person is a socially embedded biological being with a past and a future; persons normally live in a society, take on different roles, entertain relationships, work, and take leisure. Suffering occurs when any of these aspects is seriously affected and the unity constituting the person threatens to dissolve. For example, relationships with family or friends are withering away, bringing grief and loneliness; roles – as a father, husband, nurse – cannot be maintained, destroying self-respect; work is no longer possible, injuring self-esteem; control is lost and life begins to lose its meaning. Persons who suffer feel deprived of past abilities and a meaningful future; they see themselves as "coming apart," as losing their integrity.

A story might be helpful to illustrate what Cassell takes this loss of integrity to mean. The suffering the woman in this example experienced is not related to pain but to the increasing inability to live her carefully constructed life as the person she had made herself into over the years.

> Marcy Thompson was sixty-two when she became so severely impaired by advancing cancer of the ovary that she chose to die. She was determinedly single and had led a life of books, with which her apartment was filled. With her only family, a sister and nieces, she was distant by preference. Although generally alone, she had been and remained in a long love relationship. Her cancer was discovered after it had spread, and she refused chemotherapy (having researched the topic thoroughly). She stopped working as an editor a few months before her decision because of weakness and fatigue, but she continued to read and write commentary, attended only by a home health aide. Pain, although present, was adequately controlled. She found existence intolerable when she could hardly walk, could no longer read or write critically, and was not, in her estimate, a partner to the man she loved, so she decided to die.[7] (2004, p. 75)

His account leads Cassell to the following definition of suffering: "Suffering occurs when an impending destruction of the person is perceived; it continues until the threat of disintegration has passed or until the integrity of the person can be restored in some other manner.... Most generally, suffering can be defined as the state of severe distress associated with events that threaten the intactness of the person" (1991, p. 33).

To sum up Cassell's view, symptoms – "disturbances in structure or function of any part, organ, or system of the body" – give rise to sensations that are subjective in the sense that they can only be experienced by the person affected by these symptoms. The actual quality of the sensation and the impact of functional losses are mediated by the meaning the symptoms have for this particular person, sometimes a meaning others can understand only if they take up that person's point of view, and this is a second sense in which sensations can be said to be subjective. If the symptoms worsen and come to betoken a condition dangerous for one or more aspects of patients' personhood, they experience a threat, and suddenly, at a point relative to them and therefore not clearly predictable, their lives lose meaning and they themselves their integrity. And that, according to Cassell, is the hallmark of suffering.

TWO DUTCH SOURCES ON SUFFERING

In 1998, the Dutch physician M. M. Beijk published a short article entitled "Unbearable Suffering. What Is It, What Causes It, and Who Determines It?"[8] She had noticed that the interpretation of the concept "suffering" varied widely among physicians practising euthanasia, and she wanted to reduce the presumed disagreement by listing the different aspects of its meaning.[9,f] In that way she hoped to enable the patient to describe his or her suffering more accurately and, consequently, the physician to understand it more easily and to honor the request for euthanasia more readily.

Beijk's list contains five aspects, which are further subdivided into different facets. These aspects are

i. diagnosis and prognosis;
ii. symptoms and complaints, such as pains, shortness of breath, cramps, dizziness, falling, and diarrhea;
iii. loss of function, for example, sight, balance, urinating and defecating problems, and the capability to perform everyday activities, such as cooking, eating, washing, and getting dressed;
iv. personal factors, notably character and biography; and
v. situational circumstances, particularly housing and access to care.

If you compare the facets listed under (ii) with those listed under (iii), you find a considerable overlap. Falling and dizziness are summed up as symptoms, just as diarrhea and constipation, whereas loss of balance and stability, as well as problems due to diarrhea and constipation, count as functional losses. I believe the idea underlying her list can be faithfully rendered in the following way. Complaints are unpleasant sensations such as pain, itching, shortness of breath, nausea, and drowsiness originating in bodily symptoms. Functions are either biological functions, such as sight, balance, memory, and digestion, or social functions necessary to maintain oneself as a social being, such as the capability to fend for oneself, to move around, to work, and to keep up relations with family, friends, and colleagues. As to the relation among these aspects, Beijk remarks that the seriousness of a disease is determined primarily by symptoms and functional losses, whereas the capacity to bear it depends on personal and situational factors.

Beijk describes the nature of suffering rather indeterminately as "a subjective experience differing from pain." She adds the qualifier "subjective" to indicate that only the patient is in a position to tell whether he or she is suffering: "Unbearable suffering" is suffering experienced as unbearable by the patient. She warns us not to think of her list of aspects as an attempt to "objectify" the amount of suffering needed to count as unbearable; that would amount to an arrogant presumption on the part of the physician. Only patients can know whether they suffer; about the quality of their own experiences, they themselves have the final say.

A second important Dutch source on suffering is the annual reports from the Regional Review Committees. A physician who has performed euthanasia

[f] D. van Tol has convincingly shown that this is indeed the case (see 9, van Tol 2005).

or assisted in suicide must submit a report to the local coroner, who in turn informs one of the Regional Review Committees. On the basis of these reports, the members of the committee decide whether the physician has satisfied the six criteria of due care. If so, the case is closed; if not, the committee may either ask the physician to provide a fuller account or refer the case to the public prosecutor. By far the most difficult for the committees is to ensure that the physician has fulfilled the criterion of unbearable suffering. Like Beijk, the committees blame the practical difficulties of this criterion on the subjective character of suffering.[10] By "subjective," they mean determined by patients' own perspectives, their physical and psychological strength, their personalities, beliefs, values, and norms. Suffering still bearable for the one may, therefore, be unbearable for the other.

On the committees' account, however, suffering is not subjective through and through, which is to say that it is not completely determined by the patient's perspective, as Beijk seems to maintain, but only partly so determined. For that reason, suffering can be objectified at least to a certain extent in the opinion of the committees. What they mean by "objectified" can be gleaned from the requirement that the unbearableness of the suffering must be recognizable for a physician with a normal capacity to empathize. Their samples of cases show that this recognition comes in degrees: It is almost a matter of course in the case of malignant diseases accompanied by intense, intractable pain; in such cases, meaning and interpretation hardly have any role to play. It may be much more difficult in the case of progressive degenerative diseases, such as Alzheimer's disease and multiple sclerosis, whereby patients may be permanently bedridden or totally dependent on others even for their day-to-day activities; and it may be essentially contested in cases in which suffering consists in loss of dignity or fear of future suffering.

If you compare these two Dutch accounts of suffering with each other, it's hard not to be struck by the similarities. In both, suffering is described as a subjective experience, originating in bodily symptoms or functional losses. Exactly which causal role a given symptom or loss plays will depend on the patient's situation, biography, and point of view, and it may, therefore, differ from one person to another. For this reason, a physician trying to assess the suffering of a patient must adopt the patient's point of view and interpret the bearing of those symptoms on the patient from that perspective. In fact, the two accounts seem to differ from each other on one point only; according to the committees, suffering is at least partly open to objectification, whereas Beijk contends that any attempt at objectification would be preposterous. But surely even this difference is merely terminological; in both accounts, a number of aspects are listed that can be (objectively) recognized by a physician as contributing to the suffering, and both stress that the weight of these aspects can be properly determined only from within the patient's (subjective) point of view. At the most, then, they differ in their view about how accessible one person's point of view is to another, to what extent, that is, empathy is possible.

This generalized "Dutch" account in turn tallies well with Cassell's, except for the fact that his account is embedded in a richer theory of the person. In particular, they all claim that the difficulty in determining whether somebody else is suffering is due to the fact that suffering is subjective. But since they use the term *subjective* in a number of different ways, and since the term moreover is a source of confusion in its own right, it is necessary to sort out these different uses in order to be able to assess that claim.

THE SUBJECTIVITY OF SUFFERING

Subjective has at least two different meanings, both akin to "private"; it can be used to refer either to private "ownership" or to private access. That feelings, experiences, and mental states in general are private in the first sense means that they can only be had by the subject, their "owner." And since to have pain is the same as to feel pain, this is equivalent to saying that I am the only person who can feel my pain. Private access can be seen as following naturally from private ownership; if I am the only person who can feel my own feelings, I am the only person who can know them. If suffering were indeed private in either of these two senses, the criterion of unbearable suffering could not serve as a public criterion on which to base life and death decisions. The fundamental question, then, is what exactly "subjective" in these two senses amounts to, in particular whether either kind of privacy disqualifies the criterion of unbearable suffering for practical purposes.

Take private ownership as a starter. It seems almost self-evident that nobody else can have the same feeling as I have, that nobody can feel what I am feeling. But on further reflection, this claim is not as straightforward as it first seems to be. "The same" can refer to two different kinds of identity, qualitative and numerical. If two men are said to wear the same shoes, what is meant is probably that they wear the same brand of shoes, of the same color, size, and so on. The shoes are qualitatively identical – you could not tell the two pairs apart – but numerically distinct – each man wears his own pair. On the other hand, if two men are said to smoke the same "joint," what is meant is probably that there is one single joint of marijuana that they smoke together. This is the most probable reading, but not the only possible one. The first two men could be very poor and share one pair of shoes, and the second could very well be smoking two numerically distinct but qualitatively indistinguishable joints. For some values of x and y in the sentence "x is identical with y," however, this ambiguity is ruled out. If two colors are said to be identical, there is no further question as to whether they are qualitatively or numerically identical; the same holds for literary genres, professions, and, more to the point, for experiences – the only possible identity in these cases is qualitative identity.

That two persons could not have the same feeling, then, is nonsensical if "the same" is taken to mean numerically identical, while if taken to mean qualitatively identical, it is simply false. Feelings and experiences are identified by their description, not by their owner. I can have a pain that is throbbing, but not a pain that is mine. And if your feeling and mine have the same properties, if they satisfy the same description, then they are both instances of the same feeling, say nausea, just as two poems with the same formal properties are both, say, a sonnet. And as this last example makes clear, qualitative sameness allows for a certain vagueness; depending on the rhyme scheme, we call a sonnet either Italian or English. The two poems need not have exactly the same properties for both to be a sonnet, nor do two feelings have to answer to exactly the same description for both to be instances of the same feeling. So in a clear sense, it is very well possible for two persons to have the same feeling, or more generally, to be in the same mental state.

Granted, then, that you and I can have the same feeling; could we also know each other's feelings, or are feelings private in the sense that I can know something about my feelings nobody else can? It seems as if Cassell and Beijk take privacy in the very strong sense of "infallible" when they write that the only way to learn whether suffering is present is to ask the patient; unbearable suffering is unbearable whenever the patients say it is. If they meant this literally, the criterion would be a sham; there would be nothing for physicians to examine or ascertain once they had asked their patients whether they suffered unbearably. At the very best, something like that might be true for "raw feelings." It is hard to imagine what it would be for me to be mistaken about my own headache or dizziness, but suffering is not such a raw feeling. Cassell, Beijk, and the review committees all stress that suffering is dependent on situation and biography, on a personal point of view. The claim that I am suffering is a judgment, based on an interpretation of my present situation, against the backdrop of my beliefs and values, my fears and hopes, and these can be more or less realistic. At the very least, such judgments are open to examination and clarification.

Even if patients are not infallible in their judgments about their suffering, however, there remains a sense of "privacy" in which subjects have "privileged access" to their feelings. You may be able to know what I feel, but I know my own feelings in a way in which you can only know your own feelings. I don't have to find out that I am in pain, whereas for you that is the only possibility to assure yourself that I am, and this asymmetry still has to be explained. To find out whether I am in pain, you must observe my behavior and listen to what I say. Suppose these were the only ways that I could come to know whether I was in pain. I would have to observe myself, and if I were in doubt, I would ask myself whether I was in pain and await the answer. Nobody behaving in this way would be recognizable as a person. Persons are the primary source of information about their feelings, but only if their words are not based on observation.[g,11] We are in a privileged, albeit not infallible, position vis-à-vis our own experiences. I

[g] Norman Malcolm is very clear on these matters. Obviously, "these matters" refer to Wittgenstein's private language argument (see 11. Malcolm 1977).

know my own feelings directly; others observe them in my tone of voice and my gestures, or they know how I feel because I tell them.

Normally, our words, gestures, and bearing express our feelings and thoughts very well. It remains the case, however, that people differ in the way they express their feelings. What if a man was badly wounded but did not complain of pain? Would we say that he had less pain than people normally do in these circumstances, or would we say that he behaved stoically? There is no way to tell in general, because here two criteria clash: the wound pointing in one direction, the inhibited expression in another. But in those cases in which we know the person well, we can tell, and that is the reason physicians must inform themselves about their patients' biographies when they have to assess suffering.

The upshot is that we should reject both the claim that because feelings are subjective nobody else can feel what subjects feel, and the claim that nobody except subjects themselves can know what they feel. The rejection of the first claim turns on a distinction between numerical and qualitative identity, and once the only proper sense in which two feelings can be said to be the same is identified, there is no conceptual bar to two persons having the same feeling. The rejection of the second claim turns on the distinction between two ways in which feelings can be known: directly and indirectly, and on the additional fact that neither of these ways is infallible, more particularly, that the first is not.

UNBEARABLE SUFFERING

The subjectivity of suffering, then, does indeed complicate the application of the criterion of unbearable suffering, without making it in principle unsuitable or arbitrary. But the difficulties and controversies due to the fact that suffering is subjective are further allayed by the requirement that the patient must suffer unbearably. None of the authors I have discussed differentiates between suffering and unbearable suffering. This is a shortcoming especially in the Dutch sources, since the Dutch law requires the physician to ascertain that his or her patient is suffering unbearably, not that the patient is "merely" suffering. What practical difference does this additional requirement make?

Suppose a friend of yours tells you that she has run the marathon in 3:14:05. You might be impressed and reply, "Wow, that's pretty fast!" If you think about it, that is a rather puzzling remark. She gives you a precise figure and you answer with a vague description. Normally, it's the other way round. She could have told you that she had run the marathon quite fast and you could then sensibly have asked her how fast exactly. Then her answer, 3:14:05, would have given you information you did not have before. But in what sense can adding something as vague as "pretty fast" to a precise figure contribute anything to your little conversation? Analogously, what can a term as vague as "unbearable" add by way of information about suffering to a list of carefully described symptoms, functional losses, personal characteristics, and social circumstances?

In neither of these cases do the vague terms add any empirical information, but of course, then again that is not their function. Instead, they serve as a kind of evaluation.[h,12] In the case of "fast," this is straightforward. Professionals run the marathon in just over two hours; three and a half hours for an amateur is a very good result, and just over three hours is exceptional. You know that it is exceptional, if you do, because you know what time it takes to run a marathon for different categories of people. Within the relevant comparison group, your friend's performance is outstanding. "Fast" means faster than most others within that group. "Wow, that's pretty fast!" expresses your admiration for your friend's excellent performance as, say, a 50-year-old, female amateur.

Since "fast" is vague, there is some room for disagreement about where to draw the line between "Wow!" and "Not bad!" But the contested range is rather narrow, and there are clear cases on both sides. Nor is it of any great importance where exactly the line is drawn. Moreover, no one can lay down the correct application of this word authoritatively; every competent and adequately informed speaker is equally qualified. Furthermore, the line will move as results improve. At the first Olympic Games in modern times, held in Athens in 1896, Spiridon Louis ran the marathon in 2:58:50. Sixty years later at the games in Tokyo, Abebe Bikila ran it (barefoot) in 2:12:12, and in 2011, Patrick Makau set the new world record at 2:03:38. The references of "Wow" and "Not bad" have tracked the change: "Wow" back in 1896 has become at best "Not bad" in 2011.

The case of "unbearable" is different in a number of respects. *Unbearable* likewise refers to a norm, and if suffering is classified as unbearable, certain actions are sanctioned that would otherwise be forbidden. In this case, a physician would be allowed to perform euthanasia, given that the other criteria of due care have been met as well. So it is immensely important whether a patient's suffering can be validly described as "unbearable." But in this case, the norm is not established as straightforwardly as in the case of "fast." It is a social norm, laid down in the Euthanasia Act, after 25 years of public debate to which the Dutch Association for Voluntary Euthanasia (NVVE) and the Royal Dutch Medical Association (KNMG), and others, have contributed.

As it stands, "unbearable" is a vague, "open" norm. To be sure, there are paradigmatic cases of unbearable suffering that literally everybody can agree on, but there are also borderline cases for which nobody can confidently claim that the suffering is either unbearable or that it is not. Such cases are sometimes taken to court, and if they end up in the Supreme Court, the sentence passed will authoritatively specify the meaning of unbearable and make the open norm a little less open. Many of the most important euthanasia cases that have been taken to the Supreme Court involved the meaning of the concept of unbearable suffering. In the *Schoonheim* case (1984), unbearable suffering

[h] I owe this to Frank Veltman (see 12. Veltman 2002).

was adopted for the first time as the fundamental ground for euthanasia and assisted suicide. In the *Chabot* case (1994), the court established that psychological suffering could in principle fall within the scope of unbearable suffering. And in the *Brongersma* case (2002), suffering that did not originate in a clinically diagnosable disease, either somatic or psychiatric, was ruled out as a justifiable ground for euthanasia, even though the court acknowledged that suffering could in principle be unbearable whatever its origin.[i]

It is not only courts that have this normative linguistic power, however. Since 1999, the five Regional Review Committees have annually published their judgments on a number of controversial cases, and since 2006, all judgments are published on the Internet.[j] Taken together, they constitute a depository of semilegal jurisprudence, in which authoritative interpretations of controversial cases are laid down in accordance with the open social norm that serves as a regulative ideal for these interpretations. For example, since 2005, the Regional Review Committees have accepted that fear of future suffering can be an element that makes actual suffering unbearable, provided the fear is realistic and the future is not too distant. This is relevant particularly for patients suffering from dementia in an early stage. Another example of the gradual circumscription of "unbearable suffering" is the rejection of the applicability of this criterion on comatose patients. As a consequence, euthanasia performed on patients in deep coma cannot satisfy all the criteria of due care.

Unbearable, then, does not mean "I can't bear this any longer." Rather, it means "We, the Dutch political community, don't require you to bear this any longer." The tipping point at which suffering becomes unbearable is not directly determined by the physician's assessment of the seriousness of the symptoms and losses, nor by the meaning the patient attributes to them. It is a point determined by a social norm in which all these aspects are taken into account and balanced in accordance with our shared understandings of suffering and also the point at which it becomes incompatible with leading a meaningful life. Only in a limited sense can physician and patient be said to decide whether the patient is suffering unbearably. They can only do so on terms that are the outcome of an ongoing public debate. It is necessary, but not sufficient, therefore, that a physician with a normal capacity to empathize is convinced that the patient is suffering unbearably from the patient's own point of view. The physician must, of course, ensure that the patient make the request on the best information available and in accordance with the desires and values he or she really has, and generally that will involve some give and take between the two of them, preferably including the patient's family as well. But in addition, the physician must be convinced that the patient's suffering meets the norm the Dutch political community has set, or is setting, for unbearable suffering.

[i] For more on these cases, see Chapter 3 in this volume.

[j] Accessible at: http://www.toetsingscommissieseuthanasie.nl.

It is only because "unbearable" is a normative concept that suffering can function as a public criterion at all. It was commonly feared, especially before the *Brongersma* verdict, by which the Supreme Court constrained the criterion to suffering caused by a clinically diagnosable disease or disorder, that once a subjective criterion had been introduced, the only way to know whether it applied would be to ask the patients themselves.[k] In practice, the consequence of introducing a subjective criterion would be that patients would suffer unbearably whenever they said they did. In fact, both Cassell and Beijk explicitly hold that view, although, I must add, Cassell also seems to hold the opposite.

I have already given some theoretical reasons to allay these fears, and I now want to strengthen my argument by adducing some nonstandard but real life examples from the Dutch euthanasia debate that show how the public norm implicit in the concept "unbearable" constrains the interpretation of the criterion of unbearable suffering. There is no real work to do for the criterion in standard cases where the patient is suffering from, say, amyotrophic lateral sclerosis (ALS) or incurable cancer accompanied by intractable pains and extreme fatigue. More than 90% of the Dutch population is of the opinion that euthanasia is justifiable in such cases. It is only in nonstandard cases that the criterion is put to the test.

In 1996, a man convicted for murder and sentenced to eight years imprisonment demanded in summary proceedings that the state pay a psychiatrist to examine him. He suffered severely from being found guilty of murder inasmuch as he considered himself not guilty. This suffering, he claimed, was unbearable and without prospect of improvement and left him with no other option but death. He had attempted suicide several times and failed and now wanted assistance to ensure success. As a first step, he needed a psychiatrist, who confirmed that his suffering met the criteria of due care. His request was not granted. The judge explained that although Dutch jurisprudence does acknowledge that psychic suffering can count as unbearable and without prospect of improvement, Dutch law does not recognize a right to physician-assisted suicide.[l] Moreover, since the convict had entered an appeal against the decision, the criminal procedure was not yet over, and hence his condition could not be classified as being without prospect of improvement.[13]

One wonders what the judge would have said if the convict had not entered an appeal and if he had not been sentenced to eight years but to lifelong imprisonment, which in the Netherlands is, indeed, lifelong. Could not that be classified as without prospect of improvement? Another possible line of reasoning would be to hold that imprisonment is a punishment, and as such it is meant, among other things, to inflict harm on the convict, but not harm

[k] For the Brongersma case, see Chapter 3 in this volume.

[l] For psychic suffering, see Chapter 3; for patient rights, see Chapter 4.

that amounts to unbearable suffering. If a convict could nevertheless make a convincing case that he or she was suffering unbearably, that would be a reason to change the conditions of detention, rather than to grant him or her assistance in suicide.

My second case comes from a TV program about euthanasia and assistance in suicide.[14] To illustrate the "enormous problems" the suffering criterion gives rise to, a general practitioner in Amsterdam told about an old lady living on her own who had visited him some months earlier and then declared her wish to die once her old dog would be dead and gone. Some weeks later the dog died, and the woman returned to the GP and repeated her request, "Do you remember, doctor, what I asked you the last time I was here?" He did, and it took him three months to talk her out of her request and to convince her to get a new dog, which she eventually did. It's clear that he took the woman's suffering very seriously. And rightly so, I believe.

It's not exactly a picnic to live alone in old age with all the ailments it brings in its wake, when all your friends are dead and your children are too busy elsewhere with their own lives to have much time to visit their old mother. For people in such circumstances, a dog can seem to be a real friend, the last one who really cares about them. I can very well imagine that this GP had a hard time convincing the woman that another dog could be a perfect replacement for her old companion. In effect, then, the GP, notwithstanding what the woman told him, was not convinced that she suffered unbearably from the loss of her pet. She *thought* she did, but the GP, and I can safely add, we, the Dutch political community, don't endorse that view. We don't think that a human being can have a relation with a pet that is so meaningful and unique that a like relationship is not possible with another pet.

My third example was given by an expert witness in the *Brongersma* case who strongly opposed the justifiability of assistance in suicide in cases where the suffering did not originate in a medically classified illness or disease.[m] The opposite view, he claimed, would lead to euthanasia requests from, for instance, people unable to pay off their mortgage, and it would leave the doctor without an answer in such cases. But that is too hasty. Citizens are allowed to take out a mortgage on a house if they have enough financial security and, as we have seen in the United States lately, such transactions involve a certain risk. If people cannot pay the interest and redemption, they have to sell their houses and look for something less expensive, and if they really fall on hard times – I don't want to make light of poverty – we have different kinds of social services they can fall back on. That is the way the Dutch community alleviates this kind of suffering, unbearable or not, and physicians have no role to play in this scenario.

[m] I am (almost) certain that it was the expert witness Spreeuwenberg who mentioned this example at the session for the Court of Appeal in the *Brongersma* case.

CONCLUSION

If my analysis of "unbearable suffering" is convincing, it is impossible to assess suffering, whatever its cause, with strictly medical professional knowledge only, nor will it do to add to this knowledge a fair amount of empathy. Of course, to assess suffering adequately, a physician must always interpret the patient's (objective) symptoms and losses from his or her (subjective) point of view, against the background, that is, provided by his or her biography, beliefs, and values. But taken on their own, these background conditions are not sufficient for a physician to enable the patient to ascertain whether the criterion is fulfilled. He or she must also grasp the public norm concerning unbearableness. Only this practical knowledge warrants the distinction between suffering that the Dutch political community considers to be unbearable and suffering that it considers everybody capable of coping with, whatever the patient may say.

References

1. Hartogh, Govert A. den. 2007. The Dutch euthanasia law: Is mercy enough? *Tijdschrift voor Gezondheidsrecht* 31: 180–198.
2. Pans, Esther. 2006. *The Normative Foundations of the Dutch Euthanasia Law*. Nijmegen: WLP.
3. Bennett, M. R., and P. M. S. Hacker. 2003. *Philosophical Foundations of Neuroscience*. Malden, MA: Blackwell.
4. Cassell, Eric J. 1991. *The Nature of Suffering and the Goal of Medicine*. New York: Oxford University Press.
5. McKeown, Thomas. 1976. *The Role of Medicine*. Oxford: Basil Blackwell.
6. Wall, Patrick. 1999. *Pain: The Science of Suffering*. Great Britain: Weidenfeld & Nicholson.
7. Cassell, Eric J. 2004. When suffering patients seek death. In *Physician-Assisted Dying*, ed. Timothy E. Quill and Margaret P. Battin, 75–88. Baltimore: John Hopkins University Press.
8. Beijk, M. M. 1998. Unbearable Suffering: What Is It, What Causes It, and Who Determines It? *Medisch Contact* 53: 825–827.
9. Tol, D. van D. 2005. Borderconflicts. Ph.D. diss.,University of Groningen.
10. Regional Review Committees. 2003. Annual Report 2003: 20. Regional Review Committees for Euthanasia (1998/2005) Annual Reports are accessible at: http://www.toetsingscommissieseuthanasie.nl.
11. Malcolm, Norman. 1977. The privacy of experience. In *Thought and Knowledge*, ed. Norman Malcolm, 104–132. Ithaca, NY: Cornell University Press.
12. Veltman, Frank. 2002. The difference between *vague* and *not precise*. Amsterdam: Vossiuspers.
13. Judgment passed by the president of the court, the Hague, 28 October, 1996. 1997. *Tijdschrift voor Gezondheidsrecht* 21: 248–250.
14. Spraakmakende Zaken; Ned. 2, August 7, 2007.

22

Assessment of Unbearable and Hopeless Suffering in Evaluating a Request to End Life

Gerrit K. Kimsma

INTRODUCTION

In this chapter I shall describe how Dutch physicians assess the suffering of patients who have requested a physician's active aid in dying. Unbearable suffering is the central condition for acceptable physician-assisted death (PAD), second only to the request itself. I shall focus on the legal norms for acceptable euthanasia first, and then examine how the Royal Dutch Medical Association (KNMG) and the Euthanasia Review Committees (ERCs) address suffering. The next step will be to analyze the possibility of adequately assessing suffering in general. Finally, I will focus on how the assessment of suffering changes in a climate that allows euthanasia. My thesis is that the optimum assessment of suffering depends upon the development of a deep reciprocal physician–patient relationship after a patient has requested help in dying.

SUFFERING

The concept of suffering has played a key role in the Dutch euthanasia debate, particularly with respect to medical-legal analyses and decisions. Court decisions have laid the groundwork for conditions under which euthanasia is acceptable. However, it is important to realize that the court decisions depended heavily on the norms of medical science and medical ethics. These medico-legal norms and conditions were stipulated in the Dutch Euthanasia Act of 2002.[1] The evolving conceptual framework of legal thinking about these norms and conditions can be characterized in four words: objectification, individualization, abstraction, and medical disease classification.[2] Each of these norms has been defined in the ongoing legal jurisprudence over 30 years, as part of the process of decriminalizing euthanasia. Each is connected to one of four landmark cases. The first norm is from a regional court (Leeuwarden, 1974) and the other three decisions (1984, 1994, 2002) are from the Dutch Supreme Court, the so-called Hoge Raad.[a]

Jurisprudence and the law are based on two fundamental convictions: It is *possible to assess the suffering* of a patient who asks for euthanasia; there is room *within the professional ethos of physicians* for a *justifiable obligation to honor the request*. A physician may be excused for ending a life if that physician feels an obligation to help a patient die actively and is experiencing a conflict of medical duties – namely, to alleviate the patient's suffering and to protect life. In addition, according to a 1984 policy decision of the KNMG, there is no principled medical professional objection to ending the life of an incurable, seriously ill patient when and if the conditions of the law, the so-called criteria of due care, have been satisfied.

How should these "legal ingredients" be understood as they apply to a proper assessment of suffering?

Objectification implies that a physician should construct an argued case. The norms and consecutive steps of the argument should be made transparent, and the final decision should be made in agreement with the patient on the basis of the facts and perceived dilemmas of the situation.

Individualization focuses on defining the physician's conflict of duties in terms of the facts of the case and the individual patient. This individualized focus allows for a lot of latitude, if it can be justified by the facts of a case. There are, however, certain limits that are non-negotiable. A physician will be excused for taking a life only when there is a voluntary request and when the assessment procedure includes a psychiatric evaluation concerning any doubt about a patient's competence or if there is a history of psychiatric disease.

Abstraction implies that it is not the source of suffering – that is, physical or psychic – that determines whether euthanasia is justifiable; rather, it is the seriousness and depth of the suffering. This abstraction is not without limits, however, and those limits are determined through classification.

Classification focuses on the requirement that there be a *clinical* diagnosis that is within the domain of medicine in order to provide a basis for the physician's appeal regarding a conflict of duties. A patient who claims to suffer unbearably because of certain life experiences or loss of meaning in life will not qualify for euthanasia. That is essentially the significance of the term *classification*. We shall demonstrate how this term functions with respect to the policies of the KNMG and the conception of suffering employed by the ERCs.

THE MEDICAL ASSOCIATION'S DESCRIPTION OF THE ASSESSMENT OF SUFFERING

The KNMG published guidance on physicians' duties to assess suffering in 1984, in 1995, and in an addendum in 1998. The KNMG's work is the first effort by a

[a] See Chapter 12 on Euthanasia Review Committees.

professional medical body to come to terms with a physician's perceived duty to assess suffering, and to develop a conceptual framework that encompasses the individual patient's experience of suffering and the physician's obligations in treating severely suffering patients. The KNMG focuses on the physician's obligation to objectify suffering, turn it into an intersubjective agreement with the patient, and be able to communicate about it – thus satisfying the conditions of objectification, individualization, abstraction, and classification.

The KNMG's pragmatic, but broad and balanced, view toward the suffering that justifies euthanasia is reflected in how that suffering is described in the policy. The adjectives used in 1995 were "durable," "unbearable," "serious," and "hopeless." Each of these terms has a certain overlap with the others. Admittedly, a certain measure of subjectivity seems to be unavoidable given patients' differences in their pain experiences and their abilities to accept the inevitable end of life.[3] The KNMG focused more on patients' experiences and less on differences in physicians' perceptions. Although physicians look at suffering in a professional, objective way, the KNMG was of the opinion that the physician must integrate the individual patient's experience into that perspective. Thus, the physician must arrive at a balanced evaluation that rests on a mutual assessment of the suffering:

> The unbearable and hopeless nature of someone's suffering is very much dependent on individual norms and values, meaning that its evidence may not always be immediately perceptible [in Dutch, *invoelbaar*; in German, *einfülbar*] to someone else. Although the subjective experience of the patient carries much weight, the Board maintains the opinion that there should be in principle an "intersubjectively unbearable situation," i.e., that the patient's experience must also be immediately perceptible [*invoelbaar* in the original Dutch text] to the responsible physician. In the end, because how durable, unbearable, and hopeless an individual's suffering is cannot be directly accessible for evaluation and verification, the patient's experience is always decisive. The physician must "empathically perceive" [*invoelen*] – i.e., be able to experience and yet assess and objectify – the suffering to be able to concur with a request for euthanasia.[b]

With respect to the cause of suffering, either somatic or psychic, the KNMG's policy states:

> Dispute about the nature of suffering obscures rather than clarifies the debate.... Whether the cause of suffering is deemed to be psychic or somatic, it remains the case that the suffering is primarily the subjective experience of this particular patient. The cause of the suffering does not determine how the suffering is experienced. If the suffering cannot be alleviated, it is irrelevant whether its origin is psychic or somatic. Nonetheless, according to the Supreme Court, extreme caution is warranted if and when the suffering does not originate demonstrably from a somatic disease or affliction and only exists in experiences of pain or loss of functions and

[b] 3. KNMG 1995, 26.

the suffering insofar as its seriousness and hopeless nature, especially, is more difficult to assess.[c]

Thus, whatever the physician perceives and verifies through communication must adequately reflect the patient's experience of suffering.

THE IDEAS OF THE EUTHANASIA REVIEW COMMITTEES ON SUFFERING

How do ERCs look at suffering? In their 2007 Annual Report, the ERCs described the concept of suffering that forms the basis for their work and how physicians should look at it.[4] A physician's report must satisfy two substantive conditions: the presence of a voluntary and well-considered request and the presence of unbearable, hopeless suffering "without prospect for improvement":

> The physician must find the patient's suffering to be palpably unbearable and must convince the committee of this. The committees are well aware that the question of suffering can sometimes be a difficult one for the physician to answer, and have therefore focused on it in more detail in this report.
>
> Suffering is a complex experience, like pain, love, hope or despair. It is a fundamental part of human life, and can often be recognized as such more readily than it can be put into words.
>
> Any description of suffering is therefore a reconstruction of components of suffering to form as complete a picture as possible, based on what the suffering patient says and on [the physician's] observations of the patient. In that sense, suffering is an "intersubjective experience" that can to some extent be communicated, and hence assessed. As the Royal Dutch Medical Association has stated, "assessments by physicians are based on the assumption that suffering is to some extent palpable [*invoelen*]."[d,5]

It is important to reflect on the term *invoelen* (in German, *einfühlen*), which is key to understanding physicians' assessment of suffering. In the Dutch discussions of euthanasia, *invoelen* has the meaning of "recognition by feeling." It may be best translated as "to grasp and understand intuitively and rationally after identifying with the object of perception," rather than "palpable." I will return to this subject later.

The report then continues:

> To understand and communicate suffering in connection with the end of life, we often use a conceptual framework based on the notion of "the person in medicine," in which people are seen as physical, mental, social and spiritual/existential beings. Suffering is then classified according to whether it has a physical, mental or existential cause. People's differing perceptions of suffering caused by similar factors are described as "subjective," which usually implies that they are beyond other people's

[c] 3. KNMG 1995, 27.

[d] 5. Euthanasia Review Committee 2007, 16 ff.

ability to comprehend. Reflecting on what suffering means also involves facing the fact that the most frequently used conceptual framework has its limitations. The medical concept of the human being is in itself sufficiently broad and abstract to identify the most common symptoms of disease and abnormal behavior, but it is too limited to help us understand all the main elements of a phenomenon as complex as suffering. Finding a definition of suffering means describing an experience that involves a threat to intact existence and the decay or disintegration of the personality.

It should be remembered that all suffering is existential, regardless of the cause, because people who suffer are existential beings. The perception of pain is based on a mind that can perceive it, and in that sense all suffering – even suffering that has a physical cause – is mental suffering. Without a mind to perceive suffering, human beings cannot suffer. This means that suffering is not "subjective" in the sense described above, but it is linked to a subject or person. It is thus by definition personal: "bodies do not suffer, persons do."[6] Besides the physical, mental, social and existential aspects, this concept of the individual includes the notion of man as a being with a perception of time and expectations of the future, a being whose life is informed by a need for meaning or meaningfulness. And it is these very aspects, such as the loss of future prospects and the perception that life no longer has any meaning, that are reflected in many requests for euthanasia when patients indicate why life is now unbearable for them.

The requirement that the patient's suffering be "unbearable with no prospect of improvement" does not make it easier to reach a conclusion, but it does not make it impossible. All the aspects of a particular person's suffering can be brought together to form a whole that in its *totality* is unbearable for this patient.

Philosophical Positions

Is it possible to assess suffering adequately?

There are countless descriptions of and ideas about suffering, but "the majority of definitions of suffering are too narrow and simplistic, conceptualizing suffering only as degree of physical and/or psychological pain."[7] All of these discussions share two fundamental features: that suffering is a universal human experience, [8] and that suffering entails a prima facie duty to relieve it.[9] Suffering is a "lived experience" of the whole person, not an isolated medical event, and is much more than pain. There seems to be a general agreement with Eric Cassell's definition of suffering "as a state of distress induced by a threat of the loss of intactness or the disintegration of a person from whatever cause"; further, "suffering is a consequence of personhood – bodies do not suffer, persons do."[10] The duty to alleviate suffering rests on two questions: First is an epistemological question: Can someone else grasp/understand/assess the suffering of another human being? Second is a moral question: If persons suffer and others can empathically perceive the response, is there a moral obligation to relieve suffering? And if so, what are the nature and limits of such a duty? These two questions define the morality of suffering in health care.

UNDERSTANDING THE SUFFERING OF ANOTHER HUMAN BEING

Is it possible to understand and objectify suffering – that is, can we get a clear picture of the suffering of a patient? The answer is that we can, but the issue is how correct this picture is. The KNMG maintains that physicians should be able to *invoelen,* "sympathize to a certain extent," in order to be able to concur with a request for euthanasia. There is a limit to the possibility of assessment. We cannot feel exactly what another person experiences, but we can approach it and come close to an adequate assessment. Let us try to narrow down some existing ideas on the possibility of an assessment: How close can one come to the suffering of another human being, in general and in medicine?

We usually think of suffering – or love, or despair – as an experience that we can recognize, especially when it is communicated. However, most people would probably agree with Cassell's statement that "[suffering is necessarily individual. We *cannot* know the origins of suffering within the sufferer."[10] But suffering is not *only* individual. Suffering is an experience that we share because we are from one and the same human tribe.

Cassell argues that it is possible to engage in someone's suffering on the basis of *compassion* and *transcendence* in human relationships, because we are not atomistic individuals incapable of engaging in each others' experiences. There is a world that we share. But there is no clear mirror image or reflection of the experience of suffering; there is always a "veil" between our experience and that of another. Observing the experience of suffering is not the same kind of activity as reading a thermometer or listening to a heart murmur. The observation of suffering implies a certain emotional commitment, even though some physicians tend to disagree. For example, Thomas Natsoulas takes an extreme position: "A physician who wishes to alleviate a patient's suffering may need to be intensely aware of the suffering in order to determine its nature and source, yet the physician need not be engaged in sympathizing."[11] That is, the patient's suffering does not have to "move" the physician "to want to help the other.... [T]he physician's intense awareness of the suffering of another may be no more affective than the physician's awareness of street directions to a medical conference."[12] I disagree.

M. E. Duffy's research reveals the different factors that shape the ways in which health-care professionals experience a patient's suffering. He found that nurses' inferences about patient suffering were "significantly related to their own socioeconomic and cultural backgrounds, patient ethnicity and patient diagnoses, but not to nurse age, marital status, education, experience, specialty practice, or patient gender."[7] If that is true, then there are certain barriers or confounders to a clear assessment of suffering. Some, such as Jamie Mayerfield, claim that such barriers are dependent upon sociological and psychological differences – that is, that there are unconscious and even "deeply irrational" factors at work.[9]

One of the most common responses to the suffering of others may well be denial, which reflects an effort to protect ourselves and our emotions. That type of reaction may be normal in daily life, especially when the quantity of mass media exposure numbs our ability to acknowledge suffering. But this type of numbing or denial does not occur when we enter into relationships, especially those in which we have the obligation to confront and try to alleviate the suffering of others. Such confrontation causes anxiety and provokes reactions that are both rational and irrational. It forces us to acknowledge the existence of the other's suffering, as well as our own vulnerability and mortality. Although it is possible to become numb to suffering in daily life and to deny this anxiety, that isn't possible once there is a connection between the observer and the suffering human being. Our response is shaped by what we see, as well as the confrontation between "our unconscious [and] its deepest fears."[e]

The effect of this unconscious barrier is a tendency to minimize suffering, which creates "a formidable obstacle to accurate moral understanding. It leads us to underrate the evilness of suffering, and consequently the urgency of eliminating it."[f]

Denying the anxiety provoked by suffering is impossible in a professional relationship that implies an obligation to alleviate that suffering. Doctors deal with such anxiety by maintaining a certain distance that enables them to confront the patient's suffering, without succumbing to denial. While the suffering is palpable and the physician can "sympathize to a certain extent," there is a cost: Though recognized, the suffering is minimized.

In psychiatry, this phenomenon is known as *transference* and *coutertransference*. In psychiatric practice, the terms refer to the psychiatrist's conscious and unconscious attitudes and feelings toward his or her patients, and the projections of patients onto the therapist. But the phenomenon is not limited to psychiatry; in fact, it occurs in all medical decisions that are filled with emotion, especially in the area of terminal illness and in the face of suffering.[13] Some have concluded that the risk of countertransference makes it impossible to assess the suffering of a patient who requests assisted suicide or euthanasia. As Francis Varghese and Brian Kelly, for example, argue:

> The subjective evaluation by a doctor of a patient's "quality of life" and the role of such an evaluation in making end-of-life decisions of themselves raise significant countertransference issues. Inaccurately putting oneself "in the patient's shoes" in order to make clinical decisions and evaluations of quality of life leave the patient vulnerable to the doctor's personal and unrecognized issues concerning illness, death and disability.[g,14]

[e] 9. Mayerfield 1999, 105.

[f] 9. Mayerfield 1999, 105.

[g] 14. Varghese and Kelly 1999, 92.

Given these formidable obstacles, why then does the Dutch medical profession believe that adequate assessment is possible at all?

FOR PURPOSES OF ASSESSMENT: THE DIFFERENCE BETWEEN A *REQUEST* FOR HELP IN DYING AND THE NECESSARY CONDITION OF A DEEPER *RELATIONSHIP*

Two considerations are crucial for understanding how physicians can accurately assess a patient's suffering. One involves the consequences of a patient's request to end life; the other reflects the fact that physicians do not "put themselves in the patient's shoes," but instead enter into a new phase in their relationship with the patient. In societies in which ending a life is not allowed, suffering remains a "quality" or characteristic *of the patient* – that is, something physicians everywhere have a moral obligation to alleviate as much as possible, up to and including the provision of palliative sedation. In the Dutch context, a patient's request to die engenders a relationship that goes beyond the normal professional patient–physician relationship, in which the suffering becomes, at least in part, a function *of that relationship*. That assessment of suffering, which leads to the conclusion that "it has been enough," is only possible within a reciprocal relationship between two competent human beings. Thus, Dutch physicians refuse to end the lives of advanced Alzheimer patients, even when there is an advance directive that asks for an active end of life when and if there is no more quality to continued living. Apparently, and perhaps not surprisingly, it is impossible to help a person die when there is no reciprocal relationship, at least not in the context of health care.[h]

The obligation to alleviate suffering is universal in health care and cannot be evaded – particularly in a culture in which the professional relationship includes the option of euthanasia. That obligation requires that physicians not become as disengaged as they otherwise might, and that they be accountable for sustaining objectivity in the patient–physician relationship. A request for help with dying changes that relationship in a fundamental way, both psychologically and cognitively.

The relationship is changed psychologically because the request to end a patient's life causes the physician to be more immediately aware of, or attuned to, the patient's situation than would otherwise be the case. This is the *conditional request*: If and when —, then —. The cognitive change is based on the knowledge that the patient's suffering may lead to a request for help in dying at some point in the treatment – that is, *the actual request*.

It is crucial to correctly assess the patient's suffering at the moment of the actual request. At that moment, physicians realize that the road they take will lead to a grave decision that is not without consequences for them personally

[h] See also Chapter 14 by Hertogh in this volume.

and professionally. Patients who request help with dying compel the physician to identify with their suffering over and beyond the limits of the physician's own fears. The physician must engage in a process of rational assessment in order to agree that the patient's suffering has become so severe that it is acceptable to end his or her life. Physicians also realize they will have to tell the ERCs how they reached their conclusion about the patient's suffering and decided to act. They realize that their decision will be evaluated by outsiders.

In ordinary circumstances of care, even care for terminally ill patients, physicians are able to overcome – to a certain extent – the tendency to distort the meaning of suffering and to deny its existence. Physicians can mediate the psychological weight of experiences of suffering. They develop a level of awareness and focus that enables them to overcome their own fears and anxieties. A vast body of literature and many teaching programs document the possibility of caring well for suffering patients and addressing their suffering. However, there is a fundamental difference between caring for a suffering patient and assessing that suffering once the patient has requested euthanasia. Dutch physicians who have provided euthanasia report that they would not have been able to do so without building a more personal relationship.[15] Such relationships are fundamental in order to adequately assess the patient's suffering – not only because of greater sustained intensity and mutuality but also because of the continued level of awareness over a longer period of time.

Euthanasia is never simply an act to end a life; rather, it is a process, sometimes short – a couple of days – but more often weeks or months. There is a relationship in which the severity of suffering is continuously assessed within the context of diminishing treatment options. In this process of assessment, the treatment options play an essential role. In the end, both patient and physician must come to an agreement that there are no more options. Euthanasia is not the opposite of palliative care, but it is always an option after all palliative-care interventions have been exhausted or are no longer acceptable for a patient.

From a psychological point of view, the physician – who must go on living with the experience of having ended a life – must be convinced that in this particular case, with this particular patient, ending life was the respectful road to take. This implies the need for intimacy and knowledge of the patient as a person and as a human being with a life story, in order to understand why suffering has become unbearable for this patient at this moment – and all this must occur within the limits of a professional medical relationship.

The American anthropologist Frances Norwood observed the evolution of patient–physician relationships in her study of Amsterdam physicians treating seriously ill patients.[16] Norwood observed what she described as "euthanasia discourse" among the 25 patients and 10 physicians in her study – that is, a continuous process of discussing the patient's medical condition and impending death after a request for help with dying. Even when the process did not result in the physician's taking action to help the patient die, it enabled *patients to control their movement through the specific phases leading to termination of life.* Norwood distinguished those phases as the initial request, the discussion of treatment options, the actual request for the near or sometimes immediate future, the agreement to seek consultation, the actual consultation, and the intervention to end life. Her prospective study made it clear that patients, not physicians, initiate the shift from one phase to the next. This process is a true discourse that involves continuous deliberation and discussion.

CONCEPTUAL FRAMEWORK FOR ASSESSING SUFFERING

In the context of euthanasia, the assessment of suffering requires both *objectification and classification* and *individualization and abstraction.* The physician considering euthanasia must distance him- or herself from the patient to a greater degree than what occurs from the therapeutic perspective of "ordinary" medicine; at the same time, he or she must become closer to the patient in order to determine what suffering means for this particular person.

The physician must observe the patient's *medical* signs, symptoms, and loss of functions with a clear, objective, outsider's eye, seeing developments over time and knowing which signs will get worse or remain static. But the physician must also read the same signs, symptoms, and losses closely in order to understand their *existential* meaning for the patient.

Conceptually, then, assessing suffering in the context of euthanasia combines the analytic/empirical *and* the hermeneutic. Assessment of suffering must take signs and symptoms in the here and now into account – that is, a synchronic dimension – and note how they evolve over time – a diachronic dimension. The assessment must be informed by a moral anthropology that recognizes humans as beings who live in time, have awareness of time and future, and are composed of both a body and a mind that interact in many ways; it must recognize humans as both individuals – persons who have their own ways of experiencing the world – and social beings who interact with others and whose lives involve a social context.

The patient's suffering must be *unbearable* and *hopeless* – that is, without prospect of improvement – for euthanasia to be ethically justified. The physician must consider the suffering in relation to *time, personality, biography,* and *context* as follows:[17,18]

Suffering and Time

- Fear of *future* suffering: That is, what specific suffering does the patient fear and what is the source of this fear (the disease condition itself or the patient's imagination or past experience)? Can the fear be treated, through either psychological or pharmaceutical interventions?
- *Current* (or *actual*) suffering: that is, current symptoms, complaints, and loss of function. These include clinical symptoms, such as nausea, cachexia, fatigue, and so on; loss of function, such as the ability to walk, to care for,

bathe, or feed oneself or carry out other activities of daily living independently; and to communicate, to speak, to hear, to see, to write, and so on.

Current suffering, as we have noted, has both a synchronic and a diachronic dimension:

- *Synchronic* – that is, symptoms and so on that exist at this particular moment; and
- *Diachronic* – that is, the development of symptoms and loss of function over time.

The latter distinction is important in discussing with the patient the reality of impending symptoms that will worsen or the development of new symptoms. It may be even more important to discuss the potential development of symptoms over time in order to hear from patients where they would draw, or have drawn, a line, while recognizing that patients' perspectives and preferences are not stable, that people later in the course of illness tend to adapt to situations that they would not have – or thought they could not have – in earlier phases.

Suffering and Personality

To find out why a particular human being concludes that "enough is enough," it is necessary to find out how a person feels about particular symptoms. This often reflects the patient's personality and directly relates to his or her personal conceptions of dignity, one of the major reasons patients ask for an end to life. The loss of the ability to walk means a great deal for an independent, active person coping with the effects of a disease. If a person is used to reading and writing, the most important factors may be loss of vision or hand function. On a more physical level, incontinence and the loss of privacy in matters of personal hygiene can be an immense burden for someone who needs physical distance – as compared to someone who does not experience the intimacy of personal care as negative.

Suffering and Biography (Personality over Time)

A patient's biography provides additional insight into the limits of his or her endurance. Important biographical details include the individual's professional life, marital relations, religion, and, most significantly, how he or she has coped with disease in the past. One needs to understand personal conceptions of dignity – that is, how the patient would cope with the loss of independence and being forced to live a life of dependence on others. The loss of partners or parents and other shocking or violent experiences also play in role in assessing the patient's suffering.

Suffering and Context

Under this heading, the focus is on context of care: the living situation, the team of caregivers, the need for care versus the ability to provide care, and the feeling of being a burden to others.

In general, context by itself almost never qualifies as sufficient grounds for concluding that a patient's suffering is unbearable. It can, however, be important in the patient's own assessment of the limits of endurance and when they have been reached. One example of the relevance of this criterion is observed in patients with chronic neurological diseases who have maintained their independence over a long time with additional help from professional and family caretakers. They may find that forced admission to institutional care is an absolute limit they do not wish to accept.

"Hopeless" Suffering

The term *hopeless*, meaning without a prospect of improvement, has a legal and a medical connotation. The legal connotation applies to the medical diagnosis and treatment: A patient's suffering is hopeless if there are no more medical options to reverse a patient's condition and the disease will lead to an inevitable death. From the medical perspective, there is an additional meaning that focuses on the individual patient's experiences and feelings. During the course of disease and treatment, patients react in a personal and individual way to the symptoms and loss of functions when there are no options to heal. In addition, they experience loss of meaning in life and loss of appetite for living. Each person has his or her own moment in time when this loss of meaning reaches a point at which "enough is enough." At that point, the individual will ask for an active end to life – that is, the "actual request." It is striking to notice that if and when that moment has arrived, patients tend to become insistent on ending their lives. It is a significant indication of the way the patient–physician relationship usually evolves that the *patient* initiates the next step, but has enough respect to wait for the physician to come to an agreement.

This "waiting for the physician to agree" becomes apparent when, for example, patients refuse palliative measures that physicians believe might alleviate their suffering. Such options are usually determined by the intervention's potential to alleviate suffering versus its side effects for the individual patient.

REFLECTIONS, OBJECTIONS

Patients are able to describe why they have come to a decision that their suffering is no longer something they can endure. They base their decisions on how long they have struggled with their disease, their personalities, particularly in the present context, and the absence of chances for improvement.

The physician's conclusion that the patient's suffering is unbearable is reached through communication with the patient. The physician is not the final, unilateral arbiter. Rather, the intention, and the grounding presumption, is that there should be – and most often is – an intersubjective agreement between patient and physician.

Conceptual frameworks that are methodologically sound can result in desired and intended effects. But when the framework is novel, its use can – as might be expected – result in strong reactions and criticism. We found this to be the case when we began training consultants to use the aforementioned framework for assessing suffering, with the goal of ensuring some uniformity in applying the framework.[i] We observed that every physician has his or her own personal way of assessing suffering – for example, using references from daily practice, *treating* pain and symptoms, and looking at the here and now of usual pain assessment. These methods do not usually include a more conceptual construction that encompasses notions of time, personality, biography, and context, as well as the "medical" aspects (symptoms, loss of function, etc.). This framework can be integrated into a physician's approach, but it is not as straightforward as learning a new medical intervention. The process is inhibited by emotions and attitudes that appear to be indications of the general and medical professional ambivalence toward suffering.

Perception of Assessment as Unethical

Physicians have told us that they must overcome primal reactions when assessing suffering after a request for assistance in dying. They have described assessment as "almost unethical" from a certain perspective. The assessment of another person's suffering in order to judge whether that suffering is enough to ethically and legally justify a desired death was experienced as being disrespectful to another human being. Some went so far as to say that such evaluations or assessments are "almost" unacceptable invasions of a patient's inner life.

This hesitation reflects ambivalence toward a closer relationship, and fails to give enough intellectual credit to the societal dimension and the societal stake in ending a life. If society had no stake in the decision to terminate life, assessing the patient's suffering would be solely an interpersonal matter, in which society and social values were reduced to zero. Two objections to this reduction are important because they reflect the unique constellation of personal and societal values that interact in decisions to provide euthanasia.

The first objection is that asking someone for help with dying implies *an involvement of that person* (the physician), and thus the need to recognize that person *as a moral agent* with his or her own set of values. A physician who ends the life of a human being must be able to live with that decision; if the decision is to be morally acceptable, the physician must feel caught in a moral dilemma between ending unbearable and hopeless suffering and protecting life. If the dilemma is not recognized, it leads to undesired prolongation of meaningless suffering. It is only when the physician becomes truly involved, in order to establish the presence of that type of suffering, that the action becomes one of compassion.

[i] See Chapter 14 on consultants.

The second objection is that it is a crime to deliberately end a life, no matter what the circumstances. This view has been reflected in the euthanasia debates all through the ages. Until very recently, the only "official" means by which a physician could help a terminally ill patient die has been through "passive euthanasia" – that is, through the use of interventions intended to alleviate suffering but that have a possible but unintended effect of shortening life.[j] Within this framework, the physician was not viewed as the actor; rather, the disease was the cause of death.

This issue of intention is a so-called gray area. Even when physicians stop life-sustaining treatments, or shorten life by increasing doses of narcotics with the intention of reducing pain or suffering, they do not have to confront their decisions because they never "intended" to shorten life. Formal procedures for euthanasia move away from this self-absolving approach; they "call a spade a spade" and require physicians to assume responsibility for their decisions and actions when they accede to a patient's request to die. In order to absolve physicians from an act that would be a crime if it were performed by anyone else, Dutch society has demanded transparency from physicians.

Concern That Assessment May Be Subjective, and Thus Arbitrary

There are some other objections to the assessment of unbearable suffering, even among supporters of euthanasia. One concerns the supposedly arbitrary nature of assessment, expressed in the value-laden term *subjective*. "Subjective" determinations, it is argued, have lesser stature than "objective" ones, and may be arbitrary. They may even lead to undesired – and undesirable – differences in the conclusions reached by different physicians and patients, despite similarities in patients' diseases and symptoms. Insofar as objectivity – that is, independent of personal choices and coloring – is the desired norm, every assessment becomes suspect and carries the risk that patients will be treated unequally.

This accusation of arbitrariness can be countered, however. For one thing, every assessment is based on information and input from both the treating physician and the patient, and is confirmed by the patient's medical history. At the very least, then, every assessment is "intersubjective." More importantly, every assessment is a construction of facts and conclusions that make the judgment transparent. This construction provides insight and is open to critical analysis. This level of "accessibility" in assessments *can* be reached and can serve as a general norm.

Moreover, from the perspective that recognizes suffering as inescapably individual, it is almost self-evident that individual persons, with own their life

[j] The terms *passive* or *active* in connection with euthanasia are no longer used in the Dutch debate because they add insufficient discriminatory value.

histories and personalities, will differ in their reactions to suffering, no matter how similar their medical conditions. Such differences in response to suffering should be deliberately integrated into the joint, intersubjective conclusion reached by patient and physician. The transparency and validity of this conclusion is evaluated by the question asked of the physician during the legally required consultation: "Why do you think that the suffering of this patient has become unbearable?"

CONCLUSIONS

I have argued that assessment of suffering in medicine, in general, is possible but can get caught up in psychological issues that often lead to failure to recognize and treat suffering. The key difference in the assessment of suffering in the context of euthanasia is that such a request changes the physician–patient relationship in a fundamental way, rendering it more personal. This different, more "connected," less distant relationship becomes a condition for the adequate assessment of suffering and for the possibility of ethically ending the patient's life. In such a relationship, the assessment of suffering has "objective" elements, with respect to observable symptoms and loss of functions. The intersubjective conclusions reached by physicians and patients, with respect to what the suffering means to patients and their ability to endure it or to decide that "enough is enough," are even more significant. Most Dutch physicians, patients, and families experience this type of connection, and physicians see this level of involvement as part of their professional attitudes and the medical ethos.

References

1. The Termination of Life on Request and Assisted Suicide (Review Procedures) Act (Review Procedures for the Termination of Life on Request and Assisted Suicide and Amendment of the Criminal Code and the Burial and Cremation Act) of 2002.
2. Pans, Esther. 2006. *De normatieve grondslagen van het Nederlandse euthanasierecht* [The normative foundations of the Dutch jurisprudence and law on euthanasia]. Thesis, Vrije Universiteit, 81ff. Amsterdam: WLP.
3. KNMG (Royal Dutch Medical Association). 1995. Standpunt Hoofdbestuur (Position paper of the Board).
4. Regionale Toetsingscommissies Euthnanasie (Regional Euthanasia Evaluation Committees). 2007. Volume IIb, 14–16. Den Haag: Koninklijke De Swart. For an English translation see: http://www.euthanasiecommissies.nl.
5. Euthanasia Review Committee (ERC). 2007. Annual Report 2007, 16ff.
6. Cassell, E. J. 1992. The Nature of Suffering: Physical, Psychological, Social, and Spiritual Aspects. In *The Hidden Dimension of Illness: Human Suffering*, ed. Patricia L. Starck and John P. McGovern, 3. New York: The National League of Nursing Press.

7. Duffy, M. E. 1992. A theoretical and empirical review of the concept of suffering. In *The Hidden Dimension of Illness: Human Suffering*, ed. Patricia L. Starck and John P. McGovern, 299. New York: The National League for Nursing Press.
8. Starck, Patricia L., and John P. McGovern. 1992. The Meaning of Suffering. In *The Hidden Dimension of Illness: Human Suffering*, ed. Patricia L. Starck and John P. McGovern, 25ff. New York: The National League for Nursing Press.
9. Mayerfield, Jamie. 1999. *Suffering and Moral Responsibility*. New York: Oxford University Press.
10. Cassell E. J. 1992. The Nature of Suffering: Physical, Psychological, Social and Spiritual Aspects. In *The Hidden Dimension of Illness: Human Suffering*, ed. Patricia L. Starck and John P. McGovern, 9. New York: The National League for Nursing Press
11. Welie, Jos. 1998. *In the Face of Suffering: The Philosophical-Anthropological Foundations of Clinical Ethics*. Omaha, NE: Creighton University Press.
12. Natsoulas, Thomas. 1988. Sympathy, empathy, and the stream of consciousness. *Journal for the Theory of Social Behavior* 18: 169–195.
13. Stein, Howard. 1987. *The Psychodynamics of Medical Practice: Unconscious Factors in Patient Care*. Chicago: University of Chicago Press.
14. Varghese, Francis T., and Brian Kelly. 1999. Countertransference and assisted suicide. In *Countertransference Issues in Psychiatric Treatment*, ed. Glen O. Gabbard, M.D., 85–117. Review of Psychiatry 18. Washington, DC: American Psychiatric Press.
15. Clark, Chalmers C., and Gerrit K. Kimsma. 2004. "Medical Friendships" in assisted dying. *Cambridge Quarterly of Health Care Ethics* 13: 61–67.
16. Norwood, F. 2005. Euthanasia talk: Euthanasia discourse, general practice and end-of-life care in the Netherlands: The role of family in euthanasia decision making. Ph.D. diss., University of California San Francisco and Berkeley.
17. Kimsma, Gerrit K. 2000. Het lijden beoordeeld: een voorstel voor een conceptueel kader [The assessment of suffering: A proposal for a conceptual frame]. *Medisch Contact* 55: 1757–1759.
18. Kimsma, Gerrit K. 2003. Objectivering van de zorgvuldigheidseisen inzake het verzoek en het lijden: aanpak, valkuilen en verslaglegging [Objectifying the conditions of prudence with respect to a request and suffering: Approach, pitfalls and reporting]. In *Levensbeëindigend handelen van een arts op verzoek van een patient* [Life ending by a physician after a request from a patient], ed. Johan Legemaate, and R. J. M. Dillmann, 77–107. Houten: Bohn Stafleu van Loghem.

PART VI

OVERVIEW

23

The Regulation of Euthanasia

How Successful Is the Dutch System?

Govert den Hartogh

Euthanasia[a] and physician-assisted suicide have been legal in the Netherlands since 1984, first by judicial legislation and since 2002 by statute, if enacted by a doctor who meets a number of requirements of due care and makes it possible to assess whether he or she met them. How successful is this Dutch model?[b] The answer to that question of course depends on what we understand "success" to mean. In this chapter, I will try to assess the extent to which the Dutch model is successful *on its own terms*. I will therefore start in §1 by explaining the underlying morality of the Dutch law, which informs both the substantive and procedural requirements of due care. This will give us the frame of reference we need for judging the success of the system.

Of course, many people will not be happy with these moral foundations of the legal system themselves because on their view, they do not sufficiently respect either the sanctity of human life or the autonomy of patients. For such people, the system is inherently flawed because it is either too liberal or too paternalistic. Even for them, however, it will be of some interest to have the system evaluated on its own terms because a common view of foreign observers has always been that it has failed as such.[1,2,3,4,c] In §2 and §3 I will discuss the main points of criticism, which concern the reporting rate and the number of cases in which patients' lives have been ended without their explicit request. In addition, in §4 I will consider the criticism that what doctors consider to be

[a] Although I am not particularly fond of this piece of verbal legislation, I use the term *euthanasia* in the sense that is by now common in the Netherlands: ending a person's life on his or her explicit request. Ending life in the person's (assumed) interest but without request is not included.

[b] I will not explain the model; this has been done extensively in other chapters of this volume (see Chapter 2 by Legemaate and Chapter 3 by Weyers).

[c] All using data from the national survey reports of 1991, 1996, and 2003; see § 2. Similar judgments have been made by the Canadian Special Senate Committee on Euthanasia and Assisted Suicide 1995, and by the U.S. Supreme Court in *Vacco* v. *Quill*, 521 U.S. 793 (1997).

terminal sedation should often be seen as euthanasia (and reported as such), and in §5 the criticism that the whole system of monitoring and control is only a façade, because it never leads to the criminal sanctioning of any doctor violating the requirements.

Another criticism is that the actual practice as it has developed since the introduction of the consultation requirement and the Regional Review Committees is too restrictive, that it excludes people from access to a relatively humane death who should be eligibile in terms of the law itself. I will discuss this problem and proposals to deal with it in the final sections.

1. THE MORAL FOUNDATIONS OF THE DUTCH EUTHANASIA LAW

People who defend the justifiability of euthanasia or physician-assisted suicide under certain circumstances almost invariably argue in favor of, and by appeal to, some radical revision of commonsense morality. And opponents likewise believe that in addition to pointing out slippery-slope concerns, their only task consists in defending those same tenets of commonsense morality that the other party wants to revise. In this way, it has been argued by most advocates, prominently Ronald Dworkin and the other authors of the 1997 "Philosopher's Brief,"[5] that the prohibition of euthanasia conflicts with people's right to self-determination, which should allow not only a person to end his or her own life but also others to do this on their request. It has been argued, for example by Peter Singer, that the prohibition of euthanasia rests on a mistaken belief in the sanctity of life. Others, beginning with James Rachels in 1975, have attempted to show that there is no morally relevant distinction between killing and letting die; hence, anyone who allows doctors to abstain from life-prolonging treatment should accept euthanasia under the same conditions. Many defendants of the prohibition, for example John Finnis, have appealed to the distinction between death as a means and death as unintended side effect, the so-called doctrine of double effect. Whether or not one accepts this doctrine or its application to this case as an essential part of commonsense morality, it is clear that something like it is subscribed to by traditional medical ethics, because it allows for palliative treatment with a possible life-shortening effect. Hence, this whole family of distinctions has also come under attack, for example from John Harris.[5,6,7,8,9]

Studying the underlying morality of the Dutch euthanasia law, we could ask which of these revisions of commonsense morality have been adopted by it. The answer turns out to be: none. The morality of the Dutch law is a completely traditional one.

This can be shown either in a historical or in a systematic way, by studying the decisions of the courts from 1984 on and the *travaux préparatoires* of the 2002 law, or by reconstructing the most plausible moral rationale of the actual provisions of the law. Both give the same result. The historical account has recently been provided by Esther Pans.[d,10,11] The aim of this section is to provide the reconstruction.

FOUNDATIONS 1. From the beginning of the Dutch revolt against Spain during the sixteenth century, the rebels discussed among themselves the justifications for their actions. Did they act *pro religione* or *pro libertate*, to protect the true religion or the ancient freedoms of towns and provinces? A similar discussion has gone on among advocates of the legalization of euthanasia in the Netherlands, from the beginning of the discussion about the subject, which can be dated exactly to 1969. This time, the battle cries were self-determination and mercy. During the first 10 years, both motives were appealed to more or less equally, occasionally by the same authors. Since that time, it has been self-determination that figures most prominently in the rhetoric of advocates, as well as in public opinion. If you only dare to use the term *mercy*, you will immediately be seen as an intolerable paternalist. I remember well that a lady who asked me a question about a talk I had given suddenly started to stamp her feet, crying "I don't want any mercy." That is a sentiment that many people will recognize.

There has never been a complete consensus, however. Notable exceptions include medical authors, in particular those who have been associated with the Royal Dutch Medical Association (KNMG).[e,12,13] This is important because the views of the association, in the Dutch political tradition of finding agreement among elites, tend to be much respected by both the courts and the legislation. Moreover, as we will see, public opinion is not very consistent in stressing everyone's right to decide the time of his or her own death. Not even the Dutch Association for Voluntary Euthanasia (NVVE) is fully consistent. For long years, every item of its monthly journal contained a sad story of a person who had to die miserably because no assistance in dying had been given. The primary response such stories aim to evoke in the reader does not seem to be "what a shame that the autonomy of this patient was not respected" but, rather, "what a pity that the patient had to suffer that much."

Nevertheless, with the exception of the doctors, almost every Dutch citizen who has thoughts about the matter tends to think that the law, as it has been codified by the 2002 statute, is founded on the right to self-determination, not on a principle of mercy. Remarkably, the reverse is true. The right to self-determination has, it is true, an essential role to play, but only as a side constraint, not as the basic justification. Of course, it is not acceptable to shorten the life of a competent patient, or a patient who can express any decision at all, if he or she does not request this action. But that doesn't mean that the law permits the action *because* of the request.

[d] Pans summarizes her findings in Chapter 4 in this volume. This interpretation of the law is by now more or less generally accepted.

[e] Even though the drafters of the bill were personally sympathetic to the principle of self-determination, by and large they implemented the view of the KNMG.

At first sight, it may seem that the euthanasia law puts both principles on an equal footing, each finding its expression in one of the two basic requirements of due care. The requirement that the patient make a voluntary and well-considered request is obvious because this is seen as a condition for the request being autonomous. And the requirement of unbearable and irreversible suffering points to the circumstances in which a proper appeal can be made to mercy. However, if the right to self-determination had been more than a side constraint, the second requirement could not have been made. If you want to respect a person's autonomous decisions, you should do so without any regard to the reasons for which they were made. For example, it follows from competent patients' right to self-determination that they can refuse any medical treatment, even if it promises to prolong life. Of course, they are allowed to refuse on good grounds; they don't need any special right for making that decision. The right implies that their refusal has equal authority in case their grounds are questionable. To have the authority to decide means that your decision stands, even if it is the wrong one to make. Hence, if the right to self-determination were to be the founding principle of the law, it would exclude other substantial requirements besides those concerning competence.

This argument can perhaps be withstood. A first counterargument could be that seemingly paternalistic requirements can sometimes be justified by the difficulties involved in establishing competence. In this way, the legislator could have insisted on the requirement of unbearable and irreversible suffering because that would be the only case in which no doubts concerning the voluntary and well-considered character of the request remained. This view, however, has never been advanced by any court nor during the parliamentary debate about the law. It is interesting to note, however, that this view was advanced during the parliamentary debate about the Belgian 2002 law.[14,f] It is a possible argument, but it carries a burden of proof that no one until now has attempted to meet, not even in the Belgian case.

Another possible way to show that an additional requirement is compatible with the right to self-determination as the basic justificatory principle would be to argue that it is only in cases in which a person suffers unbearably from a medical condition that cannot be expunged or alleviated that a doctor can have any involvement. But this raises the fundamental question of why the exception that the law introduces to the prohibition on euthanasia and assistance in suicide only applies to doctors. If self-determination is the leading idea, then this is hard to understand.

[f] I suspect that for similar reasons, the state of Oregon's Death with Dignity Act (1997) restricts the option of physician-assisted suicide to patients diagnosed with a terminal illness and a life expectancy of less than six months. The Swiss organizations that offer assistance in suicide also make additional requirements. For example Exit Deutsche Schweiz requires not only that the wish to die be deliberate and stable but also that the requester suffer from a disease with a hopeless prognosis and the suffering be unbearable or an unreasoanble disability be present (Exit statutes, Article 2).

The additional requirements made by the law show that it doesn't take the right to self-determination as its basic justificatory ground. This also tells us something about the rhetoric dominating the debate, for even if some participants to that debate prefer other additional requirements to the ones insisted on by the legislator, for example the irreversible loss of dignity, few participants insist on no additional requirements being made at all.[g] As for public opinion, 68% of the Dutch people agree with the statement that everyone has the right to decide about his or her own death, but only 15% agree that the means for ending one's life should be available for everyone who wants to die, whether severely ill or not.[15,16]

FOUNDATIONS 2. The Dutch legal development is deeply influenced by the Supreme Court's pathbreaking *Schoonheim* verdict of 1984. The court argued that Dr. P. L. Schoonheim had had a "conflict of duties" and therefore could appeal to necessity or *force majeure*. In the decision itself, the conflicting duties had not been specified precisely, but obviously we should think of the duty of everyone to respect human life and the professional duty of a physician to alleviate or prevent suffering. In succeeding decisions this was made explicit. The duty opposing the duty to respect human life could not have been a duty to respect autonomy, for that is a negative duty only: not to interfere with the execution of someone's self-regarding decisions. Such a duty can always be completely fulfilled by doing nothing at all. Hence, it cannot conflict with any other negative duty. The right to self-determination by itself does not imply a duty of assistance for anyone, and in any case, a *duty* to assist anyone in fulfilling a wish to die has never been recognized in Dutch law. (It is debatable whether it has been recognized in Belgian law.)[h,17]

FOUNDATIONS 3. In order to derive even the *permission* to assist, we have to go beyond the right to self-determination itself. This is something advocates of the right, for example within the Dutch Association for Voluntary Euthanasia, seldom realize. The additional premise that we need is the Volenti principle: *Volenti non fit iniuria*, or the consenting person cannot be wronged. However, within Dutch law (and European law generally), the Volenti principle is not taken to apply to the most fundamental, so-called inalienable human rights: the right to life, to bodily integrity, and to personal freedom. In respect to these rights, the law subscribes to a form of *indirect paternalism*[i,18,19]

As for the right to life, this is clear from the two articles of the Dutch Criminal Code, 293 and 294, which still forbid taking someone's life on his or her explicit and earnest request, and assisting that person in killing him- or

[g] See §8 in this chapter.

[h] Nor in Belgian law, although there has been some debate about this (see Adams in 17. Griffiths, Weyers, and Adams 2008).

[i] In my chapter of *Medical Ethics at the Dawn of the 21st Century*, I have discussed whether indirect paternalism is subject to the same objections as direct paternalism (as J. Feinberg asserts; see 19. den Hartogh 2000).

herself. The euthanasia law has left both articles in force, only adding an exception for physicians who satisfy the requirements of due care. If the Volenti principle applied to the right to life, it would have been impossible to restrict the exceptions to physicians. Accordingly, the duty that is supposedly in conflict with the right to life is not a general moral duty but only a professional duty of doctors.

As for the right to bodily integrity, it is clear that the Volenti principle applies to relatively minor infringements of it, as for example taking a sample of your blood in the course of a criminal investigation, or perhaps even for donation of a kidney by a living person. But it does not apply to major infringements, and, moreover, it does not apply to medical action generally. The so-called law on the contract of medical treatment,[j] in spite of talking the language of contract, is clear about this point: A competent patient always has the right to refuse any treatment, but cannot demand any treatment that in the professional opinion of the doctor is harmful to him or her on balance. The doctor, as the law states, always has to conform to the professional standard. If only for this reason, all talk about health care as a market like any other and patients as care consumers is basically mistaken. The same applies to the inclusion of a person in a medical experiment: His or her consent is not enough. The risks involved should always be minor, and in proportion to the importance of the experiment, and the consent of the participant is no defense for infringement of these requirements. Lastly, as a matter of unwritten law, consent is not a defense for a crime against personal freedom either. If a man is found chained in your cellar, you will not escape a prison sentence even if you can show a signed document confirming that person's consent to his treatment. Anyone who believes that a voluntary and well-considered request should be sufficient for justifying euthanasia can be asked the question: Should a person also have the power to sell him- or herself into slavery if it is done voluntarily? If not, what is the difference?

That the Volenti principle does not apply to the most basic human rights has clearly been stated by the European Court for Human Rights in two landmark British cases: the *Spanner* case regarding bodily integrity and the *Diane Pretty* case regarding the right to life.[k] The aim of such rights is not only aim to protect spheres of personal sovereignty.

The recent euthanasia law was presented as a codification of the court-made law already in place, nothing more and nothing less. For that reason, the ministers who proposed the law at first did not even find it necessary to explain its moral foundations, though in the course of the extensive parliamentary debate

[j] Wet op de Geneeskundige Behandelingsovereenkomst (WGBO), in force since 1995.

[k] *Laskey, Jaggard & Browm* v *UK*, February 19, 1997; *Pretty* v *UK*, April 29, 2002. Article 2 of the European Convention on Human Rights, recognizing the right to life, is said in this last verdict to be "unconcerned with issues to do with the quality of living or what a person chooses to do with his or her life."

they did provide that explanation.[10,17] Of course, the conflict of duties ceased to function as a relevant legal figure, because this had only been a specification of *force majeure* as a general justificatory basis for making exceptions to any legal norm, and for these exceptions the law did now provide a general formulation. Even in this respect, the law in a way did not change the legal situation, for a paradoxical aspect of the court-made law had been that the courts had already built a system of norms, including requirements of due care, on this essentially casuistic foundation. But except for this formal aspect, which the courts had already given up de facto and which the new statute necessarily had to give up de jure, the notion of a conflict of duties has a substantial aspect that the codification has left fully intact.

This is most prominently apparent in the fact that euthanasia is not considered to be "normal medical action." Normal medical action is covered by the so-called medical exception: The provisions in the criminal code about violation of bodily integrity have an implied reader saying: "doesn't apply to physicians acting in accordance with the professional standard." If a doctor amputates your leg in order to prevent gangrene from spreading throughout your body, he or she is not supposed to be fulfilling the delict description of severe bodily injury, not even with a justification. The norm forbidding such injury simply doesn't apply. The medical exception can be relevant to the prohibition of killing as well. For a physician can use pain-killing medicine and other palliative means in order to relieve the suffering of a dying patient, even if this foreseeably will, or may, shorten that patient's life. In evident cases, it may be his or her professional duty to act that way. Such an action doesn't count as euthanasia or murder; it is covered by the medical exception, and the death of the patient will be classified as a natural one.[l]

In the case of a conflict of duties, however, neither of the conflicting norms is set aside by the other; both norms are supposed to continue to apply, even if only one can be satisfied. That even the norm that will not be satisfied is still valid and applicable, in a sense, is shown by the existence of substitute duties, in this case in particular the duty to report one's action and thereby to submit it to external evaluation. But most prominently it appears in the fact, which I already referred to, that it can never be a professional duty of the doctor to grant a patient's request for euthanasia. It is at best a justifiable result of weighing the conflicting duties, the alternative way of weighing them being equally acceptable under the law. That euthanasia is not a form of normal medical action also explains why this form of action is subjected to a special system of evaluation that involves not only physicians but lawyers and ethicists as well. Euthanasia is subject not only to professional standards but also to special societal regulations.

[l] As we will see in §2, this cannot be explained because in such cases, the doctor doesn't "intend" the death of the patient.

When a doctor chooses palliative means that may shorten a patient's life, he or she should, if possible in dialogue with the patient, consider the best interest of the patient. What is more important to this patient, suffering less or living longer? If it is euthanasia under consideration, the weighing requirement is a different one: The patient's suffering should be unbearable and irreversible. Other interests of the patient, for example avoidance of being a burden to others, do not count at all. One could say that all medical action is a form of beneficence, but it would be odd to call it a form of mercy. To act from mercy, one must be moved by the suffering of someone else that is directly experienced. The justification of euthanasia doesn't follow from the normal professional duty to act in the interest of the patient, for this duty conflicts with another one, and this means that more is needed to tip the balance.

FOUNDATIONS 4. These considerations also tell us something about the other conflicting duty, the duty to respect human life. I have already argued that a right like this one does not protect a sphere of personal sovereignty, for then the Volenti principle should apply to it. But it now turns out that what is protected by the right to life is not merely a personal interest in continued living, for then some form of weighing this interest against other interests should be allowed. In protecting human life, the law is not only concerned with the personal value of the life, the value it has for the person living that life; it is also concerned with an impersonal element.[m] I will refer to this as the taboo on killing.

This taboo is extremely important in the experience of doctors, of Dutch doctors who do not a priori reject euthanasia in all cases no less than of any other doctor. Even if such doctors are convinced that it is in the best interest of a patient to die, they have to overcome considerable inner resistance in order to accept a request for euthanasia from that patient; it will usually cost them sleepless hours during the night. The reason is that they really experience the situation as involving a conflict of duties. If they could achieve the same result by abstaining from treatment or by an action that they could, perhaps with a certain amount of self-deception, interpret as a form of palliative care, they would greatly prefer such an alternative.[n] For similar reasons, most doctors prefer terminal sedation to euthanasia, even if the result of both decisions is essentially the same from the perspective of the patient: the end of his or her conscious life. And as far as we know, no doctor will end the life of a patient in an advanced stage of dementia, even if that patient has clearly requested this in an advance directive that is recognized as valid by the law.

[m] On this point, my interpretation of the law differs somewhat from that of Pans (Chapter 4). She points to statements of the drafters of the bill during the parliamentary debates, suggesting that it is the personal rather than the impersonal value of human life that requires protection. But in that case, there would not be a conflict with the duty of the doctor to mitigate suffering.

[n] See §3 in this chapter.

It is both a difficult and a neglected task of ethics to explain the taboo on killing in secular terms.[o,20,21] For some authors, it is nothing but an atavistic remnant of a theistic worldview that still has some grip even on people who have given up that worldview. On my view, only two attempts to explain it without explaining it away deserve serious consideration. On the first view, the taboo is implied in the recognition of the moral status of the human being, in a similar way as it is incompatible with the dignity of the person to become a slave, even if this would be, though hard to imagine, both a person's choice and his or her interest.[22,23,24] I am not so sure, however, that it is really incompatible with the dignity of a human to be granted death if this is both one's choice and one's interest.[25,21] I would, therefore, prefer the second account. According to this account, such taboos are not so much a matter of the rightness or wrongness of certain actions but, rather, of the authority to make certain decisions. The prohibiting norm intends to take away the power to involve the life of another human being in a weighing of interests, any weighing of interests, and the reason may be that we don't trust one another to exercise that power.[26,27,28] This is confirmed by the fact that doctors who are prepared to accept a request for euthanasia are often accused of "playing God." and to some extent may have similar feelings themselves. There are dangers involved in having the option to kill another person, even in that person's interest and with his or her consent, and we tend to believe that these dangers are more important than the risks involved in not having that option.

If this is correct, it can explain another characteristic of the Dutch euthanasia law: that euthanasia and even assistance in suicide are only allowed to doctors. If it is dangerous to have people decide about life and death, we can restrict the danger by restricting the category of people who have that power. Doctors do not normally have any personal interest in the death of their patients, and in executing their professional duties they often have to weigh the interest of the patients' continued living against other interests. Indeed, the very fact that doctors have the authority to decide on palliative care with possible life-shortening effects should already be seen as a first inroad on the taboo on killing. The second step is then only a short one, in particular if the action allowed by it is not seen as normal medical action and is subject to a strict system of evaluation.

Some time ago, I had to explain the underlying morality of the Dutch euthanasia law to a group of Poles who had come to the Netherlands on the invitation of the Ministry of Foreign Affairs in order to obtain inside information about both the euthanasia law and the practice regulated by it. When I had finished my argument, one of my guests threw his arms in the air in a gesture

[o] According to Fred Feldman, "this ... is one of the most notorious scandals of moral philosophy: moral philosophers have not managed to explain why it is wrong to kill people" (see 20. Feldman 1992).

of despair, crying: "Here we have a representative of the most liberal legal system in the world, and he talks like a Polish Catholic priest." He had gotten the message.

FOUNDATIONS 5. In order to assess the Dutch model, one other point of view is very important. In almost all countries in the world, including even some of the countries that have legalized euthanasia or physician-assisted suicide, the majority of doctors are opposed to such legalization. That doesn't mean, however, that all of them believe that they are never morally justified in making such decisions; many doctors recognize that there may be exceptions, that is, cases in which no other humane alternative exists. But on their view, that is only a matter of their personal conscience, and the law should simply look away. And in many countries the law does. In Belgium, for example, before the introduction of euthanasia legislation, no physician had ever been prosecuted for either euthanasia or physician-assisted suicide (or the ending of a patient's life without request), although those practices occurred regularly.[p,17] In other countries, for example in the few cases that have come to court in the UK or Canada, doctors have been acquitted or given very light sentences. The main function of the legal prohibition in such countries seems to be to send a moral message, to reinforce a norm that is commonly known to allow for exceptions.

The approach of the Dutch model is the opposite. One of the main aims of the law is to ensure that the behavior of doctors in this area should be open to view, "transparent" as it is usually called.[q] This is seen as a requirement of integrity in itself, but also as a precondition of a monitoring and control system that ensures that doctors take account of the criteria of due care, which have been derived from the underlying morality of the law.

2. THE PROBLEM OF THE REPORTING RATE

In 1990, the Dutch government commissioned a group of social health-care researchers led by Prof. Paul van der Maas to study the frequency and circumstances of medical decisions with a possible life-shortening effect. Their report, published in 1991, showed that the number of cases of euthanasia and physician-assisted suicide was lower than most observers had expected: 2.1% of all deaths (annually 2,700 cases). Quite similar results were reported at about the same time in the doctoral dissertation of Gerrit van der Wal, who had concentrated his research on the province of North-Holland. In 1996, 2003, and 2007, similar reports were published, based on research (in 1995, 2001, and 2005) by the combined groups of van der Maas and van der Wal (Universities

[p] It is argued on pages 511–512 of *Euthanasia and Law in Europe* that this is the main reason why Belgian doctors opposed the euthanasia law: It imposed regulation on them where they had absolute freedom before (see 17. Griffiths, Weyers, and Adams 2008).

[q] This is rightly stressed by Kennedy in Chapter 1.

of Rotterdam and of Amsterdam). In the meantime, similar research projects were undertaken, though not quite on the same scale, in Belgium and a number of other European countries, which give us some basis for international comparison.[29,30,31]

Although the results of the first report had been received in the Netherlands mainly with sighs of relief, these same data provided critics of the Dutch euthanasia model elsewhere with heavy ammunition. The same is true of the data of the second report and to a lesser extent of the third one.[r] These criticisms were not completely fair, in the first place because they did not (and could not) compare the Dutch data with similar data for other countries, the authors often tacitly assuming that in their own countries actions that are forbidden by law do not happen either, and in the second place because they suggested causal relations between the data without offering any evidence in proof. From the beginning, the most scandalous data concerned the reporting rate and the number of cases in which a patient's life had been ended without his or her explicit request. It seems reasonable to interpret these data as failures of the system on its own terms. A low reporting rate means that the aim of transparency has not been achieved and, hence, that we cannot be sure about the extent to which the requirements of due care are being met. Indeed, we should be suspicious that they often are not, for why not report if they are? And if patients are killed without having made a request at all, let alone a voluntary and well-considered one, that seems to point to an even more alarming disregard for the notions of due care underlying the system. That figure has therefore been widely used as proof of the existence of a slippery slope.

As for the reporting rate, that is, the percentage of cases of euthanasia and assisted suicide (EAS) that had been reported to the proper authorities as cases of unnatural death, this rose from 18% in 1990 to 80% in 2005. During that time, two major events would have influenced the percentage. In 1998, the government installed a reporting procedure that required doctors to report directly to one of five Regional Review Committees, consisting of a lawyer, a doctor, and an ethicist (or their deputies).[s] And in 2002, the euthanasia law took legal force, which largely gave statutory recognition to the legal situation as it had been developed by the courts since the epochal *Schoonheim* case of 1984, but clarified this legal situation at some minor points. From this time on, the review committees only reported their decisions to the public prosecutor in cases in which they had concluded that the doctor had not satisfied the criteria of due care laid down in the law.[t] The first change may have been responsible for the (disappointing) rise in the reporting rate from 41% to 54% between 1995 and

[r] To my knowledge, they have not been revised by any of the critics after the publication of the fourth report, which, remarkably, drew very little international publicity anyway.

[s] See Chapter 12 by Kimsma and van Leeuwen.

[t] From 1998 to 2002, in no case that had been reported as "careful" by the committees did prosecution take place.

2001,[u,17] the second for the (rather spectacular) rise to 80% in 2005. Although the legal situation had not really changed, apparently many doctors only trusted "the law" when its rules had the authority of statute, not merely of case law.

All of these reporting rates, including the last one, require some scrutiny, however. Starting from 1990, the researchers have always used their own classification system of the relevant medical decisions, based on the following questions to the physician: 1) Has the death of the patient been caused by the use of a drug that has been given by you with the explicit aim of shortening the life of the patient (or to assist the patient in doing so him- or herself)? 2) Has the decision to do so been taken on the basis of an explicit request of the patient? If the answers to both questions were positive, the case was classified as one of euthanasia or physician-assisted suicide. Hence, given a life-shortening effect of the action (as assumed by the doctor) and a request of the patient, it was the "explicit aim" of the doctor that made the difference.[v,3] If the doctor reported that he or she had merely taken into account the possibility of the effect but had not aimed at it, the action was classified as alleviation of symptoms with a foreseeable life-shortening effect (15% in 1990, 24% in 2005). To complicate affairs, the researchers also gave physicians the option to state that they made the decision with the shortening of the patient's life as a second, additional aim (4% in 1990, 1% in 2005). These cases were also classified as alleviation of symptoms, rather than of euthanasia.[w]

It is an odd fact of the Dutch discussion that for more than a decade, these definitions have hardly been criticized, not even by lawyers. I know of only one exception.[x,32] It has been quite common during this period to say that the definition of euthanasia was based on "the" principle of double effect.[y,33] In

[u] It is even possible that this change by itself had no direct positive impact on the reporting rate at all, because doctors at first wanted to know how the committees would proceed (see 17. Griffiths, Weyers, and Adams 2008).

[v] John Keown claims that all cases in which the doctor had stopped or not started treatment "with the explicit aim of shortening the life of the patient" should be classified as cases of euthanasia (see 3. Keown 2002). He doesn't pause to consider whether these decisions are in any respect, including patients' refusal of treatment, medical futility, or even the intention of the doctor, different from the decisions to stop or not to start treatment made by doctors in the UK and elsewhere.

[w] A minor problem is that the questions are not mutually exclusive: A second aim can be as explicit as the first one.

[x] An exception is 32. Griffiths, Weyers, and Bood 1998, in particular their Chapter 4. Part of the explanation may be that during this period, almost no expert in criminal law wrote on the subject.

[y] It is highly debatable whether there is really one such principle. In most cases in which it is invoked, the primary aim of the action and the merely foreseen side effect concern different people. In such multiperson cases, the principle is closely related to the Kantian injunction not to treat people as a mere means but always also as ends in themselves (see 33. Quinn 1993). In the case of actions with life-shortening effects, however, both effects concern the same person, which makes it difficult to understand why they cannot be balanced. Significantly, pain relief seems to be the only one-person case in which the principle is being invoked as a standard.

recent years, however, it has been almost generally recognized that this definition of euthanasia differs from the legal one.[z,11,34] To be sure, one requirement for an action to be punishable to the full extent in Dutch criminal law is that its deplorable result should be "intended." But in any case in which the actors are aware, or can reasonably be held to be aware, that the result will occur, they are supposed to intend it, whether it is their primary aim, a means of achieving this, or only a by-product of their actions that they were merely prepared to take into the bargain.

Nevertheless, the law does not take all cases in which a medical action has foreseeably resulted in a shortening of the patient's life to be cases of euthanasia. The criterion for making the relevant distinction, however, is not the subjective intention of the doctor but the existence of a medical indication. In any case in which the medical action is justified by a palliative aim, and the possible life-shortening effects cannot be considered to be disproportional, the case is not a case of euthanasia. In such cases, what the doctor did is held to be "normal medical action," which is not only permitted by the law (the so-called medical exception) but may even be a professional duty.

It will turn out to be relevant to my discussion in a later section to point out an implication of these definitions. If the doctor either uses dosages of medicine beyond what is indicated for a palliative aim, or uses even proper dosages in a case in which the life-shortening effects of his or her action should be considered disproportional (in relation to that aim), the action, given a request of the patient, should be classified as a case of euthanasia.[aa]

If we now look at the number of cases classified as euthanasia in the 2007 report, we find that in 74% of these cases (roughly 1,800), the doctor used muscle relaxants and/or barbiturates. For these cases, taken as a separate category, the reporting rate is 99%, which, given the margin of error for such figures, is indistinguishable from 100%. On the other hand, in 18% of the cases (roughly 400), the doctor had used morphine or one of its derivates, and these cases had almost never been reported.[bb] The same is true of the 1,350 cases in which the doctor reported having had two aims.

[z] The point has not yet been recognized, however, by the researchers themselves (see 33. Quinn 1993), with a mistaken appeal to the authority of the Report of the State Commission 1985, and by Onwuteaka-Philipsen, Chapter 7 in this volume. In the legal chapters of the 2007 report, on the other hand, written by or under the supervision of J. K. M. Gevers, the point has been fully recognized (see 34. Regionale Toetsingscommissies Euthanasie 2007, in particular pp. 238–239, proposing to include the definitions of the State Commission into the law). Since 2006, this same definition has been used in the Guidelines for the Proceedings of the Review Committees.

[aa] See §4 on the borderline between euthanasia and terminal sedation.

[bb] In addition, in 7% of the cases, benzodiazepines have been used. These cases are never being reported either, and probably indicate a mistaken belief concerning the possibly lethal effect of these drugs. (Some of these cases, however, might conceivably be cases of terminal sedation, which really should be considered cases of euthanasia; see §4.) The percentage of cases

How many of these (400 + 1350 =) 1,750 cases should we count as cases of euthanasia under the proper legal definition?[cc] Only in 250 of those cases does the doctor report to have used a higher dosage than necessary for the aim of symptom alleviation. Hence, as far as we know, the other cases are all covered by the medical exception. Next, in how many of these 250 cases did the doctor not only think that he or she had shortened the life of the patient but actually did so? The answer is that we don't know.[dd,34] What we do know, however, is that doctors still tend to overrate the life-shortening effects of morphine. In order to remain effective, the dosage of morphine should normally be increased regularly because of a habituation effect. (This also means that we cannot read off a life-shortening effect from the final dosage reached.) It has now been established that even quite substantial increases of the dosage do not have the life-shortening effect traditionally attributed to them, perhaps even the contrary.[ee,35,36,37,38]

So we may conclude that the number of cases in which morphine has been used and which should properly be classified as cases of euthanasia is decreasing and lower than 250, possibly much lower. It is reasonable to assume that both of these facts can, at least partly, be explained by the secure legal availability of the option of euthanasia. Another part of the explanation probably is the increased awareness of the availability of the option of terminal sedation. Doctors who want to end the suffering of their dying patients no longer need to go for the morphine route, and they know this.

Why then do they still occasionally use this route? Recent research has suggested an interesting explanation. The use of morphine is often not followed by immediate death, and even if it is, there is still room for doubt about the causal nexus. This is probably the very reason why doctors do not classify their own actions as euthanasia. It allows them (albeit with some amount of self-deception) to entertain two thoughts at the same time: I am doing something for my patient, I am not letting him or her down, and: I am not killing him or her ("by the needle").[ff,39,17] Doctors may still occasionally be attracted to this gray area precisely because of its grayness.

in which morphine had been used to execute an explicit intention to shorten life was 41% in 1995 and 23% in 2001 (= 1,550 and 875 cases, respectively).

cc The objection could be raised that subjective intention, even if not legally, is morally relevant, either as a matter of professional or at least of personal ethics. I don't think it is, though I cannot argue the point here. It is worth observing, however, that reports of intention are very unreliable. It is particularly hard to say of two effects of one's action (which are both welcome) whether or not both were intended.

dd One intriguing datum from the 2007 report is that the average dosage of morphine used during the final 24 hours is much higher (265–285 mg) than the median dosage (180 mg), which suggests a small number of exceptionally high dosages. When the time lag between the administration of a higher dose of morphine and the death of the patient is more than several hours, as it is in most cases, it is particularly difficult to ascertain a causal link.

ee Hence, it is something of a mystery why the number of cases in which doctors ascribe a life-shortening effect has increased.

ff See Chapter 13 by Willems. This also explains why these doctors do not classify their own action as euthanasia, even if they report the explicit intention to shorten the patient's life.

One other conclusion is worth mentioning: The reporting behavior of doctors is as good as we can possibly expect it to be. It therefore makes no sense to call for further improvement of the reporting rate. The cases in which proper euthanasia agents have been used are all being reported; the others are never reported and will never be reported. Even if doctors realized that cases in which they think they shortened the life of the patient by using a clear overdose should have been classified as euthanasia and hence reported, they would not do so, because they would then also realize that they had not acted in a professionally responsible way.[gg,40,41] We should not call on these doctors to come forward and report[hh,42], but rather to change their behavior: to alleviate symptoms and shorten life both by proper means in proper dosages.

3. ENDING LIVES WITHOUT REQUEST

The other scandalous figure of the national survey reports has always been the number of cases of life-shortening actions without request. This is a very heterogeneous category of cases, including termination of life of severely defective newborn babies.[ii] But the largest group seems to concern dying patients who are too "far away" to be able to communicate clearly with the doctor and have not made a previous request, but who are still in a state of severe suffering. Often this figure has been interpreted as a corroboration of slippery-slope fears: Doctors do this because their moral aversion to killing has been eroded by the practice of euthanasia.[jj,3,43] But no evidence for this causal nexus has ever been offered. It could as well be that the figure would have been substantially higher but for the legal availability of the option of euthanasia, which normally enables the doctor to communicate openly and timely with patients about the use of that option. This explanation is to some extent confirmed by data from research in other countries, in particular in nearby Flandres.[kk,30,31,44,45,17] Before

See also Chapter 7 by Onwuteaka-Philipsen. I do not deny that some of these doctors may be mistaken about this.

[gg] For a case in which a doctor who used morphine was judged by a review committee not to have satisfied the criteria of due care, see Annual Report 2004, 30–32 (case 15) and Annual Report 2005, 35–36 (case 15).

[hh] As Onwuteaka-Philipsen does in Chapter 7 in this volume. In recent years, the number of reported cases of euthanasia and assisted suicide (EAS) has risen, from 1,815 in 2003 to 2,636 in 2009. One possible explanation suggested by the Annual Report of 2008 is that the number of doctors using morphine instead of muscle relaxants has further decreased. But that number was already so small in 2005 that it can at best explain only a small part of the increase in reported cases.

[ii] See Chapter 8 by van der Heide.

[jj] For an example, see 3. Keown 2002, or 43. Linacre Centre for Health Care Ethics 2004/2005 for evidence presented to the Select Committee of the House of Lords on the Assisted Dying for the Terminally Ill Bill.

[kk] In a comparative study of six European countries, Agnes van der Heide and her colleagues found higher rates of patients' lives ended without request for Flandres (1.5) and Denmark

the introduction of the euthanasia law in 2002, the number of cases in which the doctor ended the life of a patient without an explicit request was relatively much higher than the same number in the Netherlands (and also much higher in Flanders than the number of cases of euthanasia). Perhaps the explanation is also confirmed by the substantial decrease in the Netherlands of the figure between 2001 and 2006, from 900 to 550 cases, although this can also be attributed to the increased awareness of the availability of the option of terminal sedation as an alternative.

There is one other point about this figure to be made, and this again concerns the means used: in 1995, muscle relaxants in 18%, morphine in 59% of the cases; in 2005, muscle relaxants in 23%, morphine in 59% of the cases.[ll] That in the majority of the cases morphine has been used invites the same comments I made about euthanasia: We cannot be sure that a life-shortening effect actually occurred and have reason to be somewhat skeptical about that. And even if it did, we also cannot be sure that an overdose had been used, that is, a dosage exceeding the existing indications for symptom alleviation.[mm,11]

I do not suggest that the figure does not indicate any problematic practice at all. If there is no explicit request of the patient to have his or her life ended or to be assisted in ending it, in the dying stage (and at least 81% of the 550 cases concern cases in which the patient had a life expectancy of less than one week) only palliative measures should normally be considered for ending severe suffering, including terminal sedation as the means of last resort. Ending the life of the patient could only be an option in the very few cases in which communication with the patient is out of reach but he or she still has a life expectancy that excludes terminal sedation as an option, or in the even fewer cases in which terminal sedation cannot be used for medical reasons.[nn,17] So there is still a real problem here, but it is of very modest proportions. And this problem, like the problem of the unreported use of morphine generally, should probably not be seen as the dire result of legalizing euthanasia, but rather as a relic of a prelegalization practice.

(0.67) than for the Netherlands (at the same time, 2001: 0.6; see 30 van der Heide et al. 2003). Seale found a rate of 0.3 for the UK, slightly lower than the Dutch rate (0.4) in 2005 (see 31. Seale 2009). For the relevance of these comparative data see 44. Otlowski 2001; 45. Smith 2005; and 17. Griffiths, Weyers, and Adams 2008).

[ll] The mysterious figures of 2001 (2% use of muscle relaxants) warn us that we are in an area of very small numbers, which doesn't allow strong conclusions anyway.

[mm] Accordingly, in 91% of the cases classified by the researchers as termination of life without a request, the doctors involved do not use that classification themselves (see 11. Onwuteaka-Philipsen et al. 2007). Most of them may be right about this.

[nn] In such cases, the doctors should use proper euthanasia agents, and have the courage of their convictions to report their actions, on a plea of necessity. In the case of newborns, some doctors have done this and have been acquitted by the courts (see Chapter 19 by Sauer and Verhagen and 17. Griffiths, Weyers, and Adams 2008).

4. THE BORDERLINE BETWEEN EUTHANASIA AND TERMINAL SEDATION

In addition to this traditional gray area, in recent years a new gray area has developed, on the borderline between terminal sedation and euthanasia. Before discussing it, I have to defend my use of the very term *terminal sedation*, which has been outlawed in the Netherlands, because some people seem to have confused it with *terminating sedation*. The problem is that the alternative term *palliative sedation* has been officially defined in a broad way, which includes any form of sedation at the end of a patient's life, whether deep or superficial, whether temporary, intermittent, or permanent. The problem with sedation I want to discuss, however, arises only in cases in which sedation is deep enough to induce a coma, and is intended to last until the end of a patient's life. Because we need a word for this particular form of sedation, I will stick to the internationally common and appropriate term *terminal sedation*.[46]

Terminal sedation is properly administered by using benzodiazepines, in particular midazolam (dormicum), and midazolam has no life-shortening effect when used in proper dosages or even larger ones. Therefore, terminal sedation by itself does not shorten a person's biological life, even if it ends his or her life as a conscious subject. However, if the decision has been made to start terminal sedation, the question arises whether the patient should be given artificial hydration, and the usual policy in the Netherlands is not to do so. If the patient dies within a few days afterwards, this will be a result of illness, not of dehydration, but if death takes longer to arrive, this conclusion is no longer sure. In such cases, one could suggest that the combined policy of terminal sedation and abstaining from hydration amounts to the shortening of a patient's life, and hence, if it happens on the request of the patient, to euthanasia.

Mainly because of this worry, the Royal Dutch Medical Association has developed a guideline for "palliative" sedation. One of the requirements for starting terminal sedation formulated in the guideline is that the patient have a life expectancy of no more than one to two weeks. Of course, the estimation of a patient's life expectancy beyond two or three days is very unreliable, and so even if doctors tend to overestimate rather than underestimate life expectancy, the requirement does not ensure that no terminally sedated patient will ever die from dehydration.[oo] This is justified in the guideline by the argument that if the decision to start terminal sedation is made on good grounds – that it is the only way to end "refractory symptoms" – artificial hydration would be a futile treatment. I agree that it would be, because it would not add anything to

[oo] This means that without dehydration death would have occurred later, not that the underlying illness is not a causal factor at all in causing death at the time it occurs.

the life of the patient of which he or she is the conscious subject. But the argument mistakenly assumes that in deciding about the first step of the procedure, terminal sedation, we can abstract from the second step, abstaining from futile hydration, and vice versa. There is no problem with terminal sedation because it has no life-shortening effects by itself and is justified by refractory symptoms, and there is no problem with abstaining from artificial hydration because it is only a form of letting die, justified by futility. Neither of the actions is a form of killing, and so the combination of the two cannot be a form of euthanasia. But if that is a valid argument, it is hard to see why a requirement concerning the maximum life expectancy of the patient is needed at all.[pp,47,46]

There is no doubt that if we sedate a healthy person, and from that moment on do not artificially provide fluids, we kill that person. We should consider both actions together as elements of one policy. If the effect of that policy is the shortening of the person's life, on the killing/letting die divide the combined action falls on the side of killing. The same is true if the person is fatally ill but does not die from illness (alone) but as a result of dehydration.

It is true that if a patient with a neurological disease, who cannot swallow, refuses artificial hydration, the doctor who accedes to that refusal does not kill that patient. But in that case the patient is dependent on artificial hydration as a result of illness, not because of anything the doctor has done. In the case of terminal sedation, however, the patient needs artificial hydration for survival (for more than one to two weeks) because of the sedation. That is why the two actions have to be considered together.

We have seen (§ 2) that other forms of palliative care that have life-shortening effects, however exceptional, should be seen as falling on the "killing" side of the killing/letting die divide as well. They may be justifiable nevertheless. This particular form of palliative care with possible life-shortening effects should be assessed in exactly the same way. It may be justified when there is no other way to alleviate severe suffering, and when the life-shortening effect, no more than a few days at most, cannot be considered disproportionate.[qq]

If that argument is accepted, however, it follows that if the patient's life is foreseeably shortened by a substantially longer period, the policy should be

[pp] The Report of the AMA Council on Ethical and Judicial Affairs on Sedation to Unconsciousness in End-of-Life Care of 2008 argues in a similar way: Sedation does not shorten life, and patients or their surrogates "with guidance from their physicians should separately decide whether they … want to maintain, withhold or withdraw life-sustaining interventions (including nutrition and hydration)" (see 47. American Medical Association 2008, 5). The report states a requirement of proportionality, but does not apply it to the extent of life shortened by the combined decision to sedate and not to provide hydration. Consequently, it formulates no restriction on life expectancy; it only restricts sedation into unconsciousness to "terminally ill patients." If my argument in this section is sound, the report justifies a form of euthanasia, contrary to its stated intention.

[qq] During the second week, it may be impossible to identify the cause of death, but there is a substantial and increasing probability that death is at least partly due to dehydration.

counted as a form of euthanasia, or, if the patient has not consented to it, as ending his or her life without a request. Admittedly, the borderline between these classifications can only be a matter of stipulation. This is precisely what the guideline provides. If this is the real reason for the requirement concerning the life expectancy of the patient, it should have been made clear that if the policy of sedating the patient and withholding artificial hydration is started (on the request of the patient) when the patient has a life expectancy of more than one to two weeks, this should be classified and reported as euthanasia. (The doctor would then be judged by the review committee not to have acted in a medically careful way.) Unfortunately, the guideline doesn't say this explicitly.

How sure can we be that the requirement concerning the maximum life expectancy is respected in practice? There are some reassuring data.[rr,34,48] On the other hand, members of Regional Review Committees report that it is not uncommon for reports of euthanasia to show that terminal sedation has been discussed with the patient as an alternative to euthanasia (and euthanasia is chosen in the end) in cases in which the life expectancy of the patient exceeds two weeks. Moreover, as regards the life expectancy of the patients, we have only the opinions of the responsible doctors to go by, which, even if sincere, are not very reliable. That very fact should be a reason to insist (and not only to advise, as the guideline does) that doctors who decide to start terminal sedation should consult an expert in palliative care.[ss]

5. MERELY A FAÇADE?

I have argued that the traditional criticisms of the Dutch model have only limited force.[tt,49] Morphine is still being used as a terminal agent, whether illusionary or not, and probably considered attractive precisely because of this elusiveness. In some cases, the life of a severely suffering patient is being ended,

[rr] The estimation of the actual time span between sedation and death given by doctors in the 2007 Annual Report of the Regional Review Committees (p. 131) is more than two weeks in 2% of all cases. In the 2003 Annual Report (p. 84), it was one to four weeks in 21% and more than a month in 6% of all cases. If terminal sedation is indeed being restricted to dying patients, that may help to explain the rising number of euthanasia cases since 2003; see note *hh*.

[ss] Other reasons include: 1) to prevent doctors from deciding on terminal sedation too early, when with sophisticated palliative care the patient could have had some additional time of conscious life without severe suffering; and 2) to give sufficient room for patients to be treated in accordance with their own values. Doctors may be tempted to offer them only the option of terminal sedation if no special procedural requirements of due care apply to that option at all.

[tt] It may be added that contrary to a rather common view, the requirements of due care over the years have only been tightened, in particular in regard to reporting and consultation. And legalizing euthanasia or physician-assisted suicide in (Oregon and) the Netherlands did not result in a disproportionate number of deaths among the elderly, poor, women, minorities, uninsured, minors, chronically ill, less educated, or psychiatric patients.

for whom, in the absence of a request, terminal sedation would have been the preferable option. But the number of these cases is small and decreasing.

In addition, a new gray area has developed consisting of cases in which doctors use terminal sedation without providing artificial hydration, even when the life expectancy of the patient should rule out this option. As far as we know, however, this practice doesn't concern substantial numbers either.[uu,50] At the same time, we see an emerging practice in which physicians who consider either euthanasia or physician-assisted suicide habitually follow the proper legal procedure. The ideal of transparency of medical decisions in this area has, therefore, largely been achieved, and certainly to a much greater extent than in any other country.[vv,17]

One could still be skeptical about this result, however, arguing that it is only an illusory achievement. Dutch doctors, one could suggest, allow themselves to be controlled because the controlling system has no bite. From 1998 until 2008, 20,283 cases were reported to the review committees. Only in 38 cases did they conclude that the doctor had not satisfied the legal criteria of careful action. Moreover, in none of these "not careful" cases did the public prosecutor decide to start a legal procedure, and so no conviction took place. The most severe measure was a conditional dismissal in which the doctor was warned that he could still be prosecuted for his misstep if he acted in a similar way again.[ww]

In making these decisions, the public prosecutor acts on an instruction that distinguishes between the procedural and the substantial criteria of due care. If a doctor has failed to satisfy a procedural requirement, for example the requirement that the colleague called for consultation be "independent," the prosecutor will consider whether, as a result of this failure, there is any doubt that the doctor has also failed to satisfy any of the substantial criteria, in particular the requirement that there be a voluntary and well-considered request, and hopeless and unbearable suffering.[xx]

[uu] At present, no international comparison on this issue is possible because we have only some data about the total number of cases of terminal sedation without artificial hydration (ca. 3% of deaths in the Netherlands, Belgium, Switzerland and Italy in 2001, somewhat lower in Sweden and Denmark; see 50. Miccinesi et al. 2006) but no data about life expectancy for any country but the Netherlands.

[vv] At this moment probably still including Belgium.

[ww] The Inspectorate of Health Care has brought two disciplinary cases, both resulting in the imposition of sanctions. Already in 2001, the UN Human Rights Committee expressed its concern about the low number (at that time only 4) of "not careful" judgments of the review committees (see Concluding Observations of the Human Rights Committee: Netherlands, July 20, 2001, at: https://www.jiscmail.ac.uk/cgi-bin/webadmin?A2=disability-research;1664686b.0107).

[xx] Clearly this should mean that in the absence of a proper consultation report, the report of the doctor of what happened can be corroborated by other independent testimony. If the judgment whether the substantial criteria have been satisfied were only to be made on the basis of the doctor's report, that would effectively undermine the consultation requirement of the law. This seems the proper way to interpret the instruction, but it is not fully clear whether it is correspondingly implemented in practice.

The criticism that the control procedure is merely ritual, all bark and no bite, threatens not only the claim that it promotes transparency but also the claim that the legal system is based on a principle of mercy. Many Dutch citizens believe that they have a moral, if not a legal, right to euthanasia, based merely on their general right to self-determination. It is only to be expected that at least some doctors share this moral view, even if they form a minority among their colleagues. So they will be prepared to accept a request for euthanasia if they are satisfied that it has been made voluntarily by a competent patient, even if they are not satisfied that his or her suffering is unbearable. For example, some cancer patients at a rather early stage decide that they prefer to avoid going through the dying process altogether, whether or not it involves extreme suffering. If it is not really assessed whether all the requirements have been satisfied, the system of control fails to achieve its moral aim.

From the beginning, opponents of the *indirect paternalism*[yy] of the Dutch legal system have maintained that it is only the patient who can, and therefore should, decide whether he or she is in a state of unbearable suffering.[zz,51] For that reason, they have claimed that this requirement should be taken in the same way as the requirement of a state of emergency in the Dutch abortion law: A woman is supposed to be in such a state if she says she is. Although the abortion law at the time of its enactment had not been formally justified in terms of women's right to self-determination, this interpretation made the law indistinguishable from a law justified in that way, and, indeed, recently the Dutch Supreme Court reinterpreted the law as implementing a right to self-determination.[aaa] It could be suggested that the review committees actually accept that the patient is in a state of unbearable suffering as soon as he or she says so. In that case, the law is not really paternalistic at all: It permits doctors to accede to any voluntary and well-considered request, even if it also permits them to make additional requirements, including requirements of their own choosing, for example, their own interpretation of the requirement of unbearable suffering.[bbb,52]

[yy] See §1 in this chapter.

[zz] Henri Wijsbek convincingly criticizes this claim (see 51 Wijsbek 2001). See also Chapter 21 by Wijsbek in this volume.

[aaa] HR 18-03-2005, RvdW 2005, 42 Kelly (*Kelly* decision). The very fact that this reinterpretation has been hardly noticed is telling. The pioneer of Dutch health law, H. J. Leenen, who during his lifetime has always championed the legalization of euthanasia in terms of respect for autonomy, had proposed the requirement of an *uitzichtloze noodtoestand*, a state of emergency without perspective, in his first draft of the euthanasia law. It is arguable that he took the abortion law as his model.

[bbb] Possibly relevant on this point is the finding by Hilde Buiting and her colleagues that 53% of doctors (57% of general practioners, 27% of specialists) reported having had problems in deciding whether they themselves were convinced of the patient's unbearable suffering. Problems to assess whether the request was well considered were reported by 23% of doctors (20% of GPs, 32% of specialists; see 52. Buiting, et al., 2008). The finding may suggest that GPs take the requirement of unbearable suffering as an independent condition more seriously than medical specialists do.

I believe that the criticism misinterprets the nature of the control procedure, and actually of any possible control procedure in this area. Being essentially dependent on the voluntary cooperation of doctors, it should not be seen as a method for catching crooks and bringing them to justice, though it can have this result accidentally. It is only marginally an instrument of the criminal law. Therefore, the essential instruments of the control system are not prosecution and punishment. The most effective instrument is the consultation requirement, in particular in the actual form it takes of the SCEN (Support, Consultation Euthanasia in the Netherlands) procedure.[ccc] Almost all consultants nowadays are SCEN consultants, who have usually volunteered because of their interest in, and loyalty to, the aims of the procedure. They teach each other through discussion and peer review, they are better informed than the average doctor about the interpretation given by the review committees to the requirements of due care, and they also tend to have an interest in their standing with these committees. The doctor who doesn't take the unbearable suffering criterion seriously enough cannot expect to get a SCEN consultant who shares his or her attitude.

In addition, the committees in about 6% of the cases ask either the doctor or the consultant or both for additional information. Most of these questions concern the unbearable suffering criterion. In about 10–20 cases each year, they are not satisfied with the answers they get and invite the doctor for an interview. Most doctors experience this as a kind of informal penalty itself. The committees can inform the doctor about minor flaws in his or her behavior without arriving at a "not careful" judgment during these interviews, in the considerations preceding the judgment, or in a letter accompanying it. All in all, the best way to interpret the control mechanism is as a learning system through which the criteria of due care are being interpreted and the doctors receive feedback on the propriety of their interpretation. It seems likely that such a system has a greater impact on the behavior of doctors than a system that restricts itself to meting out punishment in the few cases of transgression that are brought to its attention.[ddd,17,11]

Let me give some examples of the way in which the criteria of due care have been interpreted during this process. For a time, the committees held that only a doctor who is responsible for the treatment of a patient can grant a request for euthanasia or physician-assisted suicide, but later on they decided that it is enough for the doctor to have a relationship to the patient enabling him or her to make proper decisions about the requirements of due care. It has been suggested that at least for all dying patients, there is always an alternative way to avoid severe suffering: terminal sedation. Patients have the legal right to

[ccc] For explanation, see Chapter 11 by Kimsma.

[ddd] Eighty-six percent of Dutch doctors agree with the statement that the system improves the carefulness of medical action (see 11. Onwuteaka-Philipsen, et al., 2007).

refuse this alternative if it is being offered to them, and the committees have taken the view that if they do so because of their view of a good death, doctor and patient can arrive at the conclusion that terminal sedation is not a reasonable alternative.[eee,11]

For some patients, the worst aspect of their condition is the very fact that they have become totally dependent on the care of others, even for such things as eating or going to the toilet. One could argue that these people have lived in an illusion concerning the human condition until now, never having been forced to realize that humans, because of their vulnerability, may at any time, not only on their deathbeds, need the care of others. But even if this is true, it would still be rather cruel to insist that patients learn this lesson at this stage of their lives. So it is accepted that loss of independence can be a prominent element of suffering. On the other hand, it is not accepted as such a prominent element that a patient doesn't want to be a burden on others.[fff,53] One reason may be that if this motivation is accepted, the voluntariness of the patient's request could be compromised. The committees have decided that euthanasia cannot take place if at the agreed moment the patient has irreversibly fallen into a coma, because at that moment he or she can no longer be in a state of suffering.[ggg]

A difficult topic is the extent to which fear of future suffering counts as a form of suffering. The official view of the committees is that the fear should be well founded and concern a state of suffering in the very near future. But this is an area in which everything is a matter of degree, and it is hard to judge on the basis of documents alone, as review committees have to do. Therefore, in this case as in others, the main gatekeeping function has to be performed by the consultants.

6. A WELL-CONSIDERED REQUEST

One interesting ambiguity in the interpretation of the law arises from the fact that the law doesn't use the notion of competence, in the sense in which it is commonly used in medical ethics (and explained in Chapter 15 by Ron Berghmans). When the work of the Regional Review Committees began at the end of 1998, the form that a physician had to use for reporting a case of

[eee] The government had already taken that view during the parliamentary debate about the law (see 11. Onwuteaka-Philipsen, et al., 2007).

[fff] D. L. Willems and colleagues found a significant difference between doctors in the Netherlands and in Oregon concerning their willingness to accept the patient's wish to avoid being a burden on others as a valid reason for granting a request for physician-assisted suicide (resp. 24, 9%; see 53 Willems, et al., 2000).

[ggg] At present, a committee of the KNMG is working out guidelines concerning the permissibility of euthanasia in the case of such patients. Difficult issues concern patients who are unable to communicate but still show signs of suffering and patients who have fallen into a coma as a result of reversible medical actions.

euthanasia or physician-assisted suicide contained a notorious *Nota Bene*. It stated, among other things, that cases involving patients whose capacity to express a well-considered request has possibly [*sic*] been disturbed, for example as a result of depression or dementia, should not be reported to a review committee but directly to the public prosecutor. When the law took force in 2002, the *Nota Bene* was not eliminated from the form. This means that the Ministry of Justice, which is responsible for the form, interpreted the law in the following way: When Article 293 makes it a separate crime, distinguishable from murder or manslaughter, to kill a person on his or her explicit and earnest request, it means that the request should be competently made; otherwise we still have a case of murder or manslaughter. Hence, if a request has not been made competently, the review committees have no power to decide whether the action meets the criteria of due care, including the requirement that the request be voluntary and well considered.

This interpretation has been criticized from the start.[48,54,hhh] It seems clear that a request can be made explicitly and sincerely, but not fully competently. Hence, incompetence is not a reason for denying the review committee the power to decide the case but rather a reason for the committee to give the judgment "not careful."

Recently, the minister of justice agreed to eliminate the *Nota Bene* from the form and hence has accepted this alternative interpretation. The new form was made available for use in May 2009. However, the requirement that the request be well considered is not equivalent to a requirement that it should have been made competently, in the usual sense in which this term is interpreted in bioethics and health law. A request cannot be well considered if it is not competently made, but the reverse is not true. The difference is that in assessing whether the request is well considered, we cannot fully abstract from the content of the request. We should normally make sure that patients are aware of their conditions, of the prognosis both of their diseases and of the development of their symptoms, of possible alternative ways to treat the diseases or alleviate the symptoms, with their probable effects and burdens. All this is also relevant to a judgment of competence. But in addition, the request can only be seen as well considered if it is at least intelligible that, given this relevant information, it is this particular request that is being made. It is not enough that from other evidence we know that the patient has the mental and emotional capacities that are needed to make an intelligible response to the situation as he or she knows it.

The literature on competence insists on abstracting from any judgment about the content of the decision because it wants to hold onto a clear and clean notion of ("hard") paternalism, either direct or indirect. If a person is

[hhh] In their Annual Report 2003, the review committees rejected the interpretation of the law of the *Nota Bene*.

considered to be competent, he or she has the right to make his or her own decisions, whether they are "good" or "bad" decisions. It is debated whether in that case it can ever be permissible to interfere with the execution of that decision (direct hard paternalism) or with others assisting in executing it (indirect hard paternalism), but even if it is, it is always a violation of the person's right to self-determination. If on the other hand the decision is not competently made, it is permissible, not a violation of the person's right to self-determination, to interfere with it if it is a "bad" decision. But we can only take that position if the judgment of competence itself does not depend on our assessment of the decision being a good or bad one.[iii]

I believe that in general, decisions of competence, as they are being made in practice in health care, are hardly ever made in this content-independent way. As long as the patient makes a decision that makes sense, no question of competence is raised, and if the decision is problematic, a main consideration about competence concerns *how* problematic it is exactly. My present point, however, is only that this is the way in which doctors, consultants, and review committees judge, and have to judge, whether a request for euthanasia has been well considered.

The consequence of this judgment is that the two main substantive criteria of the law, the requirements concerning the request and the condition of the patient, are not fully independent of each other. If the request is made at a moment when the burden of physical symptoms is still modest, the patient has a lot of explaining to do before his request will be accepted as well considered. The explanation should at least make the request intelligible to others. If, on the other hand, the patient is in a very pitiful condition in which the request is perfectly understandable, the fact that he or she may be unable to give the consultant an extended exposé about the illness's history and about the reasons for various decisions made along the way does not necessarily lead the consultant to conclude that the request is not well considered. The condition of the patient speaks for itself. Similarly, if such a patient has an untreatable psychiatric condition, that condition may be seen as increasing the burden of suffering and, therefore, the intelligibility of the request, rather than throwing doubt on whether it is well considered (or voluntary).[55,jjj]

[iii] This requirement is already compromised in an indirect way, when the criteria for assessing the competence of a decision are more stringent, if the decision concerns more important matters, for example, matters of life and death. Ron Berghmans (Chapter 15) in effect concedes this when he says that a judgment of competence based on this criterion is not a judgment of a capacity but of an authority.

[jjj] In many contexts, a decision is voluntary not because the agent, being who he or she is, could have made another choice, but precisely because the choice is the only one that is true to that particular person. In this case, the patient's death wish may be seen as voluntary because there is no position that he or she will ever be actually able to take that would not identify with this wish.

The fact that the law requires the request to be well considered and not merely competently made therefore confirms the priority of the requirement of unbearable and hopeless suffering, and hence the foundational importance of the principle of mercy. It is always against the background of the condition of the patient that the request will be assessed.

7. TOO RESTRICTIVE?

That the system as a whole has a clear restrictive effect on the conditions under which patients are considered to be eligible for having their request accepted is, if not shown, at least made likely by the results. They may even suggest the restrictive effect to be too large. Here we meet the second and opposite worry one can have as regards the actual working of the control system.

In order to specify this worry, we have to know, first, how often requests for euthanasia are being refused and, second, to what extent these refusals track the legal criteria of due care.

As regards the first point, the survey report of 2007 tells us that in 8,400 cases, explicit and repeated requests for euthanasia or physician-assisted suicide had been made, of which 2,425 (almost 30%) had been granted and acted upon. In almost 40% of the 6,000 cases in which the doctor did not act upon the request, the patient had died before a final decision could be reached or executed. In most of the cases in which the doctor refused to go along with the request, he or she thought that the request was either not voluntary (6% of the 6,000 cases) or not well considered (18%), or because the patient's suffering in the doctor's eyes was not unbearable (16%) or not hopeless (8%).[kkk,11] A problem with these data is that it is not fully clear what an "explicit and repeated request" should be taken to include. Often patients make a request for the near future, leaving it open to pinpoint the exact date, sometimes changing their minds from one day to the next. This helps to explain the substantial number of cases in which the patient has died before a final decision about the request could be made.

Perhaps more telling are the data from Boudewijn Chabot's recent research.[56,lll] They may be more telling because they concern people who afterwards have confirmed the urgency and stability of their death wish by going on to end their own lives. Chabot found that at a minimum, each year 1,600 Dutch people took their own lives in a planned way and after shared deliberation with friends and relatives by using deadly drugs they had collected in some way. Moreover, 2,800 people ended their lives by intentionally ceasing to eat and (in particular) to drink. Almost all of these cases were reported by

[kkk] See Chapter 9 by Pasman for additional figures from interviews with GPs and from earlier surveys.

[lll] See Chapter 20 by Chabot.

the coroner as cases of natural death.[mmm] This means that the official statistics for the Netherlands (and probably for other countries as well) only concern suicides that have been executed impulsively and without the consultation of others.[nnn] (Because these were the only suicides we knew of until now, our idea of the "normal" case of suicide is largely off the mark.)[ooo,56]

In about 50% of these 4,400 cases, the person involved had first requested assistance from the doctor but had received a refusal. About 40% would not have made the request because they anticipated a refusal, or even preventive action by the physician. Among the reasons given for the refusal: the requester was not fatally ill or not in the dying stage of that illness; the death wish had not been caused by any illness at all; and the suffering of the requester could not be considered unbearable or hopeless.[ppp]

The first reason is interesting for it is not, and never has been, a requirement of due care in the Netherlands that the patient be terminally ill or in the dying stage of an illness, however this is defined.[qqq] Some doctors may be mistaken about the actual requirements; others may knowingly add a requirement of their own.[11,rrr]

The data from these two sources (the survey report and Chabot) are only roughly comparable, but they don't seem to be fully compatible. It is hardly plausible that the large majority of the people who have been refused euthanasia or physician-assisted suicide on their request go on to end their own lives. Part of the explanation may be that patients may sometimes believe that they have made a request when this has not been perceived or remembered as such by the doctor.[sss]

What more do we know about the refusals? By far the largest group of people who successfully request euthanasia are cancer patients in the final stage of their illness.[ttt] Cancer is, of course, generally feared for the physical suffering it

[mmm] For reasons Chabot explains in Chapter 20.

[nnn] Recently, the Dutch minister of health care announced plans aimed at reducing the number of "official" suicides. Obviously he is not aware of the arbitrary character of the figure.

[ooo] We can at present only speculate whether the number of such cases is higher or lower in the Netherlands than elsewhere. It might be lower because a greater number of people with a death wish are being assisted by doctors. But it might also be higher precisely because the availability of legal euthanasia strengthens the belief that this is an area in which decisions can be made.

[ppp] These reasons are also reported in Chapter 9 by Pasman. She adds that there are alternatives for alleviating the suffering.

[qqq] It is a requirement in Oregon. In Belgium, the doctor has to satisfy additional procedural requirements if he or she doesn't expect the patient to die in the near future.

[rrr] Twenty-five percent of doctors believe that this is a legal requirement; 6% don't know.

[sss] See Chapter 9 by Pasman and Chapter 20 by Chabot.

[ttt] But the percentage is somewhat decreasing: from 89% in 2005 to 81% in 2008, according to the Annual Reports of the review committees. Part of the explanation for the rising number of euthanasia cases (see note *hh*) may therefore be that doctors are slightly more willing to consider euthanasia in nonstandard cases.

often involves, and so there is in a sense a presumption that a cancer patient will be suffering severely. The same is true for the other significant class of cases: those of neurological diseases like amyotrophic lateral sclerosis (ALS), which often involve almost complete paralysis and severe breathlessness. Euthanasia in other cases, according to the reports to the regional committees, is rare.[uuu] In the case of psychiatric illness, it is almost nonexistent.[vvv,17] Euthanasia in a beginning stage of dementia, when the patient may still be aware of his or her condition and prognosis, was reported for the first time in 2004. Since then, the number has been slowly rising year by year. Taken together, these data suggest that the requests most likely to be granted concern patients in the final stages of diseases that are known for their devastating physical symptoms. This is confirmed by the survey results.[56,www]

A further confirmation of this suggestion can be found in the results of D. van Tol's research.[39] The answer to the question of whether a given case is one of unbearable suffering obviously depends on our conception of suffering. According to one conception, the paradigm of suffering is pain: an unpleasurable state of consciousness that has a location in the body and can normally be related to a physical injury at that location ("normally," not always, because you can feel pain in your leg after it is has been amputated). Of course, it is agreed that there are other forms of suffering besides pain, for example, breathlessness, nausea, or physical exhaustion, but according to this conception, they have a similar structure. A richer conception of suffering, however, which has been articulated and defended impressively by Eric Cassell, treats pain, breathlessness, nausea, and so on only as components of suffering. Another essential characteristic of suffering, on this view, is the meaning attributed to these components by the suffering person, more specifically that they are being seen as threats to his or her integrity as a person.[xxx,57,58] Whether they are seen that way may depend on many other aspects of the person's life and personality, and of the future he or she anticipates; in that respect, this conception of suffering can be called a holistic one.

If we place people on a spectrum ranging from an "atomistic" conception of suffering that focuses on somatic symptoms only to a holistic conception, van Tol finds that many, but by no means all, doctors are to be located at the atomistic end.[59,yyy] (SCEN doctors are on average farther removed from that end of the spectrum, and members of review committees even more so.)

uuu Here one should remember that the reporting rate for EAS by proper means is in the neighborhood of 100%. So we cannot expect large numbers of other cases to go unreported.

vvv Two such cases were reported to the review committees in 2008. For some other data, see 17. Griffiths, Weyers, and Adams 2008.

www See Chapter 9 by Pasman.

xxx Cassell makes this a defining characteristic, which would imply that animals and newborns, who are unable to do the necessary work of interpretation, cannot suffer. A more plausible view is that the dimension of meaning is only essential for beings who have the required interpreting capacities.

yyy See Chapter 9 by Pasman.

This, of course, is not really an unexpected result. It is easy to feel compassion for people (or dogs) who are shriveling from pain, but it requires more sophisticated capacities of empathy and imagination to understand why people are suffering because they expect that they will not achieve the basic aims of their lives, or even feel these very aims to have been misconceived. Even people who are not lacking in such capacities may feel less sure about their judgment in the latter class of cases. And the professional training of doctors increases their disposition to focus on physical symptoms, although this is less true of general practitioners than of specialists.

Doctors are, to use a somewhat odd expression, most at ease with dying patients with clear physical symptoms, or at least with diseases known for such symptoms. This tendency has been strongly reinforced by the verdict of the Dutch Supreme Court in the *Brongersma* case (2002).[zzz] In its decision in the *Chabot* case (1995), the court had famously declared that it is not the cause but the nature of the suffering that matters, but in the *Brongersma* decision, it held that the unbearable suffering should be caused by a "medically classified disease or disorder," for only in such cases would it be a matter of professional competence to assess the severity of the suffering. This consideration itself seems to identify the suffering of the patient with his or her physical symptoms, and in any case the decision requires the doctor, in assessing the severity of the patient's suffering, to abstract from elements not directly caused by the illness. For these reasons, the *Brongersma* decision is incompatible with the holistic conception of suffering. It, therefore, understandably reinforced the tendency of doctors to focus on the medical facts: the illness as the cause of the suffering and the symptoms it causes.

Although it is sometimes suggested that the *Brongersma* decision has no authority because it was handed down before the euthanasia law took effect, this view is implausible because that law did not intend to change the existing rules.[aaaa] In any case, the review committees do not dispute this authority. Nevertheless, they have explicitly subscribed to the holistic conception of suffering, which therefore should be seen as the authoritative interpretation of that legal concept.[bbbb,34] Hence, we can conclude that in a substantial though unknown number of cases, the request of the patient is being refused by doctors who have no principled objection to the law and therefore do not refer the patient to another doctor who has none, a request that satisfied all the legal criteria as properly understood, in particular the requirement of unbearable suffering.

[zzz] See Chapter 3 by Weyers and Chapter 16 by Rurup.

[aaaa] And the Supreme Court did actually take into account the parliamentary discussions about that law. Moreover, the requirement that the patient's suffering be hopeless is usually taken to mean that the underlying illness cannot be cured, but this presupposes that such an illness exists.

[bbbb] Most clearly in the Annual Report 2007, from which the relevant passage is quoted by Kimsma in Chapter 22 of this volume. See also Chapter 21 by Wijsbek.

This is clearly problematical, both from a point of view of legal certainty and equality before the law and from the point of the view of the aims of the legal system.

Those involved include severely ill patients who are not yet in the final stage of their illnesses, as well as psychiatric patients. Probably the largest group consists of very old people who, to a high degree, suffer from the usual deteriorations of old age, in particular reduced vision, reduced hearing, and reduced mobility, who for that reason are losing their social contacts and opportunities for meaningful activity, and therefore are spending their lives with feelings of futility and loneliness. Actually, Schoonheim's patient belonged to this group. So did the patient in the following case:

A lady of 96 years had been living a very active life, including long journeys to other continents, until a year ago, in spite of suffering from cardiac decompensation and pulmonary emphysema. During that last year, she was hit by what the consultant called a cascade of medical accidents: a painful crural ulcer, a transient ischemic attack (TIA), several incidents of falling, several infections, and finally a fracture of the upper leg. None of these accidents was fatal, but together they have left her in a condition of almost total immobility, confinement to bed, and dependence on others. As a result of the underlying cardiovascular problems, the fracture, and her age, she can only look forward to decubitus problems, more infections, emaciation, possible recurrences of the crural ulcer or the TIA, and other complications. No one can predict how long it will take before she dies. She has tried to stop eating and drinking but has not been able to sustain the effort. What she considers particularly unbearable is her loss of freedom and of the management of her life.

In this particular case, both the doctor and the consultant concluded that it was a case of unbearable suffering, and the review committee agreed that they could reasonably have come to that conclusion. Obviously, the committee thought that the requirement of the *Brongersma* decision had been satisfied as well. But it is probable that in a case like this, many other doctors who have no principled objections against euthanasia, as well as a substantial number of consultants, would have come to the opposite conclusion. And it is not unthinkable that the patient in that case would have ended her own life, for example, by another and better prepared attempt to stop eating and drinking.

8. FOUR POSSIBLE WAYS OF DEALING WITH THE PROBLEM

Requests for EAS are not being granted in a substantial number of cases in which the euthanasia law would allow it. How to address this problem? In this section, I discuss four possible responses to it. A fifth option would be to break down the medical monopoly on the access to euthanasia agents.[cccc,60] But

[cccc] For some time, right-to-die societies across the world have been looking for a terminal agent that people could easily produce from publicly available resources, but this quest has not yet succeeded.

I believe that society has a proper interest in restricting this access as much as it has in restricting the access to firearms.[dddd,61]

OPTION 1. First would be an attempt to redress the physician's bias. Far more attention should be given in educating doctors about the concept of suffering and its importance for medicine. Because SCEN doctors have a broader conception of suffering than doctors generally, it might help to give patients the right to contact them directly in cases in which they disagree with the refusal of their request by their doctors.

Repealing the *Brongersma* decision would be a vital part of this enterprise. It is easy to criticize that decision. Clearly, people can be ill without their illness being medically classifiable, as medical knowledge is still far from complete. The boundaries of the concept of illness are both vague and contested. (Hence, if in consulting a psychiatrist Brongersma's doctor had asked not only for an assessment of his competence but also for a diagnosis, he could probably have easily obtained a relevant classification from the DSM IV.) More importantly, as I suggested already, even for people dying from a nasty cancer, it may be impossible to sort out neatly those aspects of their suffering that are caused by the illness and those by other causes, in particular because those effects may reinforce one another. Finally, it can be disputed whether or not extreme suffering is solely a doctor's business to the extent that it has "medical" causes. We go to the doctor for sleeping pills, irrespective of the cause of our insomnia. The reason is simply that we have a legitimate need for sleeping pills and the doctor has a monopoly in providing them, or the most effective ones. In the same way, it is incoherent for a society to entrust doctors with the key to recognizing unbearable suffering as the proper justification for euthanasia and then to forbid them from providing this way out to people whose suffering doesn't have a medical cause.[eeee,62,63]

This is all ideal theory, however. The *Brongersma* decision has been generally welcomed by the Dutch medical community.[ffff] Doctors strongly prefer to keep the domain of their concern limited to "medical" causes, "medical" problems, "medical" aims. They do not consider themselves particularly equipped to deal with existential problems. And it is true – I have already conceded it – that to the extent that the suffering of the patient is determined by physical symptoms, it is easier to assess its severity.[gggg] If a person is almost suffocating,

[dddd] In 1994, a physician left terminal agents in the house of a patient who had postponed the euthanasia. Her depressive partner committed suicide by using them.

[eeee] One of the common arguments against legalizing euthanasia is that this would be against the traditional norms governing the practice of medicine as defined by its essential aim, the promotion of health. One of the many weaknesses of this argument is that it doesn't provide us with a reason why people could not have access to terminal agents in ways that bypass "the practice of medicine."

[ffff] And therefore the report of the Dijkhuis Committee, commissioned by the KNMG, which criticized the exclusion from eligibility for euthanasia or physician-assisted suicide of people "suffering from life," was quickly shelved.

[gggg] It doesn't follow, however, that the suffering of a dying patient is completely due to the symptoms caused by the illness from which he or she is dying.

or vomiting feces, you do not need special capacities of empathy and understanding to be sure that this suffering is extreme. If his or her life expectancy is very limited, you can't help thinking that any mistake you make has only limited consequences. Another consideration, which is more than a consideration of nonideal theory, is that if the suffering of the patient can only be understood in the context of his or her life and personality as a whole, to assess the severity of that suffering requires intruding into the patient's private sphere to a larger extent than is normally required of doctors.[hhhh,64] In short, the hope that doctors will really extend the domain of their concern can only be limited. At this point we reach the outer boundary of the Dutch model of indirect medical paternalism.

OPTION 2. This may prompt the second response: We should leave the decision with people themselves. In cases outside of the medical domain, in particular in "Brongersma" cases, it should be up to people to decide whether they think that more time will add anything of value to their lives, and when they don't believe so, they should be given access to the most humane means available to end their lives. If we don't want such means to be publicly accessible, we should still submit those people to a test (possibly by a psychiatric or specialized psychological expert) of their competence, and we should take care that lethal agents cannot get into other hands (for example, by leaving it to specialized suicide consultants to provide those agents at the very moment they are wanted).

This is the view that the NVVE took for some years after the *Brongersma* decision. At the time, the NVVE did not basically dispute the existing legal regime for doctors, with its procedural and substantial requirements of due care. But, of course, you cannot really expect the proposal for Brongersma-type cases to simply coexist with that regime. It is unthinkable that doctors would submit cancer patients in the last stage of their illness to requirements that would not be imposed on "healthy" people who are said to be simply "weary of life." They would either stop following the requirements and stop reporting on them, or (more probably) refer their patients to the other procedure.

So what the proposal really amounts to is to exchange the existing legal regime and its basic reliance on a motive of compassion for another regime based exclusively on respect for autonomy. I will not enter into a fundamental comparative ethical evaluation of the two systems at this point.[iiii,19] It is sufficient to mention that such a radical change of basic orientation is not likely to happen. Margo Trappenburg had argued that the emergence of the Dutch paternalistic model of regulating euthanasia has been largely a matter of "path dependency." When the Supreme Court decided to break the existing political

[hhhh] Leenen's complaint when he observed that the review committees were not always satisfied by the declaration of the doctor and the consultant (see 64 Leenen 2000).

[iiii] For some considerations, see 19. den Hartogh 2000.

impasse in 1984, it had hardly any option in the existing law but the appeal to necessity, interpreted as a "conflict of duties," for identifying a possible legal justification for euthanasia. This implied, as contemporary critics plainly saw, a choice for compassion rather than respect for autonomy as the basic justifying principle. This choice in its turn determined subsequent developments, the specification of the criteria of careful action, the creation of the system of assessment by regional committees, and eventually the format of the 2002 law. I do not agree with Trappenburg that the choice of the Dutch model has been largely accidental,[jjjj] but I do agree that having developed in this direction for decades, it is not likely that any (Dutch coalition) government will change the course of this tanker 90 degrees.

OPTION 3. Probably realizing this, the NVVE has changed its policy. It now advocates supplementing the legal regime with another procedure that is structurally similar to the existing one. In this procedure, similar requirements of due care would be made as regards the voluntary and well-considered character of the request and the absence of viable alternatives. Independent consultation would also be required. But the person who would receive the request and go through the procedure would not necessarily be a doctor. He or she would be a member of a specially trained group of people who can be trusted to consider the existential aspects of the reasons for the request. This group could contain pastoral workers, humanistic counselors, psychologists, but perhaps also specially trained doctors. Let me call such a person a counselor. Finally, the requesting person would not be required to be in a state of unbearable suffering but, rather, in a condition characterized by an irreversible loss of dignity.[65]

One might perhaps be forgiven for being a bit suspicious of that last proposal. Maybe the NVVE is hoping to get rid of the (indirectly) paternalistic aspects of the present regime by arriving at an analog of the abortion law after all. If the person says that he or she has lost dignity, could the counselor dispute this? In the relevant documents of the NVVE, a connection is made between dignity and autonomy that suggests the contrary. It would, it is said, be insulting to people to deny that they are living an undignified life when they say so.

This view, I believe, rests on a mistake, like the similar view concerning suffering. We should distinguish between two concepts of dignity. The dignity of the person, his or her moral and legal standing in a community, is not a matter of degrees, and certainly every person who can make a request for euthanasia has it in full. It is this form of dignity that is the basis of (or perhaps, rather, partly identical to) the right of self-determination, but it is not the loss of dignity in this sense that can be the reason for the request. The dignity of a person's *condition*, on the other hand, can be a matter of degrees, and the loss

[jjjj] In my view, this is largely to be explained by the active involvement of the KNMG in the development of the criteria of due care as the conditions under which EAS would be allowed.

of it can be a motive for a death wish. But the dignity of a person's condition is not a private matter that can only be decided privately. It is, on the contrary, a social state par excellence. To lose one's dignity is to be in a state about which one should be ashamed vis-à-vis other people. And it is fully possible to be mistaken in believing that one is in such a state. In fact, we have already met an example of such a mistake: people who consider it a loss of dignity to be dependent on other people's care. (Note, however, that even if it is mistaken in this way, the perception of loss of dignity can certainly be a form of suffering.)

The basic problem of the new criterion is its relation to the old one: unbearable suffering. From the very introduction of this requirement of due care in the Supreme Court's *Schoonheim* decision of 1984, the court did recognize loss of dignity as a possible dimension of suffering. In order to be an aspect of suffering, loss of dignity has to be experienced as such, and this was later recognized by the court.[66] But, of course, in order to be the motive for a request for physician-assisted suicide, loss of dignity should also be experienced as such. In cases of EAS that are submitted to the review committees, loss of dignity is often mentioned as one of the most prominent elements of suffering. It mainly takes the following forms: incontinence, stinking wounds, fecal vomiting, loss of mental capacities or change of personality (for example, due to brain metastases or to medication), and dependence on care. In almost all of these cases, it is hard to imagine that the loss of dignity by itself would justify assistance in suicide, if it would not cause severe suffering. The one possible exception is an advanced state of dementia. It is no accident that doctors are extremely reluctant to kill such patients on the authority of an advance directive, one of the reasons being that the demented person may not be in a state of unbearable suffering.[kkkk,67,68] But this is a special and very complicated case, which I will set apart for this moment. Abstracting from this case, the criterion of the loss of dignity doesn't seem substantially to add to the criterion of unbearable suffering. Therefore, it should not be treated as a separate criterion governing its own procedure. That would have the inherent danger of reinforcing, within the existing medical domain, narrow conceptions of suffering that exclude such dimensions.[llll,65]

At the same time, the criterion is too narrow to cover the relevant dimensions of a broader, holistic conception of suffering. Think of a very old person who has almost completely lost the abilities of sight, of hearing, and of mobility and, as a result, is unable to be involved in any meaningful activity. Such a person would not have lost dignity nor necessarily perceive him- or herself

[kkkk] Another reason is the fact that it is impossible to communicate with the patient about the decision, and as a result it cannot be a truly cooperative action. See Chapter 14 by Hertogh.

[llll] According to the NVVE, it is possible that elderly people suffer a loss of personal dignity without being in a state of unbearable and hopeless suffering "in the strict medical sense" (see 65 NVVE 2007). There is no such sense.

as having lost it. Rather, it is a loss of meaning that causes suffering, perhaps unbearably.

So I see no good reason for supplementing the requirement of unbearable suffering by loss of dignity.

Should we leave that requirement as it is, but allow the category of the people covered by the exception to Articles 293 and 294 (or perhaps only 294, concerning physician-assisted suicide) of the criminal code to be extended to counselors? I have no principled objection to the proposal, though much would depend on the details of the new regime, in particular on the requirements for receiving the status of counselor.[mmmm] One possible step ino this direction, which doesn't require any change in the law, is to involve nonmedical experts in the assessment of unbearable suffering, if this has clear existential dimensions.

OPTION 4. A final option is to leave the spectrum of alternative choices essentially as it is. Dying patients with a life expectancy of no more than one to two weeks could avoid unbearable suffering that cannot be alleviated in any other way by being given terminal sedation.[nnnn,69] Both such patients and others can request either euthanasia or physician-assisted suicide and receive it if the doctor (and the consultant)[oooo] agree that the substantial criteria of due care have been met. If they don't agree or haven't been asked, such people (not necessarily patients) can act on their own initiative. The question is whether the political community wrongs them if it leaves them no other alternative for having their death wish enacted.

If we take the underlying morality of the Dutch legal system for granted, it can only wrong them if they have actually satisfied the criteria, in particular the criterion of unbearable suffering, but nevertheless find their request refused, either because the doctors use additional requirements of their own (like being in a dying stage), or because they use their own interpretations of "suffering," probably focusing exclusively on physical symptoms. Such cases, as we have seen, occur, probably regularly, even if we have no idea to what extent. (I am not suggesting that the 4,400 cases of carefully planned suicide found by Chabot all belong to this category.) It would clearly be very problematical for

[mmmm] At present, the organizations involved in counseling people with a death wish are all strongly motivated by antipaternalistic considerations. Hence, giving their members this new status might lead to de-emphasizing the requirement of unbearable suffering.

[nnnn] A separate question is whether we shouldn't allow dying patients to be sedated at the very end simply because they prefer to die in that way, even if they don't have "refractory symptoms" (see 69. den Hartogh 2006). The revised KNMG Guideline for Palliative Sedation 2009 moves in that direction by recognizing existential suffering as a possible refractory symptom.

[oooo] It is not a formal requirement of due care that the consultant agree with the doctor, but for obvious reasons it almost never happens that the doctor proceeds with the euthanasia if the consultant thinks that the criteria have not been satisfied. Nevertheless, it has happened a few times, and the review committees have judged the doctor to have satisfied the requirement of due care in those cases.

the political community to say to these people: If you are really determined, you can try to collect lethal agents by guile or deception, or by the hidden complicity of doctors who actually know how their prescriptions will be used, and often in the process involving other people in illegal forms of assistance. That would also clearly violate transparency as a basic principle of the system.

It is less clear, however, that the community cannot say to these people: If you are really determined, you can stop eating and drinking. Of course, this is not a particularly easy way out (which, wryly, may be a fortunate fact because it puts determination to the test). But the results of Chabot's research seem to show that it need not be an inhumane way, if some elementary palliative measures are being taken.[70,pppp]

If these findings can be confirmed, we could be satisfied with the status quo. As Chabot stresses, there has to be change in one respect: Doctors should become more clearly aware of the role they could have in this process, without either morally or legally being held to "assist" the suicide, and hence being coresponsible for it. The courts have already made it clear that providing proper information is not a form of assistance.[17] The same is true about providing proper palliative care, in particular mouth care.[qqqq,71] At present, many doctors who have refused a request for assistance in suicide believe that providing palliative care would be inconsistent with that refusal. Those same doctors, however, would rightly consider it their professional duty to provide palliative care to a dying patient who has not consented to further treatment, even if they themselves believe that decision to have been mistaken.

Several years have passed since I wrote this chapter, and interesting new developments have taken place in regard to the problems I discussed in § 7 and § 8. As a result of a recent change in the Dutch constitution, it is possible for a group of at least 40,000 Dutch citizens to bring a proposal for new legislation to Parliament. In early 2010, such a Citizen's Initiative was started, under the name Uit Vrije Wil (By Free Choice), with the active support of the NVVE for creating a nonmedical path to a self-chosen death for people 70 years of age and older. The initiative received 116,000 signatures within a few weeks, and in March 2011 the proposed bill was sent to Parliament.

The new bill follows the general structure of the Dutch euthanasia law, but with some important exceptions. The most salient deviation is that it proposes the creation of a new category of nonmedical professionals, to be called "providers of help in dying," who are to be trained and certified by a special organization. People 70 and older can ask these persons for assistance in ending their lives. In that case, a procedure has to be followed, including consultation and review, which resembles the procedure of the euthanasia law. But the substantial requirements of careful action are different; that is the second

pppp Relevant research findings by others are reported in 70. Chabot 2003, Chapter 3.

qqqq The most effective action the NVVE could take at solving the problem it describes in its strategy document of 2007 is to organize the availability of such care.

major deviation from the existing law. The provider of help in dying only has to make sure that a client's request is voluntary, well considered, and permanent. There is no requirement as regards his or her condition similar to that of unbearable suffering in the euthanasia law, and it is also not required that there be no an alternative solution to his or her problems. Irreversible loss of dignity is referred to as the common ground for such requests in the explanatory memorandum to the bill, but it is not mentioned in the bill itself. When the provider of help in dying has ascertained that the remaining requirements of due care have been met, a physician employed by the providers' organization will be able to prescribe the lethal drugs.

The KNMG has rejected these proposals for reasons similar to the ones I put forward in discussing Option 2 in §8. An additional criticism is that it is contrary to the professional ethics of doctors for them to prescribe lethal drugs to individuals whom they have not seen personally. But in response to the proposals, the KNMG has also reconsidered its own position. In a position paper published in September 2011, the association agrees that in most instances, death wishes of elderly people are ultimately the results of the afflictions of old age, at least to a large extent, and that in these cases, the requirement of the *Brongersma* decision has been satisfied.[rrrr] As the KNMG puts it, in these cases, the suffering of the patient has a "medical basis." It is possible for such suffering to be unbearable, and therefore, if the other requirements of due care of the euthanasia law have also been satisfied, the law permits the doctor to assist the patient in ending his or her life on his or her request. As the KNMG notes, such cases have repeatedly been reported to the review committees, and all of the doctors involved until now are considered to have acted with due care.

If the doctor doubts whether all requirements of due care have been satisfied, or is not prepared to grant the patient's wish for reasons of his or her own, one alternative option the patient could consider is to stop eating and drinking. The KNMG considers this a viable option for seniors, provided they are well prepared and receive proper guidance. On its view, it is a professional duty of physicians to provide patients on their request with adequate information about this option, and, if they decide to make that choice, with the necessary palliative care.

As a result of these developments, Parliament now has to choose between a mixture of my Options 2 and 3 (By Free Choice) and a combination of my Options 1 and 4 (the position of the KNMG). (In my text I may have underestimated the extent to which Option 1 can be realized.) It is unclear what the choice would be if all members of Parliament followed their own considered views, but in the present political constellation, it is generally expected that the law proposed by the Citizen's Initiative will not pass.[ssss]

[rrrr] Accessible at: http://knmg.artsennet.nl/Diensten/knmgpublicaties/KNMGpublicatie/Position-paper-The-role-of-the-physician-in-the-voluntary-termination-of-life-2011.htm.

[ssss] Govert den Hartogh, Death wishes of the elderly, in *Ethics and Aging* (provisional title), ed. Maartje Schermer and Wim Pinxten (Dordrecht: Springer, forthcoming).

References

1. Gomez, Carlos F. 1991. *Regulating Death: Euthanasia and the Case of the Netherlands*. New York: Free Press.
2. Hendin, Herbert. 1998. *Seduced by Death: Doctors, Patients, and Assisted Suicide*. New York: Norton.
3. Keown, John. 2002. *Euthanasia, Ethics and Public Policy: An Argument Against Legislation*. Cambridge: Cambridge University Press.
4. Cohen-Almagor, Raphael. 2004. *Euthanasia in the Netherlands*. Dordrecht: Kluwer.
5. Dworkin, Ronald, Judith Jarvis Thomson, Thomas Nagel, T. M. Scanlon, Robert Nozick, and John Rawls. 1997. Assisted suicide: The philosophers' brief. *New York Review of Books*, March 27.
6. Dworkin, Ronald. 1993. *Life's Dominion: An Argument about Abortion and Euthanasia*. London: Harper Collins.
7. Singer, Peter. 1994. *Rethinking Life and Death: The Collapse of Our Traditional Ethics*. Oxford: Oxford University Press.
8. Rachels, James. 1986. *The End of Life*. Oxford: Oxford University Press.
9. Keown, John, ed. 1995. *Euthanasia Examined: Ethical, Clinical and Legal Perspectives*. Cambridge: Cambridge University Press.
10. Pans, Esther. 2006. *De normatieve Grondslagen van het Nederlandse Euthanasierecht*. Nijmegen: Wolf Legal Publishers.
11. Onwuteaka-Philipsen, B. D., J. K. M. Gevers, A. van der Heide, J. J. M. Van Delden, et al. 2007. *Evaluatie Wet Toetsing Levcensbeëindiging op verzoek en hulp bij zelfdoding*. Fourth National Survey Report. Den Haag: ZONMw.
12. Spreeuwenberg, C. 1981. *Huisarts en Stervenshulp*. Deventer: van Loghum Slaterus.
13. Dillmann, R. J. M. 1998. Euthanasie: de morele legitimatie van de arts. In *Levensbeëindigend handelen door een arts: tussen norm en praktijk*, ed. J. Legemaate and R. J. M. Dillmann. Houten/Diegem: Bohn Stafleu Van Loghum.
14. Nys, Herman. 2007. Euthanasie: de toekomst van het belgische model. *Tijdschrift voor Gezondheidsrecht* 31: 199–203.
15. Holsteyn, J. van, and Margo Trappenburg. 1995. *Het laatste oordeel: meningen over nieuwe vormen van euthanasie*. Baarn: Ambo.
16. Rietjens, Judith A., Agnes van der Heide, Bregje D. Onuwteaka-Philipsen, Paul J. van der Maas, and Gerrit van der Wal. 2005. A Comparison of attitudes towards end-of-life decisions: Survey among the Dutch general public and physicians. *Social Science and Medicine* 61: 1723–1732.
17. Griffiths, John, Heleen Weyers, and Maurice Adams. 2008. *Euthanasia and Law in Europe*. Oxford: Hart.
18. Feinberg, J. 1986. *Harm to Self*. Oxford: Oxford University Press.
19. Hartogh, Govert den. 2000. Euthanasia: Reflections on the Dutch discussion. In *Medical Ethics at the Dawn of the 21st Century*, ed. Raphael Cohen-Almagor. New York: Annals of the New York Academy of Science.
20. Feldman, F. 1992. *Confrontations with the Reaper: A Philosophical Study of the Nature and Value of Death*. New York: Oxford University Press.
21. McMahan, J. 2002. *The Ethics of Killing: Problems at the Margins of Life*. Oxford: Oxford University Press.

22. Velleman, J. David. 1999. A right to self-termination? *Ethics* 109: 606–628.
23. Velleman, J. David. 2006. *Self to Self: Selected Essays*. Cambridge: Cambridge University Press.
24. Velleman, J. David. 2008. Beyond Price. *Ethics* 118: 191–212.
25. Hartogh, Govert den. 2009. Gij zult niet doodslaan. *Algemeen Nederlands Tijdschrift voor Wijsbegeerte* 101: 163–195.
26. Schauer, Frederick. 1991. *Playing by the Rules: A Philosophical Examination of Rule-Based Decision-Making in Law and in Life*. Oxford: Oxford University Press.
27. Schauer, Frederick. 1992. The right to die as a case study in third-order decision-making. *Journal of Medicine and Philosophy* 17: 573–587.
28. Birnbacher, Dieter. 1995. *Tun und Unterlassen*. Stuttgart: Philip Reclam.
29. Deliëns Luc, F. Mortier, J. Bilsen, M. Cosyns, R. Vander Stichele, J. Vanoverloop, and K. Ingels. 2000. End-of-life decisions in medical practice in Flandres, Belgium: A nationwide survey. *The Lancet* 356: 1806–1811.
30. Heide, Agnes van der, Luc Deliëns, Karin Faisst, Tore Nilstun, Michael Norup, Eugenio Paci, Gerrit van der Wal, and Paul J. van der Maas. 2003. End-of-life decision-making in six European countries: A descriptive Study. *The Lancet* 345: 361.
31. Seale, C. 2009. End-of-life decisions in the UK involving medical practitioners. *Palliative Medicine* 23: 198–204.
32. Griffiths, John, Heleen Weyers, and Alex Bood. 1998. *Euthanasia and the Law in the Netherlands*. Amsterdam: Amsterdam University Press.
33. Quinn, Warren. 1993. Actions, intentions and consequences: The principle of double effect. In *Morality and Action*, ed. Warren Quinn, 175–193. Cambridge: Cambridge University Press.
34. Regionale Toetsingscommissies Euthanasie. 2007. Jaarverslag [Annual Report], Den Haag.
35. Stone, Patrick, Clare Philips, Odette Spruyt, and Catherine Wright. 1997. A comparison of the use of sedatives in a hospital support team and a hospice. *Palliative Medicine* 11: 140–144.
36. Morita, Tatsuya, Junichi Tsunoda, Satoshi Inoue, and Satoshi Chihara. 2001. Effects of high doses of opioids and sedatives on survival in terminally ill cancer patients. *Journal of Pain and Symptom Management* 21: 282–289.
37. Sykes, Nigel, and Andrew Thorns. 2003. The use of opioids and sedatives at the end of life. *The Lancet Oncology* 4: 312–318.
38. Portenoy, Russel K., Una Sibirceva, Randall Smout, Susan Horn, Stephen Connor, Ronald H. Blum, Carol Sapence, and Perry G. Fine. 2006. Opioid use and survival at the end of life: A survey of a hospice population. *Journal of Pain and Symptom Management* 32: 532–540.
39. Tol, D. van. 2005. Grensgeschillen: een rechtssociologisch onderzoek naar het classificeren van euthanasie en ander medisch handelen rond het levenseinde. Ph.D. diss., University of Groningen.
40. Regionale Toetsingscommissies Euthanasie. 2004. Jaarverslag [Annual Report], Den Haag.
41. Regionale Toetsingscommissies Euthanasie. 2005. Jaarverslag [Annual Report], Den Haag.
42. Regionale Toetsingscommissies Euthanasie. 2008. Jaarverslag [Annual Report]. Accessible at: http://www.euthanasiecommissie.nl/Images/jaarverslag%20engels%202008_tcm17-19005.pdf.

43. Linacre Centre for Health Care Ethics. 2004/2005. Assisted Dying for the Terminally Ill Bill. Report II, Evidence, p. 705. Evidence presented to the Select Committee of the House of Lords. Accessible at: http://www.publications.parliament.uk/pa/ld200405/ldselect/ldasdy/86/5020336.htm.
44. Otlowski, Margaret 2001. The effectiveness of legal control of euthanasia; lessons from comparative law. In *Regulating Physician-Negotiated Death*, ed. Albert Klijn, Margaret Otlowski, and Margo Trappenburg, Gravenhage: Elsevier Bedrijfsinformatie.
45. Smith, Stephen W. 2005. Evidence of the practical slippery slope in the debate on physisican-assisted suicide and euthanasia. *Medical Law Review* 13: 17–44.
46. Battin, Margaret P. 2008. Terminal sedation: Pulling the sheet over our eyes. *Hastings Center Report* 38: 27–30.
47. American Medical Association. 2008. The Report of the AMA Council on Ethical and Judicial Affairs on Sedation to Unconsciousness in End-of-Life Care. Accessbile at: http://www.ama-assn.org/resources/doc/code-medical-ethics/2201a.pdf.
48. Regionale Toetsingscommissies Euthanasie. 2003. Jaarverslag [Annual Report], Den Haag.
49. Battin, Margaret P., Agnes van der Heide, Linda Ganzini, Gerrit van der Wal, and Bregje D Onwuteaka-Philipsen. 2007. Legal physician-assisted dying in Oregon and the Netherlands: Evidence concerning the impact on patients in "vulnerable" groups. *Journal of Medical Ethics* 33:5 91–597.
50. Miccinesi, G., J. A. Rietjens, L. Deliens, E. Paci, G. Bosshard, T. Nilstun, M. Norup, and G. van der Wal. 2006. Continuous deep sedation: Physicians' experiences in six European countries. *Journal of Pain and Symptom Managemen*t 31: 122–129.
51. Wijsbek, H. 2001. Knowing me, knowing you: In: Taking lives seriously: Philosophical issues in the Dutch euthanasia debate. Ph.D. diss., Free University of Amsterdam.
52. Buiting, Hilde M., Joseph K. M. Gevers, Judith A. C. Rietjens, Bregje D. Onuwteaka-Philipsen, Paul J. van der Maas, Agnes van der Heide, and Johannes J. M. van Delden. 2008. Dutch criteria of due care for physician-assisted dying in medical practice: A physician perspective. *Journal of medical Ethics* 34: e12
53. Willems, D. L., E. R. Daniels, Gerrit van der Wal, Paul J. van der Maas, and E. J. Emanuel. 2000. Attitudes and practices concerning the end of life: A comparison between physicians from the United States and from The Netherlands. *Archives of Internal Medicine* 10: 63–68.
54. Tholen, A. J. 2003. Levensbeueindiging en psychisch lijden. *Medisch Contact* 2: 64–67.
55. Hartogh, Govert den. 2008. When are living donations voluntary enough? In *Organ Transplantation: Ethical, Legal and Psychosocial Aspects: Towards a Common European Policy*, ed. W. Weimar, M. A. Bos, and J. J. Buschbach, 221–231. Lengerich: Pabst Science Publishers.
56. Chabot, Boudewijn. 2007. *Auto-euthanasie: verborgen stervenswegen in gesprek met naasten.* Amsterdam: Bert Bakker.
57. Cassell, Eric J. 2003. *The Nature of Suffering and the Goals of Medicine*. New York: Oxford University Press.

58. Cassell, Eric J. 2004. When suffering patients seek death. In *Physician-Assisted Dying: The Case for Palliative Care and Patient Choice*, ed. Timothy Quill and Margaret P. Battin, 75–88. Baltimore: Johns Hopkins University Press.
59. Tol, D. G. van, J. A. C. Rietjens, and Agnes van der Heide. 2010. Judgement of unbearable suffering and willingness to grant a euthanasia request by Dutch general practitioners. *Health Policy* 97, 2/3: 166–172.
60. Battin, Margaret P. 2001. New life in the asssisted-death debate in the USA: Scheduled drugs vs. Nu Tech. In *Regulating Physician-negotiated death*, ed. Albert Klijn, Margater Otlowski, and Margo Trappenburg, 49–63. Gravenhage: Elsevier Bedrijfsinformatie.
61. Weyers, Heleen. 2004. *Euthanasie: het proces van rechtsverandering*. Amsterdam: Amsterdam University Press.
62. Kass. Leon R. 2002. "I will give no deadly drug": Why doctors must not kill. In *The Case Against Assisted Suicide*, ed. Kathleen Foley and Herbert Hendin, 17–40. Baltimore: Johns Hopkins University Press.
63. Pellegrino, Edmund D. 2001. Physician-assisted suicide and euthanasia: Rebuttals of rebuttals the moral prohibition remains. *Journal of Medicine and Philosophy* 26: 93–100.
64. Leenen, H. J. J. 2000. Toetsing van euthanasie. *Medisch Contact* 55: 1090–1092.
65. NVVE (Nederlandse Vereniging voor vrijwillig Levenseinde). 2007. Nota Perspectieven op Waardig Sterven. Amsterdam: NVVE.
66. Decision in the case-van Oijen. November 9, 2002. Nederlandse Jurisprudentie 2005, nr. 217.
67. Hertogh, Cees M. P. M., Marike E. de Boer, Rose-Marie Dröes, and Jan A. Eefsting. 2007. Would we rather lose our life than lose our self? Lessons from the Dutch debate on euthanasia for patients with dementia. *American Journal of Bioethics* 7: 48–56.
68. Norwood, Frances. 2005. Euthanasia talk: Euthanasia discourse, general practice and end-of-life care in the Netherlands: The maintenance of life: Preventing social death through euthanasia talk and end-of-life care – Lessons from the Netherlands. Ph.D. diss., University of California, Berkeley and San Francisco.
69. Hartogh, Govert den. 2006. Het recht op inslapen. *Medisch Contact* 37: 1463–1465.
70. Chabot, Boudewijn. 2008. A hastened death by self-denial of food and drink. Amsterdam, 64 pp. May be ordered from Hemlock of San Diego or at http://www.boudewijnchabot.com/.
71. Gert, Bernard, Charles Culver, and K. Danner Clouser. 1998. An alternative to physician-assisted suicide: A conceptual and moral analaysis. In *Physician-Assisted Suicide: Expanding the Debate*, ed. Margeret P. Battin, Rosamond Rhodes, and Anita Silvers, 182–202. New York: Routledge.

24

No Regrets

Margo Trappenburg

Ian Buruma (author of several books on Japan and China and one on Occidentalism, co-authored with Avishai Margalit) was born in the Netherlands in 1951 and left the country in 1975, "at the height of its good times."[1] The Netherlands in the 1970s was a smug country, proud of its many accomplishments. It was a generous welfare state, taking care of the old, the sick, the disabled and the unemployed. It was a liberal progressive nation where people could be openly homosexual, sell pornography, commit prostitution, and smoke marijuana. It was a country where teachers tried to be progressive in schools, employing modern methods and allowing students room to follow their interests. It was a multicultural society in the making where immigrants from Surinam, Turkey, and the Maghreb were allowed to integrate while hanging onto their own cultural backgrounds, the then-government providing their children with language classes in their native tongue. Inhabitants of the Netherlands felt no qualms in lecturing the world: Americans about the war in Vietnam and about nuclear armament, South Africans about apartheid, South American countries about reigning dictatorships, and many Western countries about not contributing enough to the Third World. The Dutch saw their country as a shining example for all the world to follow.

Ian Buruma returned to the Netherlands in 2004, just after movie director and columnist Theo van Gogh had been murdered in Amsterdam by a Muslim fundamentalist. Buruma came back to a totally different country.

The welfare state of the 1970s has been dismantled. Although it is still more generous than the U.S. or the UK system, it now resembles the Anglo-Saxon model much more than it did 30 years ago.

The liberal policy with regard to prostitution, pornography, and recreational drugs is being reconsidered. The cabinets chaired by Prime Minister Jan Pieter Balkenende (holding office since 2002), and especially the fourth Balkenende cabinet (2007–2010) consisting of Christian democrats, Social democrats, and ministers belonging to one of the orthodox Christian parties, advocate a lifestyle that is much more chaste and disciplined than the dominant way of life among the cultural elite in the roaring seventies. The center-right populist coalition that took over from Balkenende in 2010 does not advocate a policy change in this area.

Author-psychiatrist Theodore Dalrymple reproaches the progressive elites for having raised an underclass of people who no longer take responsibility for their lives and their mistakes.[2] The soft leftish ideology of the seventies ("it's not your fault if you end up as a criminal; societal structures have made you what you are") has made them helpless and irresponsible. Dalrymple – not very popular in his native England – is a media star in the Netherlands. Whenever he pays a visit to the country, he is followed around by avid readers, among them several civil servants at the Ministry of Justice.

The Dutch attempts to change their high school educational system so as to make it more "student oriented," allowing students more leeway to study subjects of their choice and acquire certain competencies in their own way, while starkly reducing the number of regular teaching hours, was recently evaluated by a parliamentary investigative committee. The Dijsselbloem Committee concluded that the educational system had deteriorated rapidly, putting Dutch students at a disadvantage in international rankings.[3]

Dutch multicultural policy as it was practiced in the 1970s and 1980s is widely considered a huge mistake.[4] Economist Pieter Lakeman calculated that importing guest workers during the 1960s and 1970s (rather than letting ailing industries disappear), and subsequently importing their wives and children, has cost native Dutch taxpayers a lot of money.[5] The sons and daughters of former immigrants do not do as well as one might hope. Many of them still feel more connected to their parents' home country than to the Netherlands. Many of them attend primary and secondary schools frequented by a lot of other former immigrant children. School segregation is rampant in the Netherlands. It puts former immigrant children at a substantial language disadvantage, despite the fact that "black schools" get almost twice as much money per pupil as schools frequented by native Dutch students.[6,7,8]

The Dutch self-image with regard to international affairs suffered serious blows in 1995 when Srebrenica, the Bosnian capital (in the former Yugoslavia), was conquered by Serbian soldiers. Eight thousand Muslim men and boys were deported and massacred while they were supposedly being protected by Dutch United Nations soldiers. Although this genocide (the worst in Europe since World War II) could not be attributed solely to mistakes or cowardice on the part of Dutch politicians and the Dutch military (the primary culprits obviously being the Serbs, while part of the drama was caused by the international community, i.e., the UN), Dutch politicians were put to shame. The notion of the Netherlands as a guiding example for the rest of the world to follow has virtually disappeared from public discourse.

Buruma describes the present mood in the Netherlands as "hysteria," "panic," and "resentment"; the Dutch are "affronted by their own shattered dreams."[1] Political parties and citizens are seriously divided about all their former sources of pride. There is a general uncertainty about how to go on from here: what to do about the welfare state; whether and how to transform the reigning policy with regard to prostitution, pornography, and recreational drugs; and how to handle ethnic and cultural tensions.

The only heritage from the 1970s that is still widely cherished in the Netherlands is the Dutch policy with regard to medical ethical issues: euthanasia and – albeit to a lesser extent – abortion. In this closing chapter, I will try to assess whether this last bastion is a legitimate source of pride for the Dutch.

THE DUTCH DEBATE AND THE DUTCH SOLUTION

In 1993, the American philosopher Ronald Dworkin published a book on abortion and euthanasia, entitled *Life's Dominion*.[9] Its central message was that "rights talk" isn't always right. Rights talk can prevent us from understanding each other. It can make us focus on our differences instead of our shared understandings, it can prevent us from ever reaching consensus, it can lead to polarization, and it can trigger violence.

According to Dworkin, the American debate on abortion and euthanasia was clouded by rights talk. Pro-choicers talked about women's rights to end their pregnancy as they saw fit. Pro-lifers talked about the fetus's right to life. Americans advocating euthanasia talked about one's individual right to end one's life, and Americans opposing euthanasia talked about individuals' inalienable right to life. To Dworkin, this rights discourse has unnecessarily distanced Americans from one another and has led to serious polarization about both issues, an observation that has since been confirmed by Margaret Battin, who also notices a tendency to up the ante in American debate.[10] Dworkin argues that it would be much better to talk about comprehensive issues instead of rights. Pro-lifers and pro-choicers who disagree vehemently in terms of rights might find one another if they were to talk about "responsible parenting." Pro-choicers might explain that their wish to end an unwanted pregnancy does not sprout from selfishness but is closely connected to the way they want to raise a child: They feel that they owe their child a father, a home, some financial security, or a stable mother, and this is the reason why they cannot have a baby at age 17, in an insecure relationship, when they still need to be educated themselves. This is something pro-lifers might relate to, because wanting the best for one's children is an ideal that they probably share.

Similarly, advocates of euthanasia should not simply state that their lives are their own and that they should be allowed to take life or give it up as they see fit; they should explain why. For many advocates of euthanasia, this would entail talking about the wholeness of human life lived according to certain values. If one has always been independent, one can explain that becoming incontinent and unable to perform even the most simple activities oneself would be abhorrent. If one has always been intelligent, articulate, and funny, the prospect of losing one's wits and one's mind because of a brain tumor is extremely scary. If one has always been lovely and beautiful, losing one's looks because of a disfiguring disease is especially terrible. Most people do not want to die, but if death is inevitable they would prefer to end their lives in accordance with the way they have lived: independent, intelligent, elegant, and lovely until the end. Again, this might be something that opponents of euthanasia can understand and discuss, and is much better than a mere referral to one's right to self-determination.

If we look at the Dutch euthanasia debate from this perspective, we may say that it comes close to the ideal propagated in *Life's Dominion*. The Dutch debate has been amply described by James Kennedy.[11] It did not start with rights talk at all. The debate started with *breaking taboos*: Death should be part of life, it should not be put away in hospitals, we should be able to die at home, amid our relatives, and we ought to think about our funeral arrangements, and so on. Furthermore, euthanasia was seen as a possible answer to the ever-increasing possibilities of medical technology; it was to be an antidote for the power of physicians to keep people alive indefinitely, when their lives were no longer worth living for themselves. Finally, the debate was about openness. The Dutch were unhappy with a medical practice that took place in the dark. They intended to find out what was happening between doctors and patients and they wanted to establish some sort of control.[12,13]

Dying at home, the technological imperative, and openness were issues that could be debated without rights talk, and without much polarization. Although a large majority of Dutch citizens endorse a right to self-determination, self-determination did not become the leading principle in the euthanasia law.[a] Self-determination (or a well-considered request) is an important element in the euthanasia regime but it has never become a sufficient condition. The euthanasia regime has developed from jurisprudence about physicians' conflicting duties: Doctors want to keep their patients alive but they also want to alleviate suffering, and sometimes they cannot fulfill both duties simultaneously. Doctors who perform euthanasia have to be convinced that their patients suffer unbearably without prospect of improvement, and if this is not the case in the doctors' opinion, they should not perform euthanasia, no matter how serious and well considered the patients' requests.[b]

Self-determination has never become a sufficient condition; it has never been a necessary condition either. As Agnes van der Heide points out in Chapter 8: "Physicians feel that the obligation to relieve suffering sometimes takes precedence over their obligation to preserve life,"[c] and on occasion this may lead to the termination of life without a request (for patients who are

[a] See Chapter 4 in this volume.
[b] See Chapters 3, 4, and 23.
[c] See Chapter 8.

comatose, for severely handicapped newborns,[d,14] and sometimes for patients who are too sick to utter a request).

THERE ARE LIMITS

The Dutch debate on abortion (roughly from the 1960s till 1982 when the abortion law was passed) was much more polarized than the debate on euthanasia. Political scientist Joyce Outshoorn, who wrote a dissertation about the struggle for free abortion in the Netherlands, found that at first, doctors tried to establish criteria for a morally defensible pregnancy termination. Later, however, the debate was captured by women's rights groups, who changed the terms of the debate. They argued that only one person could be in charge of a woman's belly and this person was the woman herself. Despite the subsequent polarization (abortion clinics were closed by the Christian democratic minister of justice and women's rights groups showed their bare stomachs in Parliament, indicating that they were boss of their own bellies), in the end the Dutch abortion law was a compromise text. The law, which has not been changed since the early 1980s, now states that a doctor can terminate a pregnancy if the woman is in an emergency situation, after an obligatory five-day waiting period during which the woman has time to reconsider the request.[15]

One might say that although the debate did not look like the nonpolarized, comprehensive ideal described in *Life's Dominion*, the end result did. The law did not establish a right to self-determination for pregnant women; it legitimized abortion as a way out in a situation of utter distress.

In daily practice, however, pregnant women in the Netherlands can get an abortion if they so choose. Some of them are indeed in despair; to others the decision to terminate their pregnancies has to do with their vision of responsible parenthood: They do not want their child to grow up in a single-parent family, without a residence permit, without prospect of staying in the Netherlands, and so on. Foreign women who come to the Netherlands can fairly easily get an abortion as well.[16]

Although there are good reasons to consider the Dutch abortion regime a success – the number of abortions is low compared to numbers in many other countries, presumably because of the easy access to birth control means, and many of the abortions that do take place are for foreign women, who come from less liberal countries – for Christian politicians in the Netherlands, the abortion regime is, in a way, unsatisfactory. With regard to abortion, they feel that they got the wording of the law, whereas the secular, liberal-minded moral majority got the practice of abortion. An orthodox Christian television company from time to time broadcasts a program showing Dutch abortion clinics in action. An undercover journalist posed as a pregnant woman who wanted

[d] See Chapter 19.

to have an abortion because she did not want to be pregnant during her winter holiday trip; she met no opposition from the clinic's physician. In another documentary, a doctor who was interviewed about his abortion policy famously answered: "If a woman declares that she wants an abortion because it's raining, I will respect her wishes."[17]

By contrast, with regard to euthanasia, the principle of self-determination did not end up in the law, nor is it the only leading principle in daily practice. Many authors in this volume are witness to that fact. Gerrit Kimsma and Chalmers Clark describe the struggle of doctors who have to establish the "unbearable suffering" of their patients.[e] Henri Wijsbek emphasizes that it is in fact the political community that determines that we "don't require you to bear this any longer."[f] Ron Berghmans writes about the difficulties in establishing unbearable suffering in Alzheimer patients who wrote advance directives when they were still competent.[g] Mette Rurup discusses the fate of the very old who are weary of life.[h] Both Rurop and Marije van der Lee discuss the fate of depressed patients, suffering from a psychiatric disease. All of these groups will meet severe opposition from doctors and none of them will see their request granted without further ado.[i] Roeline Pasman shows that only 3 or 4 out of 10 requests for euthanasia or assisted suicide are granted in the end. Although sometimes the requests were not fulfilled because the patient died before a procedure could be started, in other cases the physician considered the request unfounded, because the patient was not fully competent or because there were other ways to alleviate the patient's suffering. Pasman shows that these figures have remained fairly constant over the past 15 years, thus providing some reassurance for critics who worry about slippery slopes.[j]

To date, the orthodox Christian television company in the Netherlands has never been able to find a physician to say that if a patient wished to die on account of the rain, his or her services would be offered. Euthanasia in practice is much stricter than abortion in the Netherlands.

Moreover, with regard to euthanasia, a system of control and regulation has been installed that functions rather well. Although not every case of euthanasia is reported to the proper authorities, the reporting rate is improving,[k] and according to Donald van Tol[18] and Govert den Hartogh,[19] the reporting rate for clear-cut cases of euthanasia is about 100%. According to these authors, doctors do not report some cases of unnatural death because they genuinely believe that those are not cases of euthanasia (they should be qualified as pain

[e] See Chapter 17 by Kimsma and Clark and Chapter 22 by Kimsma.
[f] See Chapter 21 by Wijsbek.
[g] See Chapter 15 by Berghmans.
[h] See Chapter 16 by Rurup.
[i] Chapter 16 by Rurup and Chapter 18 by van der Lee.
[j] Chapter 9 by Pasman.
[k] Chapter 7 by Onwuteaka-Philipsen.

or symptom relief with death as a side effect, or as terminal sedation). Judges are very severe on laypersons who set out to provide help in dying to people who are not eligible for euthanasia. In 2009, Gerard Schellekens, counsellor at a foundation called Voluntary Living, was put in prison because he had provided pills for an elderly woman who suffered from old-age deficiencies and who was weary of life.[20]

Whereas women do come to the Netherlands to get an abortion that they cannot obtain in their home country, patients do not come to the Netherlands to acquire medical aid in dying. It is simply too difficult to meet the eligibility criteria for euthanasia. One cannot build a proper relationship with a physician overnight. The novel *Amsterdam* by Ian McEwan describes two healthy (if unlucky) Englishmen who engage in a mutual suicide pact to be carried out by progressive Dutch physicians and nurses. Apparently, the two British men just have to fill in a form and hand over some money, and a deadly potion is provided.[21] It is probably not a coincidence that no such novel has ever been written in the Netherlands. Not many Dutch novelists write about euthanasia at all,[22,23] but if they do, they do not use it in a thriller-like plot. For example, they describe it as a minor detail in an otherwise heartbreaking story about a young mother dying of breast cancer[24] or as a source of consolation for family members who can think of their relative as dying a dignified or even beautiful (albeit untimely) death.[25] Or they express metaphysical, religious, or philosophical doubts about the whole enterprise.[26]

Whenever patients in other countries make the front pages because they seek euthanasia – patients like Chantal Sebire in France, whose face was completely disfigured because of a huge, painful, and inoperable tumor growing behind her eyeball, or Diane Pretty in the UK, who suffered from a progressive muscle disease that would cause her to suffocate in the end – Dutch commentators express some relief that this could not happen here. In the Netherlands, these patients would have been able to get medical help because they clearly suffered unbearably. Commentators usually strike a rather self-congratulatory or even smug note. But this is just about the only thing that the Dutch still feel smug about. We have our doubts about almost everything else. These are trying times in which many policy choices are considered unwise with the benefit of hindsight. Perhaps we should be allowed to be smug about our euthanasia policy, as something we managed to accomplish, something we really did right.

References

1. Buruma, Ian. 2006. *Murder in Amsterdam: The death of Theo van Gogh and the Limits of Tolerance*. London: Penguin.
2. Dalrymple, Theodore. 2001. *Life at the Bottom: The Worldview That Makes the Underclass*. New York: The Manhattan Institute.
3. Bronneman-Helmers, H. M. 2008. *Vijftien jaar onderwijsvernieuwingen in Nederland. Een beleidsanalytische studie ten behoeve van het parlementair*

onderzoek onderwijsvernieuwingen, Parliamentary Archives, Archive number TK 31007, nr. 7.

4. Trappenburg, Margo. 2003. Had het anders gekund? Over het Nederlandse integratiebeleid, in *Politiek in de multiculturele samenleving*, ed. H. Pellikaan and M. Trappenburg, 13–37. Amsterdam: Boom, Meppel.
5. Lakeman, P. 1999. *Binnen zonder kloppen. Nederlandse immigratiepolitiek en de economische gevolgen*. Amsterdam: Meulenhoff.
6. Karsten, S., et al. 2003. *Onderwijssegregatie in Amsterdam. Hoe staat het ervoor en wat willen en kunnen we eraan doen?* Amsterdam: Kohnstamm Instituut.
7. Tesser, P. T. M., and J. Iedema. 2001. *Rapportage minderheden 2001*. Den Haag:: SCP.
8. Trappenburg, Margo J. 2003. Against segregation: Ethnic mixing in liberal states. *Journal of Political Philosophy* 11: 295–319.
9. Dworkin, Ronald. 1993. *Life's Dominion: An Argument about Abortion, Euthanasia and Individual Freedom*. New York: Alfred A. Knopf.
10. Battin, Margaret P. 2001. New life in the assisted-death debate in the USA. In *Regulating Physician-Negotiated Death*, ed. Albert Klijn, Margaret Otlowski, and Margo Trappenburg, 49–66. Den Haag: Elsevier.
11. Kennedy, James. 2002. *Een weloverwogen dood. Euthanasie in Nederland*. Amsterdam: Bert Bakker.
12. Griffiths, John, Heleen Weyers, and Maurice Adams. 2008. *Euthanasia and Law in Europe*. Oxford: Hart.
13. Griffiths, John, Alex Bood, and Heleen Weyers. 1998. *Euthanasia and Law in the Netherlands*. Amsterdam: Amsterdam University Press.
14. Vermeulen, E. 2001. *Een proeve van leven. Praten en beslissen over extreem te vroeg geboren kinderen*. Amsterdam: Aksant.
15. Outshoorn, J. 1986. De politieke strijd rondom de abortuswetgeving in Nederland. Ph.D. diss., Vrije Universiteit, Amsterdam.
16. Visser, M. R. M., et al. 2005. *Evaluatie Wet Afbreking Zwangerschap*. Den Haag: ZonMW. Available at: http://www.zonmw.nl/uploads/tx_vipublicaties/WAZ_evaluatie_Definitieve_webversie_ b.pdf (accessed September 8, 2009).
17. Zembla: dezelfde conclusies als verboden EO-opnamen. 1997. *Trouw*, January 16. Available at: http://www.trouw.nl/krantenarchief/1997/01/16/2518260/Zembla__dezelfde_conclusies_als_verboden_EO-opnamen.html (accessed September 8, 2009).
18. van Tol, D. 2005. Grensgeschillen. Een rechtssociologisch onderzoek naar het classificeren van euthanasie enander medisch handelen rond het levenseinde. Ph.D. diss., Groningen University.
19. den Hartogh, G. A. 2003. Mysterieuze cijfers. *Medisch Contact* 58, 26/27: 1063–1066.
20. NVVE (Nederlandse Vereniging voor een Vrijwillig Levenseinde). 2009. Online news site of the Dutch Association for Voluntary Euthanasia, available at: http://www.nvve.nl/nvve2/pagina.asp?pagkey=105252&metkey=375 (accessed September 8, 2009).
21. McEwan, I. 1998. *Amsterdam*. London: Cape.
22. Soeting, M. 1996. Alleen als de dood onbegrijpelijk is, is hij natuurlijk: euthanasie in de Nederlandse literatuur. *De Gids* 159, 1: 49–56.

23. Soeting, M. 2005. Tussen wet en werkelijkheid: euthanasie in het licht van een romn van Willem Jan Otten en de filosofie van Merleau-Ponty. Ph.D. diss., Maastricht University, Universitaire Pers Maastricht.
24. Kluun. 2003. *Komt een vrouw bij de dokter*. Amsterdam: Podium.
25. Giphart, R. 2000. *Ik omhels je met duizend armen*. Amsterdam: Podium.
26. Otten, W. J. 1996. *Ons mankeert niets*. Amsterdam: Van Oorschot.

Index